THE
TAO
OF
DETOX

THE
TAO
OF
DETOX

The Secrets of Yang-Sheng Dao

A Practical Guide to Preventing and Treating the Toxic Assault on Our Bodies

DANIEL REID

Healing Arts Press
Rochester, Vermont

Healing Arts Press
One Park Street
Rochester, Vermont 05767
www.HealingArtsPress.com

Healing Arts Press is a division of Inner Traditions International

Originally published in Great Britain in 2003 by Simon & Schuster UK Ltd. under the title *The Tao of Detox: The Natural Way to Purify Your Body for Health and Longevity*

Note to the reader: This book is intended as an informational guide. The remedies, approaches, and techniques described herein are meant to supplement, and not to be a substitute for, professional medical care or treatment. They should not be used to treat a serious ailment without prior consultation with a qualified health care professional.

Library of Congress Cataloging-in-Publication Data

Reid, Daniel P., 1948–
   The Tao of detox : the secrets of yang-sheng dao / Daniel Reid.
      p. cm.
   Summary: "A practical guide to preventing and treating the toxic assault on our bodies"—Provided by publisher.
   Includes index.
   ISBN-13: 978-1-59477-142-2
   ISBN-10: 1-59477-142-1
   1. Detoxification (Health) 2. Hygiene, Taoist. I. Title.
   RA784.5.R45 2006
   613—dc22
                                                                              2006020481

Printed and bound in the United States by Lake Book Manufacturing

10 9 8 7 6 5 4 3 2

Text design and layout by Jonathan Desautels
This book was typeset in Sabon with Schneidler Initials as the display font

To send correspondence to the author of this book, mail a first-class letter c/o Inner Traditions • Bear & Company, One Park Street, Rochester, VT 05767, and we will forward the communication.

This book is dedicated to V. E. Irons, for getting to the bottom of the problem and showing us the way to fix it, and to Marlene and Julia, for keeping his good work going.

CONTENTS

Preface   ix

Introduction: Tissue Toxicity   1

PART 1: DETOX

1. Basic Protocols of Detox   16

2. Water: Hydration and Hydrotherapy   31

3. Physiotherapy: Massage and Soft Exercise   54

4. Air: The Breath of Life   76

5. Detox Diet and Supplements   113

6. The "Fast Lane": Fasting and Colonic Irrigation   149

7. "The Angel of Sunlight": Heliotherapy   172

8. The Eliminators: Herbal Detox   182

9. High-Tech Electro-Detox   197

PART 2: RETOX

10. The Art of Rational Retox   226

11. Retox Diet and Supplements   233

12. Advice on Smoking and Drinking   270

13. Advice on Medical and Recreational Drugs   282

14. Setting Your Detox/Retox Clocks   289

15. "Don't Worry, Be Happy, Feel Good"   296

APPENDICES

Appendix 1. Recipes and Formulas   302

Appendix 2. Suppliers   316

Index   323

PREFACE

Despite the "wonders of modern medicine," the state of human health throughout the world today continues to erode at an alarming rate. This deterioration prevails as much in the wealthy, industrially developed parts of the world as it does in poor, underdeveloped regions. America, for example, has one of the highest per capita rates of cancer mortality on earth, and the immune deficiency syndrome known as AIDS has spread to every corner of the planet, striking the rich as well as the poor, old and young alike. Debilitating diseases and chronic degenerative conditions that only a hundred years ago rarely manifested except in the weak and elderly have today become increasingly common conditions in the young and mainstream adult sectors of the population. Chronic pain and fatigue, indigestion and insomnia, hypertension and heart failure, and all sorts of other maladies are now par for the course in the lives of men and women all over the world, degrading the quality of their lives and causing untold misery.

So what's the problem here?

The problem is toxicity, plain and simple, the same sort of toxicity that attracts flies to garbage, kills fish in rivers, and lays waste to the environment, except in this case we're talking about the toxic waste that pollutes the blood and tissues of the human body. Modern Western lifestyle, particularly the highly touted "American way of life," has spread like an oil slick across the entire sea of humanity, smothering traditional ways of life that once kept the human body in a relatively healthy state of balance. Fast food and junk food, preservatives and additives, chemically contaminated air and water, mad-dash lifestyles and indiscriminate use of drugs, both medical and recreational, have all contributed to the overall degradation of human health and the relentless pollution of the human body.

Most people today take far better care of their cars than they do their own bodies. Imagine what would happen if you indiscriminately poured petrol, diesel, kerosene, propane, and a cup of sugar altogether into the gas tank of your car. That is precisely the way most people eat today, mixing meat, bread, milk, fat, sugar, and other digestively incompatible foods at the same meals and pouring them into their stomachs at the same time. And what if you never changed the motor oil, neglected to clean the filters, and let the carburetor get crusted up with soot? The result would be obvious: the fuel would burn inefficiently, producing foul-smelling toxic wastes and gases, the engine would soon begin to wheeze and splutter, vital moving parts would seize up and malfunction, and finally the whole machine would grind to a shuddering halt and need to be hauled to the nearest repair shop. All of this could be easily prevented, and expensive repair work avoided, simply by keeping the engine properly tuned, periodically changing the oil and replacing the filters, cleaning the carburetor, using the right type of fuel, and properly maintaining the vehicle on a daily basis.

Many of today's most common and deadly diseases, such as cancer, diabetes, and cirrhosis of the liver, are caused not by viruses or other germs but rather by long-term accumulation of toxins and acid wastes in the body, which create the conditions of tissue toxicity that germs require to infect the body. Similarly, most chronic degenerative conditions, like arthritis, arteriosclerosis, and immune deficiency, are acquired primarily as a result of blood and tissue toxicity produced from things that people put into their own bodies. As these acidic toxins fester and decay in various tissues, they damage organs and glands, corrode joints and arteries, enervate the nervous system, and inhibit immune response and other vital functions. This debilitating state of tissue toxicity is almost always self-inflicted, and it cannot be corrected with pills, injections, surgery, or any other "quick-fix" medical procedures. The one and only way to counteract self-toxification of the body is by self-detoxification, and the only one who can do that for you is the same person who allowed it to happen in the first place—you. As the saying goes, "It's a dirty job, but someone has to do it."

Fortunately, a systemic detox can be done simply, quickly, and efficiently. Unfortunately, life is toxic by nature, though, so just as fire invariably produces smoke and ash, so the metabolic processes of life quickly begin to "retox" your body the moment you've finished a detox program. Therefore, the secret to enjoying a long and healthy life—and being able to "eat, drink, and be merry" while also working, prospering, and remaining fit—is to practice the discipline of periodic detox and to apply the principles of "rational retox" to your daily life.

In the Far East, where people like to work hard, play hard, and enjoy every aspect of life, health and longevity have always been culti-vated as the two most precious treasures of life. Health and longevity form the cornerstones upon which the enjoyment and accomplishment of everything else worth doing depends.

Regardless of how busy people in traditional Asian societies became in their relentless pursuits of fame and fortune, food and sex, prosperity and pleasure, they always took the time to relax their bodies and rest their minds, to replenish their energies and to rebalance their systems. In addition, they designed their diets and other basic habits in ways that protected health and prolonged life, rather than choosing habits that hastened degeneration and death. By following these basic principles, traditional Eastern cultures developed a knack for healthy living that in current-day Asian cultures continues to enhance rather than dimin-ish the enjoyment of life's pleasures, and to assist rather than interfere with the demands of hard work. The Japanese, for example, who work harder by day and play harder by night than anyone else on earth, and who live with the most intense forms of modern industrial pollution, continue to enjoy the longest average lifespan in the world, simply by continuing to follow traditional ways in their personal habits. What they and other East Asian cultures have learned is the ancient Chinese art of longevity by means of toxic-damage control, a system known as the "Way of Nurturing Life" *(yang-sheng dao)*. In other words, they practiced the "Tao of Detox/Retox."

The "Way of Nurturing Life" is a comprehensive system of self-health care that is as relevant to the human condition today as it was when first developed over three thousand years ago in ancient China, and the life-prolonging benefits for those who practice this way of life are greater today than ever before. In my 1989 book, *The Tao of Health, Sex, and Longevity,* I introduced this system of self-purification as follows:

> The essential principle is to combat the debilitating, deathly effects of environmental poisons and self-pollution with the rejuvenating, death-defying antidote of personal hygiene and self-purification. . . . The purpose of regular regimens of self-cleansing is simply to stay a few steps ahead of the inexorable process of pollution and decay. "Aging" is not a matter of time alone; it is the *rate* at which we permit our bodies to decay over a period of time.

Having practiced these methods myself for nearly thirty years, I agree with their principles more than ever, and I wholeheartedly endorse this system as the best way to protect your health, preserve your vitality, and prolong your life. In the *Tao of Detox,* I present the practical and effective methods used for thousands of years in traditional East Asian cultures, methods that cultivate health and longevity through personal hygiene and proper daily care of the human body. The therapeutic powers of these ancient Eastern healing arts are further amplified by fusing them with modern technology and new health products; their basic principles are more clearly illuminated by viewing them in the light of modern medical science. By selectively blending the best of East and West in self-health care, this book presents a comprehensive system for protecting health and prolonging life by means of internal cleansing, and it introduces a variety of practical programs that anyone can learn to practice within the context of one's own daily life.

A book can only show you the way, however, while the will to follow it can only come from you. Hopefully this book will inspire that will in you.

Introduction
TISSUE TOXICITY

In recent years, environmental pollution and the poisoning of our food, air, and water supplies have become issues of major concern and hot debate throughout the world, but virtually nothing has been done to correct these problems or reverse the trend. In fact, as the population of the planet continues to multiply and the pace of industrialization continues to accelerate, the poisoning of life on earth grows more severe and widespread, day by day.

Along with this radical degradation of our living environment has come an equally swift erosion in the quality of human health: cancer, HIV/AIDS, heart disease, liver infection, respiratory ailments, nervous disorders, and a host of other maladies have spread like wildfire throughout the general population all over the world, ravaging lives in all segments of society. For all its highly touted surgical weaponry and massive arsenal of chemical drugs, conventional modern medicine has failed to defend humanity against this malignant attack on our health and longevity. Rather than protecting people from this relentless onslaught of disease and degeneration, modern allopathic medicine simply tries to manage its symptoms with drugs and surgery, and the treatment often leads to even worse symptoms later.

What modern medicine, as well as most victims of disease today,

1

fail to recognize is the direct correlation between external pollution of the environment and internal pollution of the human body. The simple fact is this: all poisons that are put into the macrocosmic ecosystems of nature invariably seep into the microcosmic biosystems of human health. External toxicity of food, air, and water always cause internal toxicity of blood, tissues, and cellular fluids, and these toxic conditions become the breeding ground for disease and degeneration. No drug or surgical procedure can correct this problem, because the cause is not germs, genes, or congenital defects. The cause is a state of toxicity in the blood and tissues of the human body, a condition known as "toxemia." If you see a festering pile of garbage crawling with flies and maggots, you don't blame the flies for creating the garbage, and you don't try to get rid of the garbage by poisoning the flies and maggots with chemicals. What you do is get rid of the garbage and clean up the mess it made. The flies and maggots then have no place left to breed, and they disappear naturally, thereby solving the problem without waging chemical warfare against nature.

The same principle applies to human health. The only real way to cure any chronic disease or degenerative condition is to eliminate the root cause by ridding the body of the toxins that pollute the blood and tissues, attract germs, and weaken resistance and immunity. That means detoxifying the internal environment of the human body, repairing the toxic damage done to vital organs, and restoring balance to all the basic vital functions. When the blood and tissues of the body have been purged of poisons, degeneration is arrested, germs cannot attack, and the body's natural healing mechanisms repair the damage and restore optimum health to the whole system. Until the world wakes up to the mortal danger that environmental pollution poses to human health and longevity and takes effective measures to clean up the planet, human beings who wish to live long and healthy lives in this world have no choice but to take their own measures to periodically detoxify and protect the inner world of their own bodies, and try to stay a few steps ahead of the constant "retoxification" process that occurs naturally in the course of daily life.

Even without environmental pollution, the human body produces internal toxins as a natural by-product of digestion and metabolism.

When glucose and oxygen are burned in the cells to create energy, acid wastes and other toxic by-products such as carbon dioxide are produced. Lactic acid, for example, is a toxic waste produced in the tissues as a result of muscular exertion. When new cells grow to replace damaged cells, the old cells are dismantled, dissolved by enzymes, and this cellular debris becomes more toxic waste that must be removed from the body. In a healthy, well-balanced body, all of this natural metabolic "garbage" is automatically eliminated from the system by the excretory organs. As the eminent American physician Dr. John Tilden writes in his book *Toxemia*, "Toxin is a by-product as constant and necessary as life itself. When the organism is normal, it is produced and eliminated as fast as produced."

A normal, healthy body will therefore naturally detoxify itself by eliminating its own self-produced toxic wastes as fast as they are produced. Toxemia occurs, and the conditions for disease are thereby created, when toxins are retained and stored in the body due to toxic overload or impairment of the body's own natural detox and elimination functions. As Dr. Tilden states, "Without toxemia there can be no disease. . . . Thus retention of metabolic toxin is the first and only cause of disease. . . . One of the first things to do to get rid of any so-called disease is to get rid of toxemia, for it is this state of the blood that makes disease possible." Dr. Theodore Baroody, author of *Alkalize or Die,* agrees emphatically with this view:

> The countless names attached to illnesses do not really matter. What does matter is that they all come from the same root cause . . . *too much tissue acid waste in the body*! . . . *It is these tissue residues that determine sickness or health!*

Retention of toxins within the body has two basic causes: one is massive toxic overload beyond natural metabolic levels due to excess exposure to unnatural environmental toxins in food, air, and water; the other is impairment of normal elimination processes due to unhealthy personal habits, exhaustion, and enervation of the nervous system caused by hyperactive modern lifestyles. In most cases, toxemia is the net result of a combination of various factors—indiscriminate eating habits and chemically contaminated food and water; smoking and drinking, a "fast-lane" lifestyle of hard work and hard play; excessive stress and insufficient rest; and so forth. But regardless of the sources of toxicity, the net result is always the same—a chronic state toxemia—and toxemia is the root cause of all disease and degeneration. Therefore, the first step in curing any disease, correcting its cause, and preventing the onset of other diseases is to detoxify the whole system, just as cleaning up the garbage is the only way to get rid of flies and maggots. After each period of intensive detox, you may then take appropriate measures to "clean up your act" in daily life, so that "retox" proceeds more slowly and less severely than before. This involves changing some of your eating habits, adjusting various aspects of your personal lifestyle, and learning a few basic rules that govern the way your body works, such as the axiom, "You are what you eat."

One of the most important things to learn about how your body works, especially with regard to detox and retox, is the way the autonomic nervous system operates. All of the body's vital functions are controlled by the autonomic nervous system, which has two antagonistic branches. One is called the "sympathetic" branch, also known as the "action circuit" or "fight or flight" response ("F or F"). This is the branch that is switched on by any sort of physical exertion, hard work, excitement, sensory stimulation, emotional turmoil, or any other intensive activity. When the "F or F" action circuit is switched on, the body's entire supply of nervous energy is consumed in active response to external conditions, emotional reactions, and sensory stimulation, and these functions burn up nerve energy faster than it can be produced. The result of such neuro-active depletion is a state of nervous exhaustion, or "enervation," which has become a chronic condition of daily life for the majority of people throughout the world today.

The other branch of the nervous system is called the "parasympathetic" circuit, and it is this branch that governs the immune system, controls auto-detoxification and self-cleansing responses, and regulates excretory functions. It is also known as the "rest and relaxation" circuit ("R and R"), because the one and only way to activate this branch and allow it to function properly is to give both body and mind a period of complete rest and total relaxation. The human body was designed to function in a healthy state of balance between these two modes of nervous response. Intensive bursts of activity in the sympathetic "F or F" action circuit are supposed to be followed by periods of deep rest and physical relaxation in the parasympathetic "R and R" healing circuit to allow the system to recuperate and rebalance itself. Whenever the nervous system is locked into the intensive action mode for prolonged periods of time, such as in modern urban lifestyles, immune response atrophies, cleansing and excretory functions are suppressed, and toxic wastes continuously accumulate in the body, setting the stage for the development of disease and decay. Only when the nervous system is at rest in the restorative parasympathetic mode can the body neutralize and eliminate toxins, process and excrete digestive wastes, regenerate its cellular structure, and restore itself to a balanced state of health and vitality.

Today, virtually everyone in the world finds themselves locked into the hyperactive, depleting, highly toxifying sympathetic branch of the autonomic nervous system, with very little time to spend in the healing, restorative parasympathetic mode. Modern lifestyle, with its "work hard, play hard" ethic, makes little allowance for sustained periods of rest and relaxation. Overwork, overindulgence in food and drink, overstimulation of the senses, and overexcitement of the emotions all conspire to keep the action circuit of the human nervous system switched on day and night, and this leads to a state of constant enervation and toxic overload. This in turn produces conditions of chronic toxemia, which is the root cause of most disease and degeneration. As Dr. Tilden puts it, "Toxemia is the cause of all disease, and enervation—an enervated body and mind—is the cause of toxemia." The only solution here is to give body and mind a prolonged period of complete rest and total relaxation, thereby switching the nervous system over to the healing mode of the parasympathetic branch and allowing the entire body to cleanse and purify itself naturally, replenish its energy reserves, and restore its normal resistance to disease and degeneration.

Let's take a closer look at the basic nature of toxemia. In a normal healthy body, the blood and most other bodily fluids should be slightly alkaline, very much like sea water, and the tissues and cells should be well oxygenated. Alkaline and oxygen are therefore the twin pillars of good health and strong immune response. Bacterial, viral, and fungal infections cannot develop in tissues that are sufficiently alkalized and oxygenated, and almost all microbes and toxins are neutralized by the presence of alkaline and oxygen elements. When internal toxicity exceeds the body's capacity to cleanse itself, however, alkaline and oxygen levels plummet, and a state of toxemia develops. This state is characterized by two primary conditions: excess acid (acidosis) and insufficient oxygen (hypoxia).

Acidosis and hypoxia are the underlying conditions that allow bacteria, viruses, fungus, and other microbes to invade and breed inside the human body. Virtually all germs that infect the human body are anaerobic, which means that they thrive in oxygen-deficient environments, such as toxic tissues. Ever since Louis Pasteur proposed his "germ theory of disease," modern Western medicine has become obsessed with the simplistic view that every disease must be caused by the specific germs that appear in diseased tissues and also believes that the cure for any particular disease is to kill the specific germ associated with its symptoms. As a result, modern Western medicine engages in an ever-escalating campaign of "chemical warfare" against germs, fought on the battleground of the human body. This approach fails entirely to account for the fact that under precisely the same conditions of exposure, some people become infected by germs and get sick, while others do not. The difference between those who "catch" germs and those who don't is that those who are susceptible to illness have lower resistance than those who don't. As the famous American physician Dr. Charles Mayo stated, "We are all afraid of germs because we are all ignorant of them. Germs are outside, what we should be afraid of is lowered resistance from within." Acidosis and hypoxia erode normal resistance and establish the conditions for germs and viruses to colonize the human body.

Viewing the situation from the garbage and fly analogy, people whose blood and tissues are littered with accumulations of toxic-debris acid wastes are the ones who become most vulnerable to infection by germs, just as garbage attracts flies. All microbes have a very narrow range of conditions in which they can survive and reproduce. The two most basic conditions that allow pathogenic microbes to colonize human tissues are excess acidity and insufficient oxygen. Any wine or beer maker can testify to the fact that the bacteria they use to ferment their products require an acid medium of very specific degree, without exposure to oxygen, to function. On his deathbed, Pasteur himself finally recanted his germ theory by admitting that "the terrain is everything." Without the specific preconditions of acidosis and hypoxia, germs simply cannot survive in the "terrain" of human tissues, just as flies cannot breed in the terrain of a sanitary environment. What this means is that the presence of germs in the blood is not the root cause of any disease, but rather a *symptom* of toxemia. Toxemia provides the breeding ground for germs and thereby becomes the root cause of all disease.

The implications of this fact find their greatest significance in the understanding and treatment of cancer. In 1931, Dr. Otto Warburg received the Nobel Prize for medicine for his discovery that *all* forms of cancer, without exception, are characterized by two basic conditions: acidosis and hypoxia. Like germs, cancer cells flourish only in acidic, anaerobic environments, in which they reproduce as rapidly as fermenting bacteria. This discovery clearly indicates that the best way to cure and prevent cancer is to alkalize and oxygenate the blood and tissues, thereby eliminating the conditions in which cancer cells thrive. However, modern medicine has totally ignored Dr. Warburg's work and has chosen instead to attack cancer the same way it attacks germs: poisoning it with toxic chemical drugs, burning it with radiation therapy, and cutting it out with radical surgery. None of these conventional cancer treatments provides a real cure for the underlying cause of cancer; in fact, they further aggravate the root cause by strongly elevating the levels of tissue toxicity, while at the same time severely damaging the body's own natural cleansing and healing responses.

A hundred years ago, fewer than one in a thousand people died of cancer. Today cancer kills one in every four people. Having clearly lost the "war on cancer" long ago, modern medicine nevertheless stubbornly continues to ignore its root causes and now claims that people get cancer due to a "genetic predisposition" to it, as though cancer were an inherited trait, like freckles and blue eyes. This is nonsense. While 5–10 percent of cancer cases may indeed be linked in some way to faulty genes, if most cancers were genetically determined, as some doctors now claim, then a hundred years ago the incidence of cancer should have been about the same as it is today, rather than 250 times lower. Mainstream medicine has taken the wrong track on cancer treatment but refuses to admit it because cancer therapy has become one of the most profitable branches of the modern medical industry. Meanwhile, these conventional therapies continue to make matters much worse for cancer patients by increasing the underlying state of toxemia that lies at the root cause of all cancer.

The fact is that 80–90 percent of all cancer cases can be traced back to basic environmental factors, of which diet is by far the most important, although electromagnetic pollution, particularly from microwave radiation emitted by mobile phones and phone towers, is becoming an equally dangerous factor. Toxins assimilated from external sources accumulate and fester inside the body, causing internal toxicity of blood and tissues and producing the conditions of acidosis and anaerobia upon which cancer feeds. The answer to cancer is to clean up the cumulative tissue toxicity that allows cancer to develop in the first place, and to stop using the human body as a dumping ground for all the toxic waste that enters the system with food, water, air, smoke, drugs, microwaves, and other external sources. There's no way to totally avoid toxic contamination these days, but you can certainly reduce your risk by making some basic changes in your diet and lifestyle and taking a few simple preventive measures, and you can certainly protect yourself from cancer, heart disease, and other life-threatening ailments by periodically flushing the poisons that cause them out of your system, rather than letting them accumulate to critical levels.

If cancer is detected early enough, before it causes irreversible damage to vital organs, it can usually be treated and cured by a combination of various detoxification methods, such as fasting and colonic irrigation, raw juice and detox diet therapy, herbal and nutritional supplements, alkalization and oxygenation of blood and tissues, and other holistic methods, without the need for debilitating toxic treatments such as chemotherapy, radiation, and radical surgery. However, if a licensed physician today tells a patient that cancer can be cured by means of blood and tissue detox, and offers to provide such a cure, the doctor will be prosecuted, stripped of his or her medical license, and potentially even imprisoned, as well. It is not "politically correct" these days for doctors to discuss the real causes of cancer or to provide real cures that work, because the profits of powerful pharmaceutical cartels and other branches of modern industry such as telecommunications are threatened by the truth regarding the real causes and cures for disease. It is therefore up to each of us to discover the truth ourselves, and to act on it by taking effective preventive measures to protect our health and prolong our lives in a world that grows progressively more toxic and "user-unfriendly."

Cancer is the final, fatal stage of tissue toxicity, but it takes a long time to develop, and long before it does, chronic toxemia takes its toll on human health in many other ways, making life miserable for millions of people who don't realize that the root cause of their misery is their own blood and tissue toxicity. In addition to providing fertile ground for infection by germs, toxemia also damages vital organs and impairs immune response, causing a wide range of degenerative ailments that grow steadily worse for as long as the state of toxicity continues. Listed below are some of the most common symptoms associated with blood acidosis and tissue toxicity:

heartburn	loss of hair
allergies	arthritis
headaches	foul body odor
festering sores	frequent colds
fungal infections	vaginitis
gastritis	depression
psoriasis	excess mucus
sinusitis	hyperactivity and anxiety
fatigue	all forms of cancer

While a variety of secondary factors such as malnutrition and harmful habits may also be contributing causes in these conditions, the root cause always remains the same—toxemia. Even if the secondary factors are eliminated, the condition will continue to manifest until the internal toxicity that allowed it to develop in the first place is neutralized and the toxins are eliminated from the system.

The one and only solution to pollution is purification. In the case of internal pollution of the human body, and the state of chronic toxemia that it causes, that means periodic purification of the bloodstream and complete detoxification of the bodily tissues. Unless you choose to live in a remote mountain cave and live on nothing but wild fruit and spring water, there is no way to avoid the accumulation of excess toxic residues in your body. As long as the amount of toxin does not exceed the capacity of your immune and excretory systems to eliminate it, health and vitality are easily maintained, but sooner or later the toxic overload of daily life in the contemporary world exceeds your body's ability to properly cleanse itself, and that is when toxemia develops and disease and degeneration begin. The worst mistake of all is to start using pharmaceutical drugs and surgical procedures to temporarily ease the symptoms of discomfort and inconvenience of the chronic diseases and degenerative conditions caused by toxemia, because that approach only makes the problem worse by increasing blood and tissue toxicity, while weakening immune response, damaging the body's internal organs, and disrupting vital functions. The only effective way to deal with toxemia is to "clean up your act" with a regular program of detox, followed by a rational approach to "retox." This means periodically purging the blood and tissues of accumulated toxic residues, then reforming the personal lifestyle habits that contribute most to acidosis and tissue toxicity.

For any detox program to be effective, you must take at least three days of complete rest and total relaxation to do it. Seven days is even better, because it takes exactly seven days of complete rest and clean living to purify the bloodstream and cleanse the internal organs. Only a prolonged period of "R&R" will allow the autonomous nervous system to switch over to the restorative parasympathetic circuit long enough to give the body a chance to completely cleanse and rebalance itself, while giving the overworked, overstimulated sympathetic action circuit a long overdue rest. Remember, effective detoxification and repair of the body can only take place when the mind is at rest and the nervous system is operating in the healing mode of the parasympathetic branch. There is no way you can do it simply by eating the right foods and taking the right supplements, while still remaining locked into the hectic activities of ordinary daily life. So unless you're willing to retreat from daily life for a while and take the time to do it right, there's not much point in trying to detox at all.

Besides purging the blood and tissues of toxic residues, a period of detox also provides other essential long-term benefits for health and longevity. One of those benefits is to cleanse and rejuvenate the entire excretory system—clearing clogged bowels and congested lungs, cleaning contaminated lymph glands and clearing blemished skin, and flushing out debris from dirty kidneys and bladder. The more toxic you become, the less efficiently your excretory organs work, and if extreme toxemia continues for too long, serious organic damage to the excretory organs can occur. Another benefit of periodic detox is restoration of maximum immunity and resistance, which depends on adequate alkalization and oxygenation of the blood and cellular fluids. Bacteria and other germs simply cannot survive in a body that is sufficiently alkaline and oxygenated. Even a microbe as aggressive as anthrax can only infect a person whose body is already in a toxic state of acidosis and anaerobia, and this explains why, under precisely the same degree of exposure, some people "catch" it and others do not. These days, with all the hazardous chemicals and microbes that contaminate our living environment, spending three to seven days once or twice a year doing a serious detox program certainly seems worth the investment of time and effort.

The basic problem of toxemia and the solution of detox are summarized in the schematic diagram below:

THE PROBLEM	THE SOLUTION
stress (environmental pollution; daily life)	rest (peace & quiet; clean living)
↓	↓
strain (physical/mental/emotional, overwork, exhaustion, worry)	relaxation (physical/mental/emotional, tranquility, comfort, support)
↓	↓
enervation (overdrive in sympathetic mode)	regeneration (rest in parasympathetic mode, replenish energy, restore vital functions)
↓	↓
inefficient elimination (bowels, lungs, kidneys, skin)	swift and efficient elimination (bowels, lungs, kidneys, skin)
↓	↓
retention of toxic wastes	elimination of toxic wastes
↓	↓
toxemia (acidosis and anaerobia)	purification (alkalization and oxygenation)
↓	↓
acute disease, chronic degenerative conditions, cancer	immunity and resistance, health and longevity

The importance of a sustained period of rest and relaxation as an absolute prerequisite for any detox program to be effective cannot be overemphasized, especially in today's fast-paced, high-stress world, where resting quietly and doing nothing is regarded as a "waste of time." As Dr. Tilden notes, "The present day strenuousness causes enervation which checks elimination, and the retained toxins bring on toxemia. . . . Rest from habits that enervate is the only way to put nature in line for healing. Sleep and rest of body and mind are necessary to keep a sufficient supply of energy. Few people in active life rest enough." This means taking a break not only from hard work and hard play but also from worry, anger, and all other forms of emotional excitement and strong sensory stimulation, all of which enervate the nervous system, inhibit immune response, and impede efficient elimination of toxins from the body.

If you cannot find sufficient peace and quiet to detox at home, or if you lack the discipline to conduct your own detox program, the best solution is to check into a quiet, comfortable spa or health resort* that has the facilities required to support an effective program of detoxification and rejuvenation. Such resorts are becoming increasingly popular throughout the world. They provide a wide range of facilities and services that not only expedite fast, efficient detoxification but also make the entire process a lot more pleasant. Look for places located in tranquil settings down by the ocean or up in the mountains, preferably those that offer facilities such as therapeutic massage, steam rooms, whirlpool baths, hot springs, raw juice bars, and other restorative health regimens. Instead of always taking "action holidays" that leave you even more exhausted and toxic than when you started, try taking a relaxing "health holiday" for a change, one that leaves you feeling thoroughly rested, totally refreshed, and completely rejuvenated. You'll be amazed how much better you feel and how much better your body functions, after allowing your system to drain out all its toxic residues, eliminate acid wastes, and restore natural balance in the blood and tissues. In the following chapters, we'll discuss the best ways to accomplish this goal.

---

*Such as the "Daniel Reid Detox & Wellness Center" in Singapore, established in March 2006. See www.danreid.org.

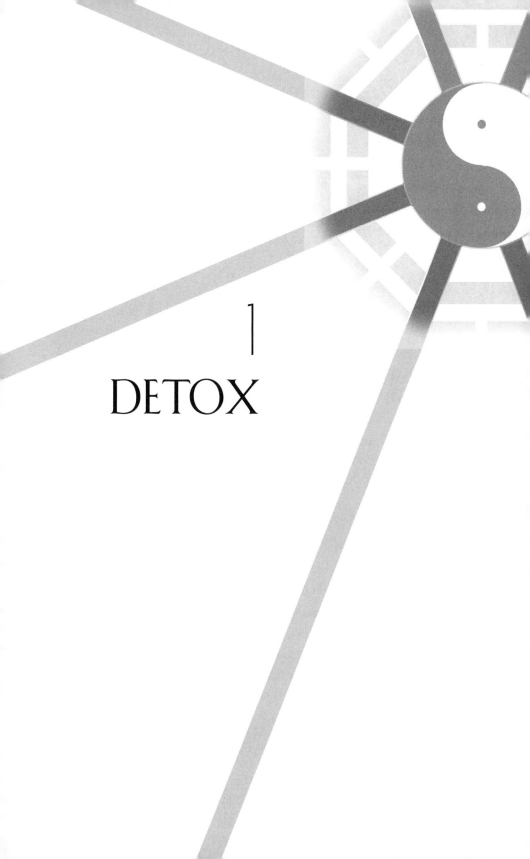

1

DETOX

1

BASIC PROTOCOLS OF DETOX

Pollution is a basic fact of life. No one is immune to it. Although the human body is designed to cleanse itself naturally of the normal waste products of digestion and metabolism, it is clearly not equipped to deal with the additional toxic overload from chemical preservatives and pesticides, pharmaceutical drugs and artificial foods, and other sources of internal toxicity that have become common in modern lifestyles. This internal pollution is the major cause of disease, degeneration, and a foreshortened lifespan.

The most fundamental principle in Traditional Chinese Medicine (TCM) is the universal law of polarity known as the "great principle of yin and yang." *The Yellow Emperor's Classic of Internal Medicine,* an important Chinese medical text written over two thousand years ago, states, "If it's hot [yang], cool it down [yin]. If it's empty [yin], fill it up [yang]." All traditional Chinese medical practices are based upon this principle of dynamic polarity. Extending it to the problem of blood and tissue toxicity, we could say, "If it's polluted [yang], purify it [yin]. If it's acidic [yang], alkalize it [yin]."

Unfortunately, like so many other dichotomies in life, the purification process is not nearly as much fun, nor as easy, as the pollution process. Therefore, most people tend to overlook the importance of self-detoxification, or they pretend that it is not necessary. To the contrary, purification of polluted blood and tissues is absolutely necessary to preserve health and prolong life, particularly in the hazardous environmental conditions that prevail throughout the world today. Periodic detoxification is the best way to purge the body of both its own natural toxins as well as the unnatural and far more dangerous toxins assimilated from external sources. By taking measures to purify their blood and tissues on a regular basis, people prevent toxemia and protect themselves from its debilitating effects, particularly the acidosis and hypoxia that make tissues vulnerable to cancer. Since acidosis and hypoxia are the primary conditions of imbalance that permit germs to breed, tissues to degenerate, and cancer to develop, periodic detox is probably the single most effective preventive measure you can take to protect your life from the entire spectrum of disease and degenerative conditions. Detox is also the best cure for most of these conditions.

FLUSHING OUT ACIDS

The first and foremost strategy in any detox program is to flush acid residues out of the lymphatic system, blood, and other bodily fluids, all of which should be slightly alkaline. Almost all toxins in the body take the form of acids, and these acids must therefore be neutralized and flushed out of the system to restore normal alkaline balance to the blood and other bodily fluids. In TCM, the blood, lymph, bile, and other essential fluids of the body are collectively referred to as jing-yi ("vital fluids"), and the condition of a person's jing-yi, particularly the bloodstream, is regarded as a primary determining factor in human health and disease.

The late V. E. Irons, one of the Western world's leading authorities on therapeutic detoxification for health and longevity, agrees with the traditional Chinese view regarding the condition of the bloodstream as a critical indicator of health and disease. As Irons puts it, "Every cell in the body is served by the blood. It nourishes the cell, replaces worn out parts, and carries away waste products." Obviously, a polluted bloodstream carries little nourishment and is already so saturated with wastes that it cannot properly fulfill its function of carrying away cellular wastes.

The same goes for the lymphatic system. The body has six to seven hundred lymph glands. About three times more fluid volume of lymph exists in the human body than blood. One of the primary functions of the lymph is to clean acid wastes from the blood and tissues, but if the lymph itself is polluted with acid wastes, then it cannot properly perform these cleansing functions. Acids interfere with the free flow of lymph within the lymphatic channels, thereby further inhibiting its capacity to cleanse the blood and tissues.

Regardless of what type of detox program you choose, you must always remember to drink at least 1¾ to 2 and ⅔ quarts per day of pure, preferably alkaline water, to neutralize, dilute, and flush away the large amounts of acids and other toxic wastes that the detox process releases from tissues throughout the body. The human body is composed of over 70 percent water. By saturating the system daily with abundant quantities of pure alkaline water, pollutants are continuously flushed from the blood and tissues and eliminated through the kidneys, bowels, and skin. As a result, all bodily tissues are "washed" and all vital fluids are replenished with fresh water. This is equivalent to changing the dirty motor oil in your car, as well as the battery, brake, and transmission fluids. The whole mechanism operates more efficiently and produces less toxic waste when dirty fluids are replaced with clean.

RESTORING PROPER PH BALANCE

The corollary protocol to flushing out acids is to restore proper pH balance in the blood and tissues. The "pH" value is a standard measure of acid/alkaline balance, calibrated on a scale of 1 (extremely acid) to 14 (extremely alkaline), with 7 as neutral. Each of our vital bodily fluids has a very specific pH level at which it functions best. Except for stomach fluids and a few others, most of our vital fluids and tissues should be slightly alkaline. Blood, for example, has a slightly alkaline pH value of 7.3 to 7.4, exactly the same as seawater. If blood pH drops below 7.1

or rises above 7.5, severe symptoms of imbalance will manifest immediately, and if pH is not quickly restored to proper balance, death follows swiftly.

Almost all forms of internal toxicity cause a state of acidosis in the body. In turn, excessive levels of acid residues in the blood and tissues suppress immune response, interfere with normal metabolism, inhibit digestion and assimilation, promote fungal arid bacterial infections, and cause all sorts of other biological malfunctions and ill health. To explain how important pH balance is throughout the human system, some of the ways vital organs depend upon proper pH balance to function correctly are listed below.

Heart

The human heart pumps about 114 quarts of blood per hour. If the blood is saturated with acid wastes, the acids can do serious damage to heart tissue as the blood passes through it, gradually causing deterioration of the heart muscle. Moreover, normal heartbeat rhythms are dependent on an alkaline environment and are therefore adversely affected by excess acid wastes in the bloodstream. And since acid wastes drastically reduce the blood's capacity to carry oxygen, the heart does not receive sufficient oxygen supplies from blood that is saturated with acids.

Lungs

One way that the body can self-regulate pH balance in the blood is by controlling the oxygen level through correct breathing. By maximizing the exchange of gases in the lungs, proper diaphragmatic breathing saturates the bloodstream with fresh supplies of oxygen, while purging it of carbon dioxide. Oxygen supports an alkaline environment in the blood and tissues, while carbon dioxide contributes to acidosis. If you permit your blood to become overloaded with acid wastes, it cannot absorb and carry sufficient oxygen from the lungs to sustain an alkaline blood and tissue pH, resulting instead in a state of chronic hypoxia (oxygen deficiency) and its twin condition acidosis, in every tissue and cell in the body. This in turn paves the way for germs and tumors to develop.

Liver

One of the liver's main jobs is to filter toxic wastes from the bloodstream. Another task is to produce many of the alkaline enzymes upon which immune response and other vital functions depend. If the blood is constantly polluted by excess acid residues from wrong eating habits, alcohol and drugs, stress hormones and other acid-forming factors, the liver eventually gets overloaded with acid wastes and becomes deeply congested with toxic debris. This overload in turn impairs its ability to filter acids from the bloodstream, so instead the body starts depositing excess acid wastes in the joints and other solid tissues, causing arthritis and tissue toxicity throughout the body.

Kidneys

The kidneys also help to filter acid wastes from the bloodstream, processing about one liter of blood per minute. This process in turn helps keep blood pH at its proper alkaline level. Excessive acid waste in the blood due to improper diet, pharmaceutical drugs, and other lifestyle factors can severely corrode the delicate tissues in which blood filters through the kidneys. It can also cause the formation of kidney stones and inflammation of the bladder and urinary tract.

Proper pH balance to the blood and tissues can be restored in basically two related ways during detox, after the acid waste residues have all been flushed out. One method is alkalization, the other is oxygenation.

Alkalization can be achieved fairly quickly by adjusting the diet to strictly limit intake of acid-forming foods, while increasing consumption of alkaline-forming items. The swiftest and most effective dietary alkalizers are freshly extracted raw vegetable juices, such as carrot and beetroot juice. Drinking lots of pure alkaline water throughout the day is another effective way to alkalize your blood and tissues quickly by dietary means. One of the primary contributing factors to chronic acidosis today is a critical deficiency of essential alkaline minerals and trace elements, particularly calcium and magnesium. The body requires the full range of essential minerals to properly regulate pH balance in the blood and tissues. For example, if the bloodstream is constantly awash with acids from sugary carbonated soft drinks, sweets and other junk foods, and calcium intake is insufficient, the body will automatically draw calcium from the bones and teeth and pour it into the bloodstream to neutralize the flood of excess acids from eating refined sugar products. Calcium is the body's most powerful and abundant alkalizing agent, and whenever the blood becomes overloaded with acids, it "borrows" calcium from bones and teeth to quickly reestablish proper pH balance in the blood. This in turn results in weak bones, which gives rise to osteoporosis, and weak teeth, which results in tooth decay. Adequate mineral supplementation is therefore a key strategy in maintaining proper pH balance in the blood and tissues, and one of the best dietary sources of balanced minerals is whole Celtic sea salt, which may be used for all culinary purposes in the kitchen and also dissolved in a glass of water as a full-spectrum mineral supplement. So-called Celtic sea salt is whole, unrefined sea salt harvested by hand the ancient Celtic way and dried naturally by wind and sand. It is from seashores that have not yet been poisoned by industrial pollutants.

Oxygenation is the other major method of quickly restoring pH balance in the blood, and the best way to utilize this method is simply by learning to breathe properly, using the diaphragm rather than the upper chest to drive the breath. Sufficient oxygenation is an essential factor for maintaining an adequately alkaline environment in the blood and tissues. Conversely, progressive acidosis of blood and tissues is always associated with insufficient oxygenation, and therefore increasing oxygen supplies to the blood and tissues is an antidote to acidosis. In addition to learning how to breathe correctly and practicing deep breathing exercises, you can also oxygenate your blood and tissues by taking various types of oxygen supplements, such as water oxygenated with ozone, a few drops of hydrogen peroxide in a glass of water, deuterium sulphate ("ESF"), ionized alkaline micro-cluster water (micro-water), and others. We'll take a closer look at some of these products in the next chapter.

DREDGING THE DRAINS

During any detox program, the organs of elimination must work overtime to process and excrete all the accumulated toxic wastes that are loosened and released from organs and tissues throughout the body. Since the organs of elimination are already overworked from dealing with environmental pollution and wrong eating habits, the extra load of toxins that are suddenly released into the bloodstream, bowels, kidneys, and skin by the detox process can put a very heavy strain on the excretory organs. It is therefore important to give your excretory systems all the supplemental support you can during detox, to ensure maximum efficiency in elimination, with minimum toxic stress to the organs.

There are four main "drains" in the body through which toxic waste products are excreted from the system: the skin, the lungs, the kidneys and bladder, and the colon. As blood and tissues grow progressively more toxic during the course of a person's daily life, these drains get clogged with toxic residues, dry mucus, dead microbes and other "biowaste." In the case of the colon, the situation is very similar to what happens to the drain in your kitchen sink: layer upon layer of grease, partially decayed food, and other debris adhere to the pipe, gradually reducing the size of the passage through which waste water flows. And since this sticky layer of waste is full of microbes and toxins, it pollutes the bloodstream by osmosis through the colon wall, allowing the poisons to circulate throughout the body.

A number of ways exist to facilitate the drainage of toxic wastes through the four organs of elimination, and to protect them from damage during the detox process, and these ways will be discussed in detail in the following chapters. Briefly, what follows are some of the primary support protocols for each of the main drains during detox.

Skin

An enormous amount of toxic waste passes out of the body through the surface of the skin, especially in hot weather when the pores remain open day and night. During detox, toxic residues become very concentrated in perspiration and can damage the skin as they pass through for excretion. Strong, foul body odor and clammy sweat are additional manifestations of heavy toxicity in perspiration during detox. Damage to skin may be prevented, as well as relieved and repaired, by soaking daily in hot baths with sea salt or Epsom salts, plus some essential oils that help draw toxic wastes swiftly out through the pores. Another effective method of facilitating skin detox is the traditional Thai herbal steam bath, which draws toxins out through the skin while also soothing skin tissue with healing herbal essences. If you're doing your detox program by the sea, daily plunges in the ocean also provide cleansing support for the skin.

Lungs

The lungs excrete carbon dioxide and other volatile gaseous wastes from the blood, while absorbing oxygen, negative ions, and other elements from the air and transferring them into the bloodstream. When the blood is highly toxic, such as during detox programs, its capacity to carry oxygen is severely reduced, and this in turn leads to a state of hypoxia throughout the system. The anaerobic state produced by hypoxia supports an acid environment, thereby creating the conditions for disease and degeneration. Therefore, learning deep breathing exercises and practicing them daily is highly recommended during any detox program. Proper breathing oxygenates the blood and tissues, thereby helping to eliminate acidosis, while also facilitating rapid excretion of carbon dioxide and other gaseous wastes that contribute to acidosis. Thai herbal steam baths are also a very effective lung support therapy during detox; the soothing herbal essences in the steam bathe the delicate lung tissues in healing vapors with every breath, while drawing toxic residues out of the lungs. It is also a good idea to keep a negative-ion generator in your room to help the lungs function smoothly and support the detox process during sleep.

Kidneys and bladder

Some of the body's most toxic wastes pass through the kidneys, which filter them from the blood and excrete them through the bladder as urine.

When these wastes are highly acidic, they can damage the sensitive kidney tissues through which they filter and can also form painful kidney stones. It is therefore advisable to drink lots of herbal teas during detox, especially those with diuretic and kidney cleansing properties, to facilitate rapid excretion and protect the kidneys from toxic damage. Another important measure to protect the kidneys and promote swift elimination is to drink between one and ¾ and two and two-thirds quarts of pure alkaline water daily, preferably ionized micro-clustered water. This water dilutes the concentration of toxins in the blood and kidneys, neutralizes acidity, and flushes poisons quickly out of the system.

Colon

Of all the excretory organs, the colon is the most abused and overloaded these days. Believe it or not, the average Western male today carries about 2⅓–2⅔ pounds of dense, rubbery, mucoid material—a thick toxic sludge—imbedded in his bowels, and none of it is ordinary feces. During a detox program, it is a good idea to eliminate as much of this toxic lining as possible from the bowels. To accomplish that elimination, the person going through detox should take ground psyllium seed shaken in water at least twice daily and should also drink plenty of extra water. The psyllium and the water gel to form a fibrous bolus that sweeps through the bowels like a broom, loosening and eliminating mounds of impacted wastes from the walls of the bowels. For even more dramatic results and a complete cleansing of the entire colon, a series of colonic irrigations is recommended, especially during the first few days of a detox program. In addition to cleansing the colon and eliminating a major source of toxins to the bloodstream, colonic irrigation triggers a strong detox response in the liver, and a major cleansing reaction throughout the body. It is impossible to describe in words the sheer volume and incredibly foul appearance of the putrid, mucoid wastes that come tumbling out of the body with a series of colonic irrigations, after festering in the bowels for years and years. It is definitely a case of "seeing is believing," and anyone who's ever done it can testify how good it feels to dump all that bad rubbish from their bodies.

If you really wish to "start at the bottom" in a progressive program to completely detoxify and regenerate your whole system, then you should definitely begin with a series of colonic irrigations to dredge your bowels of all the putrefied, partially digested debris and toxic residues that have accumulated inside over the years. This is best done in conjunction with a three-to-seven day water or juice fast. Until you do this, regardless of how well you cleanse your blood and tissues by other means, the sludge in your bowels will continue to seep toxins right back into your bloodstream. Virtually everyone today has this problem. Even a hundred years ago, the famous American naturopath Dr. Harvey Kellogg, who invented the corn flake and was portrayed in the novel and film *Road to Wellville*, noted, "Of the 22,000 operations that I have personally performed, I have never found a normal colon." V. E. Irons, who devoted his long life to promoting colon health, remarked, "About the only place you see a normal healthy colon today is in an anatomy book."

It is rather pointless to embark on a major new dietary program and spend a lot of money on expensive nutritional and herbal supplements if your bowels are impacted with toxic wastes from years of pollutants and wrong eating habits. Not only does this thick slimy lining constantly secrete toxins into the bloodstream through the bowel walls, in the small intestine it blocks the assimilation of nutrients and herbal essences into the bloodstream. Dr. Norman Walker, who lived to the age of 116 by practicing what he preached, states in his book *Colon Health: The Key to a Vibrant Life:*

> The elimination of undigested food and other waste products is equally important as the proper digestion and assimilation of food. . . . The very best diets can be no better than the very worst if the sewage system of the colon is clogged with a collection of waste and corruption.

Those who have done colonic irrigations have always remarked on how much better they feel afterwards, and how colonics often eliminate chronic conditions that defied all other treatments. Nothing facilitates internal cleansing and accelerates the detox process as effectively as colonic irrigation. If you're still a "colonic virgin" and you really wish to know how it feels to unclog your bowels and wash them "squeaky clean," you should gird your loins and take the plunge as the first big step on your own "Road to Wellville."

MOVING WATER, ACTIVE HINGES

An ancient Chinese text on human health states, "Moving water never stagnates; active hinges never rust." That means if you exercise gently every day to keep your blood, lymph, and other vital bodily fluids flowing freely and to keep your joints and other moving parts active, then your bodily fluids won't stagnate and become toxic, and your joints won't "rust" with arthritis and stiffness. Regular, rhythmic body movements are particularly important for moving the lymph, because, unlike blood, which is pumped by the heart, lymph flow depends entirely on gravity and body movement for mobility. Since the lymph must work even harder than usual to cleanse the blood and tissues during a detox program, it is important to help keep lymph flowing freely with daily exercise.

The type of exercise required during detox is very different from strenuous sports activities such as tennis, football, jogging, and weight lifting. Western field sports and other forms of "hard" style exercise produce lactic acid in the tissues and carbon dioxide in the bloodstream as metabolic by-products of muscular exertion, and this contributes to acidosis, which is always counterproductive to detox. One of the primary purposes of any detox program is to eliminate acids and alkalize the system. Hard style exercise also keeps the autonomic nervous system locked into the "fight or flight" sympathetic branch, which switches off self-cleansing and healing responses, and causes muscular tension and tightness in the joints and tendons that then interfere with the state of complete physical relaxation required for detox to proceed.

Instead of hard exercise, one should practice traditional Asian soft-style exercises, such as yoga, Tai Chi, and *chi gung,* on a daily basis throughout the duration of any detox program. Soft-style exercise has entirely different effects on the body than hard-style. The soft, slow, smooth movements of these exercises gently pump the lymph through the system, while also assisting the free circulation of blood, without causing any muscular tension and without saturating the tissues with lactic acid or overloading the blood with carbon dioxide. These gentle body movements also help dissolve and eliminate crystalline acid deposits in the joints and keep the entire skeletal structure loose and limber.

Soft-style exercises should always be practiced in conjunction with slow, deep, rhythmic breathing that fully engages the diaphragm. The combination of slow stretching and loosening maneuvers with deep diaphragmatic breathing drives blood and lymph through the body like a strong pump, facilitating rapid drainage of toxins from the tissues and swift delivery of wastes to the eliminatory organs. Deep breathing greatly enhances oxygenation of the blood and tissues, which helps neutralize acidosis and maintains a healthy alkaline environment inside the body. When breathing properly, the diaphragm descends deeply into the abdominal cavity, providing an invigorating massage to the internal organs and glands. Diaphragmatic breathing gently squeezes the internal organs like a sponge on inhalation, draining out stale blood. Then it releases the pressure on exhalation, drawing freshly oxygenated blood into the organs. This deep diaphragmatic pressure on the internal organs and glands accelerates the detox process and extends it into the deepest, densest tissues of the body.

Most importantly, deep breathing, especially when performed in conjunction with slow rhythmic body movements, immediately produces the state of physical and mental relaxation required to switch the autonomic nervous system into the healing, restorative mode of the parasympathetic branch. Detoxification and healing can only proceed when the nervous system is operating in the parasympathetic circuit, and one of the primary functions of all traditional Asian soft style exercises is to activate the body's innate self-cleansing and healing mechanisms by switching the nervous system into the calm parasympathetic mode. That is what this style of exercise is designed to do, which is why it plays such an important role in traditional Asian health and healing systems.

POLLUTION AND PURIFICATION

Pollution and purification are natural cycles of life. Like birth and death, growth and decay, and all the seasonal cycles of nature, pollution and purification follow their own natural rhythms of yin and yang phases (figure 1). The human body has its own built-in purification cycles to deal with the natural pollution produced by digestion, respiration, and metabolism, but the system is clearly not designed to handle the enormous overload of artificial pollutants in modern life. People now living on this planet assimilate more hazardous toxins in a single day than they did in an entire lifetime only a few hundred years ago. The only way to deal with this toxic overload is to assist your body's natural self-cleansing mechanisms with periodic detox programs and to adjust your daily habits, so that purification always remains a few steps ahead of pollution.

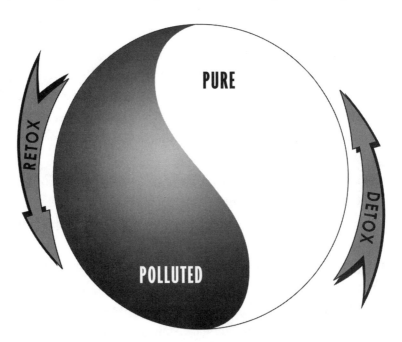

Fig. 1. The natural cycle of pollution and purification.

It should be noted that the programs described in this book are designed to rid the body of the sort of blood and tissue toxicity that most people today develop in the course of daily life from such sources as poor dietary habits, environmental pollution, chemical additives in food, water, cosmetics, and other household products, as well as moderate, occasional use of alcohol and drugs. They are not, however, designed to treat withdrawal from long-term addiction to alcohol and drugs, which usually requires additional special support for the central nervous system.

The only exception is when Neuro-Electric Therapy (NET) is used as the primary mode of withdrawal from alcohol or drug addiction, as described in chapter 9. In that case, the other detox methods presented in this book may be very effectively employed to support the drug-withdrawal process. After withdrawal is complete, these programs may be continued as a means of purifying the bloodstream and purging the tissues of toxic drug residues, to repair damage to the internal organs and to restore functional balance to the whole system so that a normal, healthy lifestyle may be resumed.

Whether you do your periodic detox work at home or at a health resort, make absolutely certain that you will not be disturbed, upset, annoyed, or interrupted from start to finish. The importance of giving body and mind a complete rest and total relaxation throughout the detox process cannot be overstated, which is why it is repeated so often in this book. You must set aside a period of at least three-to-seven days of complete peace and privacy, and you must remain, as much as possible, in a calm, quiet state the entire time. It won't work if you relax and do your detox regimens by day, then go out drinking and carousing at night, or if you work hard all day, then come home and try to detox at night. It is also a good idea to avoid watching violent films, listening to loud music, dealing with annoying people, or doing anything else that might excite your mind or stir up your emotions during detox. The moment you get excited or upset, your autonomic nervous system snaps back into the "F or F" action circuit, pumping stress hormones into the bloodstream and grinding the entire detox process to a halt.

The detox process can be accomplished in many different ways—hydration and hydrotherapy, diet and supplements, massage and exercise—but none of them will work properly for you unless you slow down and calm down long enough to allow your own natural healing responses a chance to work in complete harmony with these various supplemental programs. Half the battle is simply giving yourself that prolonged period of complete, uninterrupted rest and relaxation. The parasympathetic branch of your nervous system and the built-in healing responses that it governs will do the rest for you.

Back in the late 1960s, the hippy generation advised us all to "turn on, tune in, and drop out." Today, we would all be a lot better advised to "turn off" our normal daily habits and activities for a few days, to "tune out" the rest of the world for awhile, and "drop in" for a spell at the nearest spa or health resort to clean out, tune up, and rebalance our overworked, overplayed systems. Many adults today can't even remember what it is like to feel naturally good from the inside, so they seek a semblance of the sensation from the outside by indulging in alcohol and drugs, food and sex, money and power, all of which continuously enervate and weaken the system and end up making them feel even worse. Very few people halt their activities and retreat from the world for even as little as twenty-four hours, much less the three-to-seven days required for proper detox. For such people, a period of detox and self cleansing usually comes as a very enlightening experience, on many levels, and no one who's done it properly has ever regretted the time, effort or expense it requires. Indeed, detox may some day become the new "drugless drug" of the twenty-first century, both for its potent therapeutic healing benefits as well as for the "natural high" of well-being and good feeling it bestows.

2

WATER:
HYDRATION AND
HYDROTHERAPY

Water is the universal solvent. It is also the quintessential symbol of the Tao in Chinese philosophy. As Lao Tze states in the *Tao Teh Ching*, "Nothing is more yielding than water / but when it attacks things hard and resistant / there is not one of them that can prevail." With sufficient time and exposure, water can dissolve almost any toxin, hold it in solution, and deliver it elsewhere for elimination. Like city sewer and industrial waste-disposal systems, water is the medium required to flush waste products out of the body. Therefore, when you're detoxifying your body, you must drink extra quantities of pure alkaline water to dissolve, neutralize, and wash away all the toxins and acid wastes that the detox process releases into the bloodstream from the tissues.

Water is also the element that extracts nutrients from food, transports them into the bloodstream, and delivers them in solution into the cells for metabolism. Ninety percent of the blood and 85 percent of the brain are water; even the bones contain 30 percent water. Water is thus required for nourishment and the replenishment of vital fluids, as well as for detoxifying the blood and tissues and eliminating wastes. To do this, good quality water must be consumed daily in sufficient quantities to perform both of these essential functions properly.

Water has a unique capacity to carry energy and information, and it may be very precisely "programmed" to function as a potent and highly efficient tool for cleansing and healing the body. By using such diverse methods as electrolysis and magnetic fields, light and sound, oxygen and herbal essences, water may be energized and imprinted with specific information patterns to give it potent therapeutic cleansing and healing properties.

Today, a number of effective methods, both traditional and modern, technological ones, can be utilized to specially program water to enhance its detoxifying and purifying properties, and to improve its capacity to hydrate tissues and deliver nutrients and medicinal herbal essences into the cells. Water may be therapeutically programmed for internal as well as external use, and both applications are highly beneficial to any detox program.

INTERNAL USES: HYDRATION

Chronic dehydration has become a common condition throughout the world today. It is estimated that about 75 percent of the American population lives in a state of chronic dehydration. This in turn causes the body's natural thirst response, which is supposed to signal the body to drink water when thirsty, to be mistaken instead for hunger, prompting frequent snack binges that lead to food addictions and obesity. In a study conducted at the University of Washington, it was shown that one glass of water effectively shut off the "midnight munchies" syndrome in 100 percent of the dieters tested.

Dehydration produces a state of chronic toxemia and is one of the primary causes of daytime fatigue, sluggish metabolism, depression, and inability to concentrate. It also a major contributing factor in cancer. Several studies have demonstrated that by drinking only five glasses of pure water per day, the average person may reduce his or her risk of colon cancer by 45 percent, breast cancer by 80 percent, and bladder cancer by 50 percent. Other research indicates that drinking up to eight glasses of water daily significantly relieves chronic pain in the back and joints.

Dehydration is often the hidden cause in cases of chronic pain, including headaches, and in chronic fatigue. Dehydration dries the blood and other bodily fluids, causing cells to shrink and retain their toxic wastes. When cells are properly hydrated, they expand and become active, spontaneously cleansing themselves of toxic wastes. All bodily tissues are wrapped in envelopes of very fine membranes known as "fascia," which continuously rub against each other as various parts of the body move. All fascia require a layer of water in between them to provide lubrication as various organs and tissues rub against each other. When the body is dehydrated, this lubricating layer of interfascial fluid dries up, producing interfascial friction that causes tissue inflammation and chronic body pain. This is one of the main causes of the chronic-pain syndrome of which so many people complain these days, and for which they take billions of dollars worth of toxic chemical drugs to control pain. Yet most of this pain can usually be relieved simply by drinking sufficient quantities of pure alkaline water each day. If you drink specially energized waters, such as ionized microclustered water or oxygen water, then the therapeutic benefits of hydration become even greater and take effect faster. Proper daily hydration with good quality water is therefore the first remedy people should try for all types of chronic pain, including headaches, as well as daytime fatigue.

The water used by most people throughout the world today carries more toxic elements into their bodies than it washes out. Typical tap water contains chlorine, fluoride, aluminum, and a variety of toxic heavy metals such as lead, cadmium, and nickel. This is "dead" water, killed by chemical additives and acid elements, not the "living" water the body requires to function properly. Most commercial bottled waters are not much better, and the minerals in the so-called "mineral water" that is sold these days as an expensive gourmet health beverage are not in the ionized, microclustered form required by the cells for assimilation and utilization.

What the body requires is alkaline, ionized water that has been "restructured" into microcluster form. Only alkaline water can effectively neutralize acids in the blood and tissues and carry them away for excretion, and only alkaline minerals are beneficial to the body. Water that is charged with negative ions functions as a potent antioxidant to scavenge free radicals and prevent degenerative damage to the cells and tissues. The presence of negative ions also neutralizes all toxic substances in the bloodstream, because all toxins in the body take on a positive charge. Water that has been restructured into microcluster form passes easily through cell walls and tissue membranes, quickly hydrating the whole body and delivering essential nutrients into the cells, while also flushing out and carrying away toxic wastes. Water thus plays four fundamental roles in the body: hydration; alkalization; mineralization; and detoxification.

MICROWATER

A device has recently been developed in Japan that produces alkaline, ionized, microclustered water, known in health circles as "microwater" or "restructured water." It is a small machine about the size of a large dictionary that sits on the kitchen counter and attaches to any faucet. First the water runs through a very fine activated charcoal filter to remove solid particles and microbes. Then it enters a chamber with two titanium plates that are coated with platinum. By the process of electrolysis, all alkaline minerals held in solution in the water are drawn toward one plate, while all the acid elements, such as chlorine, fluoride, and heavy metals, are drawn to the other plate. The acid water drains out an exit tube into the sink for disposal, and the alkaline water is dispensed through a spout for consumption. In Japan, microwater has been successfully used to treat cancer, arthritis, immune dysfunction, and many other debilitating conditions, and it is now beginning to catch on in the West. Dr. Theodore Baroody, author of the aptly titled book *Alkalize or Die,* uses microclustered water as a therapeutic tool in his clinical practice and says, "It is my opinion that this technology will change the way in which all health care providers and the public approach their health in the coming years." Microwater has become so popular in Japan that bars and nightclubs now make all their ice and mix all their drinks with alkaline ionized microwater, and Japanese drinkers claim that when they mix their whisky with microwater and use microwater ice cubes, they never get hangovers the next morning, regardless how much they drink at night. That is because the negatively charged alkaline microwater neutralizes the acid by-products of alcohol metabolism and flushes them out of the body before they get lodged in the liver, brain, and other tissues.

The microwater technology does three things to water:

Alkalize: By eliminating every molecule of acid while retaining all alkaline minerals, the machine alkalizes the water with beneficial minerals. These alkaline elements serve two functions: they neutralize acids and thereby restore proper pH balance to the blood and tissues, and they mineralize the cells with beneficial alkaline minerals in ionized microcluster form.

Ionize: Electrolysis ionizes the water molecules as well as the minerals with an extra electron, giving them a negative charge and turning them into potent antioxidants that scavenge free radicals throughout the body. Negative ions also charge each water molecule with strong antitoxin properties that enable it to neutralize and carry away positively charged toxic molecules in the blood and tissues.

Microcluster: This technology also breaks the alkaline minerals and the water itself into smaller microclusters, so that they pass more easily and swiftly into the cells and tissues to hydrate, alkalize, mineralize, and detoxify the body. Ordinary water clumps in clusters of about twelve molecules each, while microwater is restructured into clusters of only five to six molecules. Similarly, the alkaline-ionized minerals are reduced into smaller molecular clusters, so that they, too, pass more easily into the cells to remineralize them.

Many good reasons support the purchase of one of these units and its use for all of your water requirements at home and at work, including cooking, making coffee and tea, and preparing ice cubes. During a detox program, drinking microwater is a great way to neutralize and flush out all the toxins and acids that drain from the tissues and bodily fluids, and to quickly rehydrate the body and keep the blood alkaline. If you use microwater for all your drinking and cooking requirements at home, it provides you with an ongoing "mini-detox" each and every day.

Microwater is a highly efficient antioxidant, and if you drink it throughout the day, it provides continuous antioxidant activity in the blood and tissues. Since free-radical damage is now commonly acknowledged in medical science as the primary cause of premature aging and tissue deterioration, drinking microwater daily can help you slow down the aging process and prevent a lot of unnecessary debilitating damage to your tissues. Many people complain that they find it difficult to drink large amounts of water, but drinking down two large glasses of alkaline microwater is both easy and pleasant, because the microclusters allow it to assimilate so quickly through your stomach and into your blood and tissues. By contrast, drinking just one glass of ordinary "dead" tap water or commercially bottled water makes your stomach feel bloated and heavy, because it just sits and pools there, like a stagnant pond, and that is why so few people like to drink water these days. Microwater solves the problem of "hydrophobia," as well as the problem of dehydration, by making it pleasant to drink sufficient amounts of water throughout the day, and its positive effects can be felt immediately. Its alkalinity counteracts the excess stomach acidity caused by modern eating habits; its microclustered minerals and trace elements provide essential nutrients that are chronically deficient in modern diets; and its negative-ion charge continuously scavenges free radicals and sweeps toxic substances from the bloodstream, enhancing overall vitality. All these benefits come at a cost that amounts to only a small fraction of what you'd pay for expensive nutritional and antioxidant supplements sold in health stores, and in the long run it is also much cheaper than buying bottled drinking water.

Other new technologies that enhance the blood-purifying and tissue -detoxifying powers of water include the "Vortex Energizer" and the "Grander Living Water System," both of which utilize water's unique capacity to transmit energy and information into the human system, by imprinting it with healing energy frequencies and wave patterns. The Vortex Energizer, developed by the Center for Implosion Research in England, is a small device that energizes water and counteracts the damaging influence of artificial electromagnetic fields in the environment. Drinking this activated water strengthens the human immune system, purifies the blood, and protects the body from toxic contamination.

The Grander Living Water System, invented by Austrian naturalist Johann Grander, revitalizes ordinary tap water by running it through a chamber in which it is exposed to sealed cylinders of highly energized water drawn from a five-thousand-year-old artesian spring in Austria. This water, which carries the natural electromagnetic properties of the earth itself, is further encoded with healing energy information by subjecting it to implosion technology and properly balanced bio-magnetic fields. As it passes through the chamber, the flowing water picks up the precise energy frequencies and polarity patterns encoded in the programmed water in the cylinders, thereby becoming identically "informed" to perform cleansing and healing functions in the body. In addition to purifying the bloodstream and detoxifying the tissues, Grander Water imparts its bio-active energies to all the vital fluids in the body, thereby enhancing immune response, improving digestion, facilitating excretion, and increasing the overall vitality and resistance of the whole system.

SEA WATER AND SEA SALT

Seawater has precisely the same pH as healthy blood and contains all of the essential minerals and trace elements, in exactly the correct proportions required by the human body. The sea is therefore an excellent source of mineral nutrients for human health, especially those rare trace elements that are generally missing in modern diets. It is also a rich source of alkalizing elements that counteract acidosis in the blood and tissues.

If you live near the ocean, one way to use seawater as a supplement is to keep a bottle of it in your refrigerator and drink a few ounces each day, diluted in a glass of pure water. Dr. Norman Walker, who lived to the age of 116 by periodically detoxifying his body, keeping his blood and tissues at proper pH balance, and eating properly, drank a few ounces of seawater daily to insure that his bloodstream contained all of the essential elements, known and not yet known, required by the blood and cells. If you're doing a detox program at a health resort near the ocean, this is a good way to help neutralize all the acid wastes that are released from your tissues by detox, and to provide your body with all the essential minerals it needs to support the detox process. It is important, however, to make sure that the water is drawn from clear, unpolluted parts of the ocean, not from coastal waters that have been excessively exposed to industrial contamination. One way to do this is to ask someone on a fishing or diving boat to haul a gallon of clean sea-water from deeper offshore waters.

Another way to tap into the sea as a source of alkalizing minerals and essential trace elements is to use whole, unrefined sea salt for all of your culinary requirements and also as a nutritional supplement. The best choice, as mentioned in chapter 1, is Celtic sea salt. The use of the word Celtic refers to an ancient northern European method of harvesting whole sea salt, a method still practiced along the Normandy coast in northern France today. This harvesting process makes it possible for all of the salt's essential elements to remain, as well as the important trace elements contained in the brine. The brine, also known as "bittern" or "mother liquor," is the thick residual fluid that remains in the salt pans after wind and sun have evaporated the water and the salt has been collected. With much of the brine's elements remaining in the harvested sea salt, the salt has a characteristic light gray color and slight dampness that distinguishes genuine Celtic sea salt from ordinary refined forms of sea salt. Commercially refined sea salt is heated and bleached and often treated with additives, to make it snow-white and to prevent clumping, but this process also strips the salt of many of its essential nutritional elements, especially the vital trace elements contained in the bittern.

Celtic sea salt contains eighty-four minerals and trace elements, including every one that is essential to human health. Its light gray color and moist crystals are the identifying traits that indicate the presence of the bittern in the salt. Besides providing all of the essential minerals required by the body, Celtic sea salt bestows specific benefits that are particularly helpful for detoxification and rejuvenation. It contains organic iodine, which, unlike the refined iodine added to industrially processed table salt, protects the body from harmful radiation in the environment and radioactive fallout in the atmosphere. The microminerals in Celtic sea salt provide the adrenal and pituitary glands with precisely the elements they require to sustain balanced secretions of vital hormones. Studies have shown that when refined table salt is used, secretions of the adrenal and pituitary glands are measurably reduced, and this results in low vitality, low motivation, and low libido.

Another type of sea salt that has become available today is Himalayan Glacial Salt, which is harvested from glaciers that were formed when the Indian subcontinent pushed its way into the Asian land mass, trapping huge lakes of seawater in the Himalayan valleys. As the water evaporated, enormous deposits of sea salt remained, and these were compressed into gigantic pink salt rocks by subsequent glacial pressures. These deposits of sea salt are the purest and most complete source of essential minerals and trace elements on earth, because they come from ocean waters as they existed many millions of years ago, before mercury and other industrial contaminants were dumped into the earth's seas. This salt is now available both in rock crystal as well as finely ground forms.

The denatured, industrially refined table salt that most people in the world use today does more harm to the body than it does good. This salt has been robbed of its synergistic minerals, trace elements, and other cofactors, leaving a denatured white substance that is 99.9 percent sodium chloride. Doctors today often advise people to drastically reduce their salt intake to prevent high blood pressure, but this advice applies only to the deleterious effects of industrially processed table salt, which contains an unnaturally high ratio of sodium and no synergistic cofactors to counterbalance the excess sodium. Furthermore, the sodium in refined table salt is hardened, and it therefore remains lodged in the body for an excessively long time, which is why it causes blood-pressure problems. The sodium in Celtic sea salt retains its natural pliant form, is less concentrated, and drains out of the body quickly. Furthermore, some of the trace elements contained in the bittern automatically neutralize and flush out excess sodium from the blood and tissues, thereby preventing it from causing any problems.

One way to use Celtic and Himalayan Glacial sea salt as an alkalizing mineral supplement is simply to dissolve about ⅓ tsp in a glass of water and drink it. This is also very helpful when you experience excess acidity in the stomach. Another way is to reconstitute the bittern, or "mother liquor," from whole Celtic sea salt, which is richly permeated with bittern, and use this as a supplement. To make your own bittern, place five to ten pounds of coarse light gray Celtic sea salt in a clean, unbleached cotton bag and tie the bag shut with a piece of string. Fill a large pot with pure spring water, and soak the bag of salt in the water for three to five minutes. Then hang the soaked bag of salt over a ceramic or glass bowl (but not metal), and let all of the fluid drip into the bowl. Funnel it into clean glass bottles, and take about one ounce of this reconstituted bittern, diluted in pure water, once or twice a day. A similar saline solution can be made simply by placing a pound of rock crystal Himalayan Glacial salt in a large jar and filling it with a liter of pure water, periodically adding more salt and water as you use the liquid brine. One or two teaspoons of the brine in a large glass of pure water is an excellent way to start each day.

Magnesium is one of the macrominerals that is most required for human health, but today more than half the population of the world suffers a critical deficiency of magnesium, including people in the richest, most highly developed countries, such as America and Western Europe. Magnesium deficiency is a major contributing factor to heart disease, and studies in the United States have shown that more than half of the fatal heart attacks there could probably have been be avoided if adequate magnesium supplementation had been administered in time. A shortage of magnesium contributes to depression, insomnia, irritability, and other problems related to central-nervous-system dysfunction. Magnesium is also one of the most important nutrients required by the body during the detox process, because magnesium is an essential element for the production of a multitude of alkaline enzymes that are required for the detoxification process. It is therefore a good idea to include some form of magnesium supplementation in any detox program, as well as in daily life.

You can prepare an excellent magnesium supplement yourself at home, using Celtic sea salt and magnesium chloride hexahydrate. Dissolve .28 ounces of Celtic sea salt in just under a quart of cold water, and seal tightly in a bottle with a cap. Then dissolve ⅖ths of an ounce of magnesium chloride hexahydrate in one liter of cold water, and cap it in a clean bottle as well. To use, mix one part of the salt solution with five parts of the magnesium solution and three or four parts of your favorite fruit or vegetable juice, or herbal tea, to make one full cup. Drink one cup in the morning and another in the evening for a period of ten to fifteen days, to correct conditions related to magnesium deficiency. The formula is also an essential support for any detox program. For ordinary use as a daily dietary supplement, one glass in the morning is sufficient.

An even easier way to get your daily magnesium chloride is to buy a bottle of magnesium oil, a viscous fluid solution of pure magnesium chloride available in the United States from globallight.net. The best way to use the oil is to fill a sprayer bottle with the fluid and add three to five sprays to a glass of drinking water two to three times daily. It may also be sprayed directly onto the skin for even more effective transdermal assimilation.

While we are on the topic of internal salt-water therapy, let's take a quick look at an ancient Indian technique for detoxifying and restoring the delicate tissues of the sinus cavity. Known as the "Neti" nasal douche, this method employs whole sea salt dissolved in warm water to gently wash the sinuses and flush out dust, smoke, air pollutants, and other toxic residues that become lodged in the sinus cavities. It is a highly refreshing cleanse that greatly improves nasal breathing, fully restores the sense of smell, and detoxifies the convoluted passages of the sinuses.

To do the Neti nasal douche, put about ⅔ tsp of Celtic sea salt into a small ceramic tea pot of about 1½ cup capacity. Add warm water at about body temperature and stir to completely dissolve the salt. Bend over forward, or kneel down, place the spout of the tea pot firmly into the left nostril, then tilt the head slowly to the right, until the water starts flowing into the left nostril, through the left sinus passage, and back out through the right sinus passage and right nostril, in a steady stream. When about half the solution is used, switch over to the other side and do the same thing. When you've finished the solution, bend over forward and rock your head up and down, then from side to side, while snorting air out your nostrils to blow residual water from the nasal passages.

OXYGEN WATER

Less than two hundred years ago, the earth's atmosphere contained about 38 percent oxygen. Today, oxygen constitutes only about 19 percent of the air we breathe, half of its former level, and a lot less than that in polluted inner cities. Oxygen deficiency has therefore become a common condition throughout the world, and it is a major contributing factor in toxemia, immune deficiency, cancer, and most chronic degeneration conditions. Since the air we breathe delivers only half the oxygen we require per breath, it is very helpful to provide an additional form of oxygen supplementation during detox, and one of the most effective ways is to use oxygenated water.

Besides its essential role as a fuel for metabolism, oxygen is also the great cleansing agent of the body. All toxins must first combine with oxygen to be carried out of the cells and tissues for excretion. Oxygen kills bacteria and viruses, neutralizes toxins, and purifies the blood, tissues, and individual cells. Unlike antibiotics, however, which kill friendly as well as harmful bacteria, oxygen kills only the harmful anaerobic bacteria that invade the inside of the body, without damaging the beneficial bacteria in the bowels and other tissues.

Brian Goulet, a health practitioner who utilizes oxygen therapy in his clinical practice, says, "Rubble, garbage, toxins, refuse, debris, and anything useless are destroyed by oxygen and carried out of the system. Just as a clean house holds little interest to passing flies, likewise any oxygen-rich body is a difficult fortress to assail." Molecular biologist Dr. Stephen Levine believes that oxygen deficiency could be the beginning phase of immune deficiency syndrome. Levine says, "We can look at oxygen deficiency as the single greatest cause of all diseases. It is believed and supported by a great deal of research, that a shortage of oxygen in the blood could very well be the starting point for the breakdown of the immune system."

One of the swiftest ways to oxygenate water to produce an oxygen supplement is to put a few drops of hydrogen peroxide into a glass of pure water. Hydrogen peroxide has the same molecular structure as water, except that it has an extra oxygen molecule. When dissolved in water, each molecule of hydrogen peroxide breaks down to produce one molecule of ordinary water and one molecule of free oxygen. These extra molecules of free oxygen enter the bloodstream and circulate throughout the tissues, thereby enriching the entire body with additional supplies of detoxifying oxygen. When you first start using hydrogen peroxide as an oxygen supplement, however, it is advisable to first consult with a health professional for specific guidance.

During detox, a small daily dose of hydrogen peroxide provides the blood with an extra boost of oxygen to deal with the overload of toxins that are released into the bloodstream from the tissues. In addition, you may take daily doses of this oxygenated water to protect yourself from the flu and other contagious diseases during epidemics. In the autumn of 1983, in the midst of an avian flu outbreak that killed over eleven million chickens in America, about one million chickens were given small amounts of hydrogen peroxide in their drinking water, and not a single one of these birds died of the disease. Another effective way to oxygenate water is to bubble ozone gas through it, but to do that, you must have a special ozone machine. Some spas and health resorts now have these devices. Drinking water treated with ozone releases even more free oxygen into the bloodstream than water treated with hydrogen peroxide, and this makes it a very useful item for internal cleansing purposes. As Dr. George Freibott of the International Association for Oxygen Therapy states, "Oxygen is a powerful detoxifier, and when its quantity is deficient, toxins begin to devastate body functions and deplete the body of life-giving energy."

One of the most remarkable oxygen supplements on the market today is a specially formulated solution of "heavy water" (deuterium sulfate) known as "ESF," which stands for "Everett Storey Formula," named after the American nuclear scientist who invented it during the 1950s. This product is sold throughout the world under license from the company that holds the patent, using various different brand names, including Cellfood, Liquid Life ESF, Hydrocell, Cellogen, and Hydroxygen.

ESF is based on a patented split-water technology. What it does is split a very small amount of the water molecules in your body to release one molecule of free oxygen and two molecules of free hydrogen, which then enter the blood and permeate the cells. As we have already noted, oxygen is one of nature's most potent detoxifiers, and oxygen levels in the air we breathe, which is our primary source, have dropped by half over the past two hundred years. ESF therefore serves to correct this oxygen deficiency by providing the body with a constant internal stream of free oxygen released from water. It also releases free hydrogen, which is an essential element for producing energy, repairing cells, and maintaining strong immune response. ESF contains microscopic, ionized forms of 78 vital minerals, 34 essential enzymes, and 17 important amino acids, all of which are carried into the cells along with the oxygen and hydrogen. ESF is therefore both a potent nutritional supplement and a highly effective detoxifying agent.

ESF should be taken three times daily (early morning, afternoon, and night) to insure a steady stream of free oxygen and hydrogen in the blood and tissues. For detox programs, or to help cure specific diseases, eight drops of ESF taken three times daily in a glass of plain water or juice is an effective dosage. For ordinary use as a daily supplement, five drops three times a day is sufficient. To order this product, please refer to the section on "Suppliers" at the back of the book.

EXTERNAL USES: HYDROTHERAPY

During detox, the skin must bear an extra heavy burden as an excretory outlet for toxic wastes, and it can easily get damaged and become blemished from contact with all the toxins that pass through the pores. The skin therefore needs special attention while the body is detoxifying itself to prevent toxic damage and to facilitate the rapid elimination of all toxins that are driven from the lymph, blood, and tissues out to the surface of the skin for elimination.

It should be noted that unlike the interior of the body, which should be slightly alkaline, the exterior surface of the skin should have a slightly acid mantle to protect the body from invasion by external pathogens. While the microbes that invade the interior of the body are anaerobic and thrive in acid environments, those that attack the exterior surface are aerobic and cannot tolerate an acid environment, which is why the skin is meant to have a slightly acidic pH value. Most people wash away this acid mantle on a daily basis, by using commercial bath soaps and shampoos, all of which contain strong alkaline detergents. This renders the skin vulnerable to infections, rashes, and other irritations. It is therefore advisable to cut down on the use of commercial bath soaps and shampoos, or to switch to milder varieties made only from pure vegetable, nut, and essential oils, without chemical additives. Another solution is to keep a bucket of the ionized acid water discharged from a microwater ionizing unit in the bathroom, and rinse your skin and hair with a few cups of this water after finishing your shower or bath. Since this acid water has been filtered, ionized, and reduced to micro-clusters, the same as the alkaline portion that you consume internally, it too is an extremely pure and potent therapeutic water but serves instead as an antiseptic acidifying agent for external use on the skin and hair.

The best way to protect your skin from damage and accelerate the excretion of toxic wastes through the pores during detox is to soak your body, or even just your feet, in hot water laced with sea salt or Epsom salt and a few drops of detoxifying essential oils. If you don't have time for a full body soak, or if you don't have a bathtub at home, just soaking your feet and ankles in a basin of hot saltwater is also very effective, for it draws toxic wastes through the lymph channels down to the feet and facilitates their excretion out of the body into the water.

HOT SALT WATER BATHS

The most popular way to prepare a hot saltwater bath today is to add a cup or two of Epsom salts to a bathtub full of hot water. Epsom salts are various forms of magnesium salts, and these are particularly effective for detoxification purposes because they stimulate lymph drainage and draw toxins out through the pores by osmosis.

You may also use coarse gray Celtic sea salt, which includes dozens of beneficial micro-minerals and trace elements contained in the bittern, to prepare a hot saltwater bath for detox purposes. To prepare a potent, sea-salt, detox bath, add three pounds of gray Celtic sea salt plus one pound of magnesium chloride hexahydrate to a bathtub full of hot water, and soak in it for about half an hour. The higher the salinity of the bath water, the stronger the power of osmosis that draws the toxins out through the skin, so for intensive detox purposes you need to use a greater quantity of sea salt, and add magnesium chloride for an extra boost of lymphatic detox. For ordinary saltwater bathing, one or two pounds of gray Celtic sea salt is sufficient to cleanse the skin and mildly detoxify the system, and the magnesium chloride may be omitted.

A particularly potent form of sea salt is available from the Dead Sea in the Jordon Valley. At 400 meters below sea level, the Dead Sea is the lowest spot on the surface of the earth, and it produces a bath salt that is extremely rich in medicinal minerals and natural detoxifying agents. This bath salt, which is available from health-product suppliers, has both detoxifying as well as healing properties, and hot Dead Sea salt baths provide highly beneficial support for the skin during detox.

Another useful skin detox product from the Dead Sea is therapeutic mineral mud. Dead Sea mud has amazing cleansing and healing powers, and it seems to work on both the physical, biochemical level as well as the energetic, electromagnetic level. To use Dead Sea mud for detox, put a sufficient amount of mud into a bowl and place the bowl in hot water to heat the mud. Smear the mud thickly over the affected part of the skin, cover with food wrap or cellophane, and tape in place with medical tape. Leave it there for about an hour, then wash off the mud, and take a hot Dead Sea salt bath. One woman in Australia reports that she cured herself of breast cancer and completely eliminated the tumors by applying Dead Sea mud packs and soaking in Dead Sea salt baths repeatedly over a period of several months. While such evidence is often discounted as "anecdotal," it is nevertheless a documented fact that it happened, and if such a cure can work once, it can certainly work again.

The therapeutic benefits of hot salt-water baths may be further enhanced by adding essential oils, which have detoxifying and healing properties, to the bathwater. Since these oils are also highly aromatic, some of their therapeutic essence is absorbed through the sinuses and lungs as the volatile vapors rise from the hot bath water. The oil of grapefruit seed and peel is a particularly good choice for helping to detoxify the lymphatic system. Sage and rosemary both have potent tissue cleansing properties, and peppermint oil may also be used for detox purposes. If you're feeling enervated and "uptight," try adding a few drops of frankincense oil to your hot saltwater bath, or a dash of lavender. Keep a variety of these essential oils in the bathroom, and experiment with different combinations for various conditions.

Another way to enhance the therapeutic power of bathwater is to use a Jacuzzi or whirlpool tub. The gentle vibratory stimulation from the water jets activates lymph drainage and boosts micro-circulation in the tissues just below the skin, thereby facilitating elimination of toxic wastes through the pores. By virtue of the piezoelectric effect, whereby any sort of rhythmic vibratory stimulation applied to a crystal substance is transformed by the crystal structure to produce an electromagnetic energy pulse, jet-water baths create a soothing, healing energy pulse deep within the body as a result of the piezoelectric effect of the vibrations in the water on the crystalline structures in bones, glands, connective tissue, and bodily fluids.

"MAGNUM" BATH

An extremely effective version of hot salt water bath for detox is what I refer to as the "Magnum" Bath. To prepare this bath, place ⅓ cup of magnesium chloride bath crystals, 1–2 tablespoons of magnesium chloride oil, and 1 tablespoon each of magnesium oxide and mica powder into a bathtub of hot water. Then soak your body in it for about half an hour. Alternatively, you can add about half those amounts to a bucket of hot water and simply soak your feet in it for twenty to thirty minutes. This method is almost as effective as a full-body bath, and it is a lot easier to do.

The magnesium chloride not only draws toxins out of the body through the skin, it also feeds magnesium into the tissues and cells of the body, thereby replenishing optimum cellular levels of this essential mineral, which is required for over three hundred vital enzymatic reactions in the human body.

The complete formula for this bath is given in appendix 1, "Recipes & Formulas," p. 303.

BATHING IN THE SEA

If you live near the ocean, or stay at a health resort by the sea, daily plunges in the ocean are another good way to provide your body with saline detox hydrotherapy. Seawater contains all of the medicinal minerals and cleansing elements found in sea salt, and therefore bathing in the sea allows the skin to detoxify and repair itself, albeit not as intensively as in a hot bath containing extra high concentrations of mineral salts added to the water. Again, be sure that the sea is clean before you jump in, otherwise you'll come out even more toxic than before. Avoid harbor waters and areas where raw sewage is disposed into the sea.

Another benefit of bathing daily in open seawater is that the ocean, which has its own vast electromagnetic energy field, naturally recharges and rebalances the human energy system whenever the body is submerged in it. This contributes significantly to the detoxification and regeneration process, and accelerates healing. In addition, the air along ocean shores is highly charged with negative ions, which also help detoxify the blood and tissues and facilitate rapid elimination of wastes. Finally, the rhythmic force of waves and currents in the ocean provides a gentle massage to the entire body, providing similar therapeutic effects as those discussed for whirlpool baths. Added together, these various benefits transform a daily dip in the ocean into an effective and pleasant therapeutic activity. No doubt that is one reason so many spas and health resorts are located by the sea.

MINERAL HOT SPRINGS

Since time immemorial, throughout Asia as well as the Western world, soaking in steamy mineral water baths at natural hot springs has been a traditional way of relaxing, cleansing, and healing the body. Today, this ancient custom is still widely practiced as a health regimen in East Asia, particularly in Japan, Korea, and Taiwan, whose mountain ranges are riddled with natural hot springs. In Japan, the mountainous southern island of Kyushu is the place to go for traditional hot-spring spas, many of which feature charming old Japanese inns with all the traditional amenities. Korea has numerous hot spring resorts in the mountains along the southern and eastern coastline. In Taiwan, the entire island steams with over one hundred hot-spring sources, from the well developed traditional hot-spring resorts of Peitou in the north to the rustic alfresco spas in the central highlands and southeast coastal region. Some of these hot springs have been operated as health spas and rest retreats for hundreds of years.

Since hot springs are usually located in rugged mountain settings that often feature waterfalls as well, a few words on the purifying power of falling water are in order here. Waterfalls produce a powerful, pulsing energy field that radiates for many meters, and the effect of this vibrant field on the human energy system, when one sits tranquilly at rest by a waterfall, is to detoxify and rebalance the entire system. Simply sitting quietly beside a big waterfall, and cultivating a calm state of mental serenity and physical relaxation, quickly clears blockages and corrects imbalances in the human energy field, and this in turn activates cleansing and healing responses in the nervous and endocrine systems. In addition, the air around waterfalls is richly charged with negative ions. Breathing this air saturates the blood with negative-ion energy, which acts as a powerful antioxidant to scavenge free radicals and neutralize toxins in the bloodstream, tissues, and cells The detox effect is swift, and it reaches the deepest tissues of the body. This form of hydrotherapy works on both the physical and energetic levels and may be utilized as an effective support for any detox program. Indeed, "sitting still doing nothing" beside a waterfall is an ancient Taoist way of practicing meditation, so you may combine your meditation practice with your hydrotherapy and reap a richer harvest from both.

HERBAL STEAM POWER

Among the most effective and pleasant ways of all to detox is to use traditional Thai herbal steam therapy, which is one of the most efficient methods of ridding the body of toxic wastes through the skin and lungs. It is basically the same set-up as any ordinary steam room system, except that highly aromatic medicinal herbs are added to the water in the boiler to produce a therapeutic herbal steam that engages both skin and lungs in the detox process. This is also a form of aromatherapy, but instead of just sniffing the aromatic essence released in the air through your nose, you immerse your entire body in it and breathe in hot damp vapor that carries the medicinal aromatic essences of the herbs deeply into your lungs, where they are quickly absorbed into the bloodstream and circulated directly to every tissue of the body, delivering their therapeutic powers to each and every cell. At the same time, the hot steam opens the pores and allows the herbal vapors to enter the skin to draw toxins out with the sweat. Thai herbal steam simultaneously cleanses the body from the inside and the outside, providing a doubly detoxifying effect as well as a very relaxing, soothing experience.

At the beginning of the twentieth century, hundreds of herbal steam facilities existed all over Thailand. Every town and village had them, and many were located on the premises of Buddhist temples, where traditional Thai medicine is still taught and practiced by monks. Herbal steam served as a primary form of healing and health care, with specific formulas for every disease and condition. Today, these herbal remedies have been replaced by Western pharmaceutical drugs, and public health in Thailand has diminished proportionately as a result. Nevertheless, you can still find traditional herbal steam facilities in most of Thailand's cities and resort areas, and you can also set up your own steam room at home.

More than seventy different aromatic herbs are used in traditional Thai steam therapy, but the primary ones are lemongrass, kaffir (a common Thai cooking herb), lime, ginger root, galanga root, basil, cinnamon, rosemary, thyme, pepper, and mint. In addition, you may also use aromatic medicinal herbs from other regions of the world, particularly those known for their cleansing, relaxing, and rejuvenating properties. The exact proportions are not particularly important, and they may be blended according to personal preference. As to quantity, that depends upon how strong you wish to make the steam and how big the boiler is in your steamer system. Generally speaking, you might use a total of 7–9 ounces of mixed fresh herbs, or 3½–4½ ounces of mixed dried herbs, for a medium sized steam boiler of 5–10 gallon capacity. Fresh and dried herbs may also be mixed together in the same batch. The lemongrass should preferably be fresh rather than dried to derive maximum benefit from this refreshing, relaxing, highly aromatic herb. Fill the steam boiler with water and let it come to a full boil before adding the herbs, which should be coarsely chopped. The herbs may be added directly to the boiling water, or else placed inside a cloth spice bag and tied shut with a string, which is then dropped into the boiling water. You may experiment with a variety of different blends until you discover the ones that suit you best. Meanwhile, as a general guideline, several classic combinations that are still commonly used in traditional Thai herbal steam therapy today are given in the "Recipes and Formulas" section (appendix 1, pages 302–3) at the back of the book.

To use an herbal steam bath for detox therapy, first drink a few cups of hot herbal tea that has cleansing or relaxing properties, such as chamomile, peppermint, sage, or ginger. Then enter the steam room and sit quietly inside for about twenty minutes, breathing deeply through the nose. Next, leave the steam room and take a plunge in a cool pool, or stand under a cold shower, to cool off the body, rinse sweat from the skin, close the pores, and stimulate the lymph and endocrine systems. Relax for five to ten minutes and then repeat the process two or three more times. When you're finished, be sure to drink at least two large glasses of alkaline water to rehydrate your tissues and remineralize your cellular fluids.

WATER SHORTAGE

Today, the supply of pure, naturally balanced water is shrinking at an alarming rate. The water situation has gotten so bad that many people now depend on bottled water for their daily drinking supplies, because the water provided by most municipal water utilities is so overloaded with chemicals.

Water's incredible solvent properties are a two-edged sword. On the one hand, water is required to dissolve and transport essential nutrients, trace elements, and herbal essences into the cells and tissues; water vapor can carry healing herbal energies into the lungs and skin; and water can neutralize and flush away virtually any toxin in the body. On the other hand, these characteristics also mean that water dissolves any toxic substance to which it is exposed in the environment, holds it in solution, and transports it wherever it goes. Thus, the more toxic the environment becomes, the more poisonous the world's water supply gets. Regardless of whether you use it internally or externally, water can either harm you by bringing dissolved toxins in solution into your body, or else heal you by dissolving toxins that are already imbedded in your system and then carrying the toxins out of the body as liquid waste. It all depends on the original quality of the water you use, how well you purify it, and whether you "program" it to nourish, cleanse, and heal your body.

Most of the water on the earth today has been seriously polluted and acidified by various artificial means, such as industrial waste, sewage, and chemicals such as chlorine and fluoride. Therefore the only way to purify and alkalize water for consumption is to use special technology that makes water fit for human health and healing. When used for intensive detox purposes, water may be specifically programmed in the various ways discussed in this chapter to enhance its hydrating and alkalizing properties, increase its cleansing and detoxifying effects, and amplify its antioxidant activity.

It is also important to remember that when taking water internally for detox purposes as well as for ordinary daily consumption, quantity is every bit as important as quality. Water can only work to cleanse and heal your body if you drink sufficient quantities each day to keep your blood and tissues consistently well hydrated and to fully replenish the water lost from the body each day with the excretion of wastes. That means you need to drink about five to eight glasses of pure water per day, depending on your individual requirements and metabolism, to prevent dehydration and keep your bodily fluids fresh and freely flowing.

3

PHYSIOTHERAPY: MASSAGE AND SOFT EXERCISE

Stagnation of bodily fluids due to insufficient movement is one of the great afflictions of modern life and a major contributing factor to chronic toxemia. The more "convenient" life becomes—with cars to replace feet, machines to wash clothes, elevators to avoid stairs, and motors to perform virtually every other chore—the more sedentary people become and the less they exercise their bodies. Like stagnant ponds, their bodily fluids become inert and turbid, losing vitality and the capacity to support life. In a section on health in the Confucian classic entitled *Spring and Autumn Annals,* compiled over two thousand years ago, it is written, "If the body does not move, essence [vital fluids] does not flow. When essence does not flow, energy stagnates." And when energy stagnates, the whole system loses power, and the first function to fail is the body's ability to cleanse and repair itself.

The human body was designed by nature to move, not to remain perpetually inert and immobile, and bodily fluids were meant to flow, not to sit still and stagnate. Some of these vital fluids, such as lymph, depend entirely on body movements for their own mobility. When you're watching television or sitting at a desk, riding in a car or standing in an elevator, your lymph stands still and your blood slows down. Whenever such immobility takes place, waste drainage halts and toxins accumulate rapidly in the blood and tissues. Insufficient exercise also stiffens the joints and tightens the tendons, congests the bowels and reduces metabolic efficiency. Activity is the principle attribute of energy and of life itself, while inertia and stagnation pave the way for decay and death.

During detox, it is especially important to keep your blood, lymph, and other bodily fluids flowing freely, to keep your joints loose and limber, to stretch your tendons and other connective tissue, and to stimulate activity in your organs and glands. There is a tendency during detox to remain inert and inactive, because the detox process makes your body feel tired, weak, and sluggish as the toxins are released continuously into the bloodstream for elimination. However, if you don't move your body and keep your fluids flowing, the toxins released from your tissues circulate in your bloodstream for a much longer period of time, making you feel even worse and prolonging the discomfort as well as the duration of the detox process.

Fortunately, if you're too lazy or too tired to mobilize your own body and move your own blood and lymph during detox, you can pay someone else to do it for you with therapeutic massage, which kneads toxins from the tissues, activates lymph drainage, stimulates glandular secretions, calms the nervous system, and tones the joints, muscles, and tendons. If you cannot afford professional massage every day, or if it is not available, you may apply self-massage techniques instead to facilitate the detox process and prevent stagnation. Alternatively, you could practice some form of traditional Asian soft-style exercise, such as yoga, Tai Chi, or chi gung, or simply go for a stroll or a swim every day, to keep your body loose and limber, to stretch and tone your tissues, and to keep your cleansing bodily fluids flowing freely.

MASSAGE

The Chinese term for massage translates literally into English as "press and rub," reflecting its two main techniques: deep tissue pressure, followed by shallow surface rubbing, applied alternately. The deep pressure stimulates vital points along the meridians and dislodges toxic deposits in the tissues. The rubbing then scatters the released toxins and facilitates their drainage through the blood and lymph. A variety of different styles of traditional Asian massage are available, and most of them work with a combination of deep tissue pressure and soothing surface palpation.

You may enhance the therapeutic benefits of detox massage by thoroughly washing your body (or having an herbal steam) before the massage, to remove dirt, oil, sweat, and toxic residues from your skin. Eliminating this greasy layer of dust, dead cells, and dried perspiration from the surface of your skin facilitates the interaction and exchange of energy between your body and the massage therapist's hands, and this in turn amplifies the therapeutic benefits of the massage and corrects imbalances in your energy field. It is important to rest quietly and remain completely relaxed throughout the duration of a therapeutic massage. Don't allow yourself to be disturbed by loud music, blaring televisions, urgent phone calls, or any other invasive distraction, and abstain from carrying on a conversation while you're receiving massage therapy. Energy always follows wherever you aim your attention, so if you focus attention on external sensory distractions during a massage, your energy will flow out to those distractions and dissipate externally. On the other hand, if you focus your attention internally, shining it like a spotlight on the parts of the body that are being massaged, your energy will flow there instead, magnifying the therapeutic power of the massage on that part of the body. Last but not least, don't forget to drink one or two large glasses of pure alkaline water immediately after every therapeutic massage, especially during a detox program. This hydration is necessary to quickly dissolve, flush out, and excrete the flood of toxins that deep tissue massage releases into the blood and lymph from every part of the body.

Traditional Thai Massage

Thai massage originated in India, but over the centuries it has also adopted some techniques from China, such as the applying of acupressure to vital points along the energy meridians. It is one of the most comprehensive and effective therapeutic massage systems in the world, combining deep-tissue massage, yoga stretches applied to your body by the therapist, acupressure therapy, joint and spine manipulation, and direct stimulation of the endocrine glands. Even the force of gravity is employed to mobilize the flow of vital fluids by holding the body in various upside-down postures. Another maneuver unique to Thai massage is the artery block, whereby the major arteries that feed blood into the legs are blocked shut by manual pressure for thirty to forty-five seconds, then suddenly released. This brings a strong wave of blood rushing warmly down through the legs, sweeping loose plaque and other debris from the walls of these arteries and providing a big boost to circulation throughout the system.

A session of traditional Thai massage, which is known as *nuat boran* and still widely practiced today in Thailand, should last for at least one hour, preferably two or three. Some of the older, classically trained massage masters in Thailand refuse to do a session of fewer than two hours, because this therapy was designed to slowly and very systematically detoxify, tone, and rebalance the entire human system, including all the organs, glands, and tissues of the physical body as well as the channels, chakras, and energy fields of the body. This takes time, and since some of the techniques are quite powerful, such as the artery block and the spinal stretches, they cannot be applied quickly in rapid succession. Instead, strong and gentle techniques are applied alternately, gradually preparing the body for the deeper techniques and giving the whole system time to adjust and rebalance itself after each major shift.

Again, don't forget to drink one or two large glasses of pure water after a Thai massage, just as you would after any therapeutic massage.

Chinese tui-na *Massage*

One of the most ancient forms of therapeutic massage is Chinese *tui-na,* literally "press and rub," as mentioned above. It is done with the ball of the thumb and sometimes with the knuckles of the index and middle fingers. Tui-na massage is performed with a single deep press of the thumb or knuckle, pushing deeply into the tissues, then releasing the pressure and immediately rubbing the surface with circular motion to disperse stagnant energy. This pressing and rubbing therapy is applied repeatedly along the entire length of specific energy meridians and nerve channels associated with the organs and tissues that require treatment. Stagnant organs and toxic tissues are activated by the deep pressure along the meridians and nerves that control them, stimulating them to discharge their toxins, recharge their cells, replenish their fluids, and rebalance their functions. The deep pressure and rhythmic rubbing gradually kneads toxic residues loose from the tissues and drives them into the lymphatic system for disposal.

Since blood vessels and lymph channels follow the same basic pathways through the body as meridians and nerves, tui-na therapy stimulates blood circulation and lymph drainage as well. This facilitates swift elimination of the toxins and acid wastes discharged from the organs and other tissues.

Tui-na massage is particularly effective for dislodging impacted toxins from nerve tissue and pushing them into the lymph channels for elimination. As noted earlier, some of the most hazardous toxic substances in the body, such as heavy metals and inorganic chemicals, have a particular affinity for nerve tissue due to its electromagnetic potential. The body's natural cleansing mechanisms cannot easily eliminate these heavy toxins, and so they cling to nerve tissues, gradually becoming embedded there and causing all kinds of maladies and malfunctions of the nervous system. Tui-na massage, applied along the entire length of the neck and spine and down along the major nerves of the arms and legs, loosens and releases clumps of toxic deposits impacted in the nerve tissues, allowing them to be dissolved and carried away for excretion in the blood and lymph. When the deep tissue pressure is released and followed by circular rubbing on the surface, fresh blood and energy flow into the tissues, repairing and recharging nerves damaged by long-term toxicity.

Some tui-na therapists begin each session with fifteen to twenty minutes of work applied entirely to the four branches of the bladder meridian, which run up along the spine, with two parallel channels on each side. This technique relaxes the internal organs, switches the nervous system into the healing mode of the parasympathetic branch, and releases tension from the muscles that support the spinal cord. These branches of the bladder meridian pass through the thick, tough bands of muscle that support the spinal cord. In most people, these muscles are usually tight as springs with nervous tension. This tension compresses the upper vertebrae and inhibits the passage of nerve signals through the spinal cord and out to the organs and glands. Tension in the nerves and muscles of the spine also keeps the autonomous nervous system locked into the hyperactive "fight or flight" responses of the sympathetic branch, thereby blocking detoxification and healing responses. By applying alternating deep-tissue pressure and circular rubbing along the full length of the bladder meridians on both sides of the spine, tension in the spinal muscles is gradually released and the entire spinal cord and all the vertebrae and surrounding connective tissues gradually relax, switching the nervous system over to the calm, healing mode of the parasympathetic branch and allowing the nerves to communicate freely with the organs and endocrine system to activate cleansing and healing responses throughout the system.

There's a special branch of tui-na massage in TCM called *hsiao-er tui na,* literally meaning "little children's tui-na." It was developed entirely for pediatric application. Most children rebel at taking bitter herbal concoctions, and they buck like broncos if a doctor tries to stick an acupuncture needle in their bodies. Pediatric tui-na was thus developed as a special branch of TCM to provide an effective means of applying medical therapy that children will accept. To make it even more acceptable for children, soothing aromatic oils are usually applied to the skin as well, to increase the therapeutic benefits of the massage and to produce a more pleasant sensation. Children are far more responsive to touch than adults, and they usually don't carry the psychic tensions that tighten the tissues of adult bodies. A relatively lighter touch may therefore be used on children's bodies than on adults, making the therapy even less invasive. Due to the softness and sensitivity of children's growing bodies, therapeutic results are usually swift and effective. A weekly or monthly "tune-up" with pediatric tui-na massage by a qualified therapist is an excellent preventive regimen for keeping young children's systems healthy and strong and counteracting the toxicity that junk food and environmental pollution produces in children today.

Japanese Shiatsu Massage

Shiatsu is a traditional Japanese therapy based on even older Chinese acupressure techniques. In shiatsu, a thumb or knuckle is used to apply deep pressure to various acupuncture points to produce a specific therapeutic effect in the organs associated with those points. This technique is especially effective when applied by a therapist who has developed the ability to "emit energy" *(fa chi)* through his or her hands, thereby boosting the therapeutic benefits of the acupressure by transferring a "turbocharge" of healing energy directly into the patient's energy system. In recent years, both shiatsu and traditional Thai massage have come to the attention of alternative health-care providers in Europe and North America, and many aspiring young healers from the Western world now spend time in Thailand and Japan learning these ancient healing arts under the tutelage of accomplished masters. If you're doing a detox program in an area where you can find a qualified practitioner of shiatsu or traditional Thai massage, you can accelerate the pace and reduce the discomfort of the detox process by having a daily treatment.

Traditional Asian Foot Massage

All Asian healing traditions include a special form of therapeutic massage applied exclusively to the terminals of major energy meridians and nerve channels located in the feet. In the West, this form of foot therapy is called "reflexology," but it is not nearly as well developed nor as effective as the ancient Asian method, which has been practiced continuously throughout the East for thousands of years.

The techniques of traditional Asian foot massage are similar to the deep-tissue pressing and surface rubbing used in tui-na but are applied exclusively to vital points on the many meridians and nerve channels that terminate in the feet. Six of the twelve primary organ-energy meridians have terminals in the feet—spleen, liver, kidneys, stomach, bladder, and gall bladder—and the main branches of the autonomic nervous system also have roots there. By stimulating specific points on the feet with deep tissue pressure, specific therapeutic effects may be produced in the related organs and glands of the body.

In TCM, cramped and misshapen feet are seen as a primary cause of chronic dysfunction in the internal organs and glands connected to the nerve and energy channels in the feet. These terminals are literally crushed by hardened tissues and bone deformities in the feet. The liver and kidneys, for example, which are responsible for filtering toxins from the blood, cannot properly perform their cleansing functions when the energy meridians and nerve endings that regulate them are pinched and blocked in the feet. Consequently, toxic wastes accumulate in the blood and tissues, and bodily fluids become increasingly acidic, producing a state of chronic toxemia that sets the stage for the onset of disease and degeneration. Deep acupressure applied to blocked nerves and meridians on the soles of the feet triggers a massive internal cleansing response in the related organs, particularly the liver and kidneys. Individuals who are especially toxic will sometimes run to the nearest toilet to pass a liter of coffee-colored urine immediately after their first treatment, or purge their bowels with a bout of diarrhea. A foul odor often exudes from their skin as well, as toxins are driven out through the pores. Clearly, this is a powerful detox therapy.

Dr. Lee Shih-min, a doctor from Taiwan who was trained in modern Western medicine, has in recent years drawn a lot of serious professional attention to his use of this ancient Chinese healing art form in America. At the University of Southern California's medical center, where Dr. Lee practiced Western medicine for many years, he was frequently exposed to the invasive and often counterproductive methods of modern allopathic medicine and radical surgery. After a while, he says, he "got so tired of all the needles, knives, and drugs" that he started studying the ancient ways of traditional Chinese medicine in search of better methods. There he discovered foot therapy and started practicing it as a sideline in his own clinic. Before long, he gained a reputation for producing "medical miracles," and foot therapy soon became his main profession, as more and more doctors and surgeons at the medical center referred their "hopeless cases" to him as a last resort. More often than not, he completely cured those patients. Initially skeptical, his medical colleagues themselves now go to Dr. Lee for treatment. It can take months to get an appointment with him. Fortunately, Dr. Lee is training a new generation of therapists in this powerful detoxification and healing technique, and hopefully it will soon become more widely available.

If you're traveling in Thailand these days, you'll notice dozens of new foot massage salons in every major city and resort area. Traditional Asian foot massage has enjoyed a big revival in Thailand recently, and most of the salons are staffed by properly trained therapists. A traditional Asian foot massage costs less than having a few beers in a bar, and it is therefore a service that most visitors can afford on a daily basis. Even if you're not doing a detox program, having a traditional Asian foot massage from time to time is a wonderful way to totally relax your body and recharge your batteries, while also cleansing the internal organs, stimulating glandular secretions, and clearing congested energy and nerve channels in the feet.

A convenient way to perform your own deep tissue foot massage is to walk barefoot on smooth round stones embedded in concrete, like little cobblestones. This technique, known in Chinese as "treading stones" *(tsai shir-tou)*, has been used for thousands of years in China and elsewhere in Asia as self-healing therapy, and its effects are fast and effective, because it stimulates points deeply imbedded in the tissues of the feet. You can easily make your own therapeutic stone walk at home by pouring one or two square meters of concrete and setting smooth round stones varying in size from a plum to a peach halfway into the wet cement, then letting it dry. To use the stones for deep-tissue foot massage, walk around slowly on the stones with bare feet, pausing to rock back and forth on your feet whenever you find points that are sore or sensitive. The idea is to soften any hard spots and to dissolve any crystallized particles that you find in your feet by pressing and rubbing those spots on the stones. For best results, you should try to do this for about twenty minutes, twice daily, for a period of one to two weeks. It is also an excellent supplemental therapy for any detox program, because it greatly accelerates internal cleansing and elimination of wastes and it stimulates healing responses throughout the system.

Nei-dzang *Internal Organ Massage*

TCM also has a special type of massage designed to directly stimulate the internal organs, facilitate their drainage of toxic wastes, and draw circulation of blood and energy into the organs and glands to repair and replenish them. Known as *nei-dzang* (literally, "internal organ") massage, this technique employs the extended tips of the index, middle, and ring fingers to probe deeply into the abdominal cavity and apply massage therapy directly to the internal organs. This direct pressure clears stagnant fluids and disperses congested energy, drives toxic residues from the organ tissues, and stimulates sluggish organs to restore normal function. It is a very effective way to relieve abdominal bloating and water retention, move clogged bowels, clear liver congestion, reduce swelling in the pancreas, and eliminate gas. Not many therapists are qualified to practice this method today, and it should only be done by someone properly trained to work in the soft tissues of the abdominal cavity, but if you manage to find a qualified practitioner, it is well worth arranging a series of treatments as a support for any detox program.

When internal organ massage is performed by a healer who has mastered the skill of "emitting energy" through the hands, it is known as *chi nei-dzang,* and the results are even more dramatic. The hands of such healers are known as "flags of energy" in Chinese, because they can wave healing energy directly into the channels of the ailing organs through their palms and fingertips, producing therapeutic effects in the energy system to amplify the physical therapy provided by tactile pressure.

Hot Herbal Oil Massage

In India, Thailand, and Bali, a form of traditional therapeutic massage using hot herbal oils and based on the principles of classical ayurvedic medicine is still widely practiced. Natural massage oils such as sesame, sweet almond, and coconut are infused with aromatic essential oils known for their purifying and healing medicinal properties and heated to slightly above body temperature. The hot medicinal oil is applied liberally to the body with a vigorous massage, driving the volatile medicinal essences deeply into the tissues, where they enter the bloodstream and energy meridians and circulate throughout the system. This type of massage is particularly effective for curing arthritis, rheumatism, and any sort of inflammation in the joints and ligaments. It also drains the lymph channels, tones the skin, and soothes the nervous system.

Chiropractic

Chiropractic is a remarkably effective medical therapy developed as an early offshoot of Western medicine and long ridiculed by conventional allopathic doctors as some sort of "voodoo medicine." But just like Dr. Lee's traditional Chinese foot-massage therapy, chiropractic is based on sound scientific principles and often produces positive results when all modern medical methods fail. The public is therefore beginning to rediscover and utilize this form of treatment, which realigns all of the major joints and bones in the body and rebalances the entire skeletal framework. Misaligned bones, especially in the neck, spine, and sacrum, can cramp and obstruct nerve and energy channels, depriving the related organs and glands of energy, and blocking nerve signals to them from the brain. By loosening up the joints and ligaments and by manipulating the bones back into proper alignment, the free flow of blood, energy, and nerve impulses is restored to all of the internal organs, thereby allowing them to cleanse and heal themselves. During prolonged periods of toxicity, the body stores many toxic wastes as crystalline deposits in the joints, gradually throwing posture off balance and pushing bones out of position. Therefore, a few chiropractic adjustments either before or during a detox program can assist the body's cleansing and healing mechanisms to function more efficiently.

SELF-MASSAGE

Self-massage is a simple, convenient technique that may be applied any time, any place, during the detox process to help keep bodily fluids moving, release tension and toxins from tissues, and relieve the minor aches and pains that arise in the body during detox. Anyone can do it, and it requires no special training.

When practicing self-massage, it is best to sit on a chair or stool with the spine straight and feet flat on the floor. Before you start, rub the palms of the hands together briskly for about thirty seconds, until they feel warm, to charge them with energy and increase their polarity. This enhances the therapeutic benefits of self-massage, especially when working on vital points along the energy meridians. Recharge the palms in this manner every two to three minutes throughout the treatment.

Acupressure

Several major energy points on the body may be effectively stimulated for detox purposes by means of self-acupressure. It is important to remain as relaxed as possible while doing this, because energy cannot flow freely through tissues that are "uptight" with physical tension. It is also best to do this technique while breathing deeply and slowly from the diaphragm, to help circulate blood and energy and keep the nervous system in the restorative parasympathetic mode.

The four most useful points for self-acupressure during detox are illustrated in figure 2 and are briefly described below:

Ho-gu ("Valley of Harmony"): This is one of the body's primary power points, and stimulation here gives a boost to the entire energy system. It is located on the large intestine meridian, in the V-shaped depression in the webbing between the base of the thumb and index finger. Press the tip of the thumb deeply into the "valley" until you find this sensitive point, then push hard on it for about ten seconds, release, rub the surface in circles, and repeat two or three times. This point stimulates the colon, relieves headaches and toothaches on the side pressed, alleviates fatigue, and improves respiration, all of which are beneficial to the detox process.

Tai-chung ("Supreme Thruster"): This point is the equivalent on the foot to the "Valley of Harmony" point on the hand. Located along the liver meridian on top of the foot, the point is tucked in between the tendons of the big and second toes, a little over an inch up from the slot between those toes. Press the thumb deeply between these two tendons until you find the point, then apply pressure in the same way as described above. This point is the most powerful one on the liver meridian, and acupressure here stimulates all liver functions, prompts liver detoxification, helps cure hepatitis and other liver disease, relieves headaches and eye aches caused by congestion and "fire" in the liver, and is also a good way to take the edge off a hangover.

Fig. 2. Four vital acupressure points for practicing self-massage therapy.

San-yin-jiao ("**Triple Yin Intersection**"): Located at the junction where the meridians of the three primary Yin organs (liver, kidneys, and spleen) intersect on the inside of the calf, this point is found one hand-width above the ankle, along the inside edge of the shin bone. Both the liver and kidneys are primary excretory organs, and pressure on this point provides strong stimulation to both. It also governs sexual energy, enhancing potency in men and helping to regulate menstrual cycles in women. It is a good point to press for an energy boost when your vitality is running low during detox.

Yung-chuan (**"Bubbling Spring"**): This is the most powerful point on the kidney meridian, located in the center of the ball of the foot, 2 inches down from the middle toe. Pressure here stimulates kidney functions and energizes the entire system. This point is also specifically effective for treating hypertension, anxiety, and insomnia, and for balancing irregular heart rhythms. In addition, this point stimulates the adrenal glands, which are attached to the kidneys, to secrete hormones that enhance vitality and to help keep the entire endocrine system in balance.

Squeezing (ya) *and Rubbing* (mo)

This technique may be applied to the flesh and joints of the neck, shoulders, arms, and legs to stimulate drainage of lymph channels, activate blood circulation, drive toxic residues from tissues, and release tension from muscles and tendons. Rub the palms together to charge them with energy, then use the fingers and thumb of the right hand to grab and give a strong squeeze to the muscles and tendons on the left side of the body, then briskly rub the surface with an open palm. Start at the neck and shoulder, work down the arm to the fingers, and massage from the top of the thigh down the leg to the toes. Then use the left hand to work on the right side of the body.

"Chi Brushing"

This method uses the charged palm of the hand as a "brush" to disperse congested energy from various tissues and organs, thereby opening circulation of blood and energy to those tissues, clearing stagnation, and draining toxins. It is also a good way to relieve minor aches in the body. After charging the hands by rubbing them together till warm, use one palm to repeatedly brush in a downward direction across the surface of the tissues you wish to treat, as though you were trying to wipe off something from the skin and sweep it away. For example, if the muscles of your arms or legs ache, brush a charged palm across the aching muscles, always sweeping downward and away from the body. This "scatters chi" (*san chi*) from tissues where energy and fluids have become congested and stagnant, relieving the pain and reducing the inflammation that such congestion causes. If you wish to clear and soothe an aching liver, use the charged palm of your left hand to reach across and brush down across the surface of the skin directly over the liver. Since this therapy works primarily on the level of energy, the clearing and soothing effects are not confined only to the physical surface where the brushing is applied; the hand functions as a sort of "energy wand" to transmit therapeutic benefits deeply into the tissues beneath the surface.

While we're on the topic of "brushing," another tried-and-true way to facilitate rapid detox by self-massage is by dry-brushing the entire surface of the body, except for the head, using a dry bath brush made with natural plant bristles. Brush briskly down the inside and outside of the arms, from shoulders down to hands, down the entire surface of the legs from hips to feet, and down the front and back of the torso and both sides of the rib cage, moving from neck down to waist. This is an excellent way to activate lymph drainage and stimulate microcirculation of blood in surface tissues. It also strips away dead skin cells and stimulates generation of new skin, which is a highly beneficial effect during detox.

Tapping (chui-da)

Rhythmically tapping various tissues of the body produces a vibrational wave that carries therapeutic stimulation deeply into the body and penetrates the bone and marrow as well. Tapping therapy has manifold benefits that assist the detox process. It scatters congested energy and stagnant fluids from surface tissues as well as internal organs, activates blood circulation and lymph drainage, stimulates glandular secretions, clears blocked meridians, and loosens toxic residues from nerves and other tissues. By virtue of the piezoelectric effect, the vibrations resonate into the crystalline structure of the bones, which transform the vibrations into energy pulses that stimulate production of white blood cells and other immune factors in the marrow. This effect strengthens immune response, thereby making the detox process more efficient.

Fig. 3. Diagrams of how the hand is held in two different ways for self-tapping therapy: A) Cupped palm for tapping meridians and energy gates. B) Clenched fist for tapping meridians and energy gates.

There are two basic ways to apply tapping therapy. One way is to slightly curl the fingers and thumb to form a concave "cup" in the palm (figure 3A). This creates a little "echo chamber" in the palm that amplifies the tapping vibrations and resonates them within the hollow cavities of the chest and abdomen, where they stimulate the organs and glands. This technique is particularly effective for dislodging toxic residues from the lungs and abdominal organs. First charge the hands, then use the cupped palm of one hand to slap and tap down the opposite side of the ribs from armpit to hip, and from the collarbone down the front of the chest and torso to the waist, then do the same thing with the other hand on the other side.

Another technique is to curl your fingers all the way down to form a fist, with the thumb pressed against the side of the index finger, rather than across the knuckles (figure 3B), and use the curled knuckles and the butt of the palm as a mallet to tap the body. This method is most effective for rattling toxic deposits loose from nerve tissue and stimulating hormone secretions in the endocrine glands. It also has a strong piezoelectric effect on the crystalline structures within the body.

A traditional self-tapping set drawn from chi gung practice may be applied as a highly effective therapeutic support during detox. It is also an excellent morning exercise to give a daily boost to immune response and to balance the endocrine system. Known as "The Three Taps" (Figure 4), this set has been introduced in several of the author's previous books, but since it is so useful for detox and only takes about ten minutes, it is worth a brief review again here. This exercise involves the rhythmic tapping of three parts of the body where important glands are located: the head and neck (pituitary); the center of the chest over the heart (thymus); and the kidneys (adrenals). Spending three to four minutes on each one is sufficient to obtain therapeutic benefits. The Three Taps are briefly explained below:

Neck and Head Tap

Rub the hands together to charge them with energy, then roll the fingers into a fist, with the thumbs pressed against the sides of the index fingers. Use the palm-side of the fists to drum vigorously along both sides of the vertebrae in the neck, alternately left and right, starting at the top of the

Fig. 4. "The Three Taps:" A) Neck, Head, and Pituitary Tap; B) Heart and Thymus Tap; C) Kidney and Adrenal Tap.

shoulders and moving slowly up along the neck, continuing up the back of the skull and over the top of the head to the hairline, then drumming back down to the neck again. Tap a bit harder and longer on the area where the neck runs into the base of the skull. The tapping vibrations reverberate through the skull into the head, stimulating hormone secretions from the pituitary gland, dislodging toxins from the tissues of the brain and the thick nerve cords in the neck, and activating circulation of blood and energy in the head. It is a great way to clear "cobwebs" from your head in the morning and stimulate cerebral functions.

Chest Tap

For this exercise, use the second row of knuckles on the fist of one hand to rhythmically rap on the breastbone in the center of the chest, directly over the heart. Time the tapping to a beat of one heavy tap followed by two lighter taps: ONE, two three; ONE, two, three; etc. This pattern specifically stimulates the thymus gland, which is located directly beneath the breastbone and whose secretions play a vital role in immune response. One of the first symptoms of AIDS is a radical reduction in the production of immune factors from the thymus gland known as "T-cells." Daily tapping on the thymus gradually increases the size of this important gland, which tends to shrink with age, and stimulates secretion of T-cells and other immune factors. This exercise also loosens impacted toxins from lung tissue and has a stimulating effect on the heart.

Kidney Tap

To tap the kidneys, use the back side of the hands to gently tap the kidneys, alternately left and right, from top to bottom, covering the area on the back from the soft tissue just below the rib cage up to the third rib. The vibrations stimulate secretions in the adrenal glands, which sit like hats on top of the kidneys and whose hormones regulate a wide range of vital functions. Chronic stress depletes the adrenals, so this is a good way to recharge them. As in all three taps, the vibrations work on both the physical level, by vibrating the glandular tissues, and on the energetic level, by virtue of the piezoelectric effect on the structures within the glands. In addition, the kidney tap dislodges toxic deposits in kidney tissues and helps break up crystallized acid wastes before they can form kidney stones. This makes it particularly effective as a kidney support during detox.

SOFT EXERCISE

Many people these days completely avoid exercise because they associate it with panting and sweating, strain and injury, toil and trouble. The popular Western notion of exercise includes such heart-racing, joint-grinding, tendon-tearing activities as jogging and weight lifting, tennis and football, surfing and skiing—activities that most people are neither fit nor inclined to do. As a result, when it comes to exercise, the population is divided into a small minority that does it, and an overwhelming majority that just watches.

In Asia, exercise has traditionally been regarded as something one does for therapeutic purposes, not for fun, and it still plays a key role in most traditional Eastern medical systems. Like all "medicine," the first principle of exercise is that it should "do no harm." That obviously eliminates any activity that strains the body, injures tissues, and leaves one exhausted. Instead, traditional Asian exercises, particularly Chinese styles, are designed to help the body repair and heal itself, to assist the blood and lymph in detoxifying tissues and excreting wastes, and to energize rather than deplete the system. Such exercises are known as soft exercise. In addition to being soft, they are also very slow and smooth.

In his great masterpiece, *Precious Recipes,* written fifteen hundred years ago, the renowned Tang Dynasty physician Sun Ssu-mo states:

The Tao of nurturing life requires that one keep oneself as fluid and flexible as possible. One should not stay still for too long, nor should one exhaust oneself by trying to perform impossible tasks. As the ancient Chinese expression says, one should learn how to exercise from nature by observing the fact that flowing water never stagnates and active hinges never rust.

Let's take a quick look at some of the basic differences between hard Western-style exercise and traditional soft Eastern-style exercise. Soft exercise focuses on stretching the muscles and tendons and loosening the joints and limbs, thereby opening all the tissues of the body to the free flow of blood and energy. Hard exercise contracts the muscles and compacts the joints, blocking circulation and retaining toxic wastes in the tissues for a long time. Soft exercises are done in conjunction with deep, slow, diaphragmic breathing, which oxygenates and alkalizes the blood and tissues, while hard exercises force the breath into a shallow, panting mode that utilizes only the narrow upper sections of the lungs. This type of fast shallow breathing in the upper lungs exposes only a very small fraction of the lungs' surface area to incoming air, greatly reducing the intake of oxygen and the discharge of carbon dioxide. As a result, the blood and tissues become increasingly acidic and oxygen-deficient for as long as the exercise continues.

That's not all. Hard exercise causes a rapid accumulation of lactic acid in the tissues, thereby contributing to acidosis. Lactic acid is a metabolic waste produced by muscular exertion, and the last thing you want to do during detox is to produce more acid wastes. By contrast, soft exercise, which requires only minimal muscular exertion, avoids the accumulation of lactic acid in the tissues, and since it is usually done in conjunction with deep breathing, it actually alkalizes and oxygenates the bloodstream, rather than loading it with acids and carbon dioxide. Hard exercise strains the heart by forcing it to race to accelerate circulation of blood to the muscles. Furthermore, since hard exercise makes the breath grow shallow, the diaphragm is not engaged in the breathing process, and therefore the heart must bear the full load of pumping extra supplies of blood through the body. Soft exercise combined with deep breathing effectively turns the diaphragm into a second heart, engaging it to help pump blood through the circulatory system by virtue of differential pressures in the abdominal and chest cavities. This takes a huge work load off the heart, and when practiced daily, the cumulative benefits to the heart can be lifesaving.

Perhaps most important, soft exercise performed in conjunction with deep, slow breathing shifts the autonomous nervous system into the calm, cleansing, healing mode of the parasympathetic branch and keeps it in this mode. This point is important because unless you take effective measures to unwind, relax, and keep the parasympathetic branch of the nervous system switched on, and the sympathetic branch turned off, for at least a few days, your body's self-cleansing and healing responses will not be able to function properly, and the detox process cannot proceed. Doing soft exercise and deep breathing for an hour or two each day is a very good way to stay relaxed and keep your nervous system in the healing detox mode.

The best type of soft exercises for detox purposes are stretching and loosening maneuvers, such as those found in yoga and in the Chinese exercises associated with Tai Chi and chi gung. Stretching the muscles squeezes stagnant venous blood out of the tissues, while the subsequent relaxation phase allows fresh arterial blood to flow in. Since these movements are always done softly, slowly, and smoothly, with minimal exertion, they do not result in the accumulation of lactic acid in the tissues, they don't race the heart, and they don't shorten the breath. Stretching also keeps the nerve and energy channels open and active and stimulates lymph drainage.

There are many good books on yoga available today, and lots of qualified yoga teachers. As for traditional Chinese stretching and loosening exercises, the author has described and illustrated several dozen of these in previous titles (see *The Tao of Health, Sex, and Longevity, The Complete Book of Chinese Health and Healing,* and *The Complete Guide to Chi Gung*). Prior to practicing these exercises, it is important to familiarize yourself with the basic principles of chi gung movement and breathing, and observe a few precautions, which is why the reader is referred to the books mentioned above for guidance.

If you simply don't like doing repetitive formal exercises, almost any type of gentle, slow activity that does not race the heart or shorten the breath, but that does move the "water" and activate the "hinges" of the body, may be done instead as a way of keeping fluids flowing and tissues toned during detox. A long stroll on the beach or a hike in the forest, paddling slowly around in a swimming pool or in the ocean, tending a garden—any such activity will do the trick, as long as you do it softly, slowly, and smoothly. If you're a confirmed "couch potato" and flatly refuse to do even that much activity, then at least you can pay someone else to keep your blood and other bodily fluids moving and your tissues active with therapeutic massage.

The bottom line is this: the blood, the body, and the breath are designed to move, not to stand still and stagnate. Anything that remains still and stagnant for too long invariably loses its vitality and starts to degenerate and decay. So the basic message here is, "Move it before you lose it!"

4

AIR:
THE BREATH OF LIFE

Most health-conscious people take a lot of time and trouble each day about the quantity and quality of the food they eat and pay only scant attention to drinking sufficient amounts of good water, while taking air and breathing almost entirely for granted. In terms of life's essential requirements, however, most people have their priorities backwards. As chi gung Master Hung Yi-hsiang of Taiwan often reminded his students, "You can live two months without food and two weeks without water, but you can only live a few minutes without air."

Air contains essential elements that are at least as important as those derived from food and water as sources of nourishment for life, and proper breathing contributes even more to health and longevity than proper eating. The fact remains, however, that very few people today know how to breathe correctly. Add to that the fact that most of the air in the world has now become as denatured and contaminated with pollutants as food and water, and it becomes clear that most people these days do not take in sufficient supplies of good quality air, depriving their bodies of the essential airborne elements that are required to sustain optimum health and vitality. Even when air quality is good, unless you breathe correctly, your body cannot properly assimilate, circulate, and utilize the essential elements contained in air, nor can it properly perform a wide range of other vital functions that are directly dependent on correct breathing.

Breath is the bridge that links body and mind. As the only vital autonomic function that can be consciously controlled by the mind, breathing may be utilized as a sort of tuning device to balance and harmonize all of the other functional systems in the body, and as a pump to replenish all the vital organs and tissues with fresh supplies of blood and energy. Thus, by consciously regulating the breath, the mind becomes capable of directly regulating the conditions and balancing the functions of all the internal organs and glands in the body. Moreover, by correcting imbalances in the human energy system and increasing the supply and flow of energy, breathing exercises manifest therapeutic benefits for the mind as well as for the body, enhancing mental clarity and improving cerebral functions, because body and mind are both dependent on the same basic energy of life.

Fifteen minutes of slow, regulated deep breathing gives an immediate boost to blood circulation, lowers blood pressure, alkalizes and oxygenates the bloodstream, stimulates glandular secretions, improves digestive functions, and activates detox and immune responses throughout the body by switching the nervous system into the healing parasympathetic mode. At the same time, it calms the mind, pacifies the emotions, and banishes stress by switching off the "fight or flight" action circuit of the autonomous nervous system, thereby stopping secretions of stress hormones such as adrenaline and cortisol.

If you doubt the direct connection between the way you breathe and the way you feel emotionally and mentally, then try this: next time you find yourself all wound up in a state of anxiety, stress, or anger, pause for a moment and check the condition of your breathing. You'll discover that whenever you feel tense from anxiety or anger, your breath grows very short and shallow and remains lodged high in the upper chest, while the diaphragm and abdomen remain frozen stiff. Now sit up straight, with spine erect, and do a few minutes of slow, deep breathing, using the diaphragm to draw and drive the breath from below and pulling air deep down into the lower lobes of the lungs, thereby causing the abdominal wall to expand. Presto! Anxiety and anger evaporate into thin air, body and mind immediately relax and release their tension, and a soothing state of calm flows like a wave through the entire system. A state of anxiety or anger simply cannot be sustained when the breath is consciously kept slow, deep, and diaphragmic, because deep breathing immediately switches the nervous system off the "fight or flight" action circuit, shutting off the secretion of stress hormones and their related neurotransmitters.

Good air and correct breathing may therefore be utilized as effective therapeutic tools to prevent and cure disease, to assist and accelerate detoxification and regeneration of the body, and to harmonize both body and mind by balancing the entire energy system. In *Precious Recipes*, the centenarian Tang dynasty physician Sun ssu-mo states:

> When correct breathing is practiced, the myriad ailments will not occur. When breathing is depressed or strained, all sorts of diseases will occur. Those who wish to nurture their lives must first learn the correct methods of controlling breath and balancing energy. These breathing methods can cure all ailments great and small.

First let's review the basic principles involved in learning "the correct methods of controlling breath and balancing energy," and see how these methods may be applied to support the detox process. Then we'll take a closer look at air itself and find out what makes it such an essential element of life, and how it may be used as a supplement to help detoxify and regenerate the body.

THE ART OF BREATH CONTROL

The key to mastering the art of breath control is to actively engage the diaphragm to serve as a pump to drive the breath. If you observe the way an animal or a baby breathes while sleeping, you'll notice that the abdomen expands on inhalation and contracts on exhalation, while the chest itself remains still. That body response is due to natural diaphragmic breathing, which is the way our bodies were designed to breathe. Due to sedentary lifestyles, poor physical posture, obesity, and the inhibiting effects of chronic stress and fatigue on respiration, adults tend to breathe high up in their chests, using the clavicles and upper ribs to suck air into the narrow spaces at the top of the lungs, rather than using the diaphragm to draw the breath down toward the abdomen and fill the large lower lobes of the lungs with air. Clavicular, upper-chest breathing, which is extremely inefficient, is an emergency response to anxiety and stress, and it is the mode of breathing associated with the hyperactive "fight or flight" instinct. For most adults today, this mode has become their habitual way of breathing.

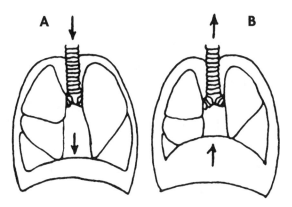

Fig. 5. Using the diaphragm to drive the breath: A) Inhalation; B) Exhalation.

In proper diaphragmic breathing, the diaphragm descends downward into the abdominal cavity on inhalation (figure 5A), expanding the lower lungs and allowing them to draw air deep down into the spacious chambers of the lungs' lower lobes. On exhalation (figure 5B), the abdominal wall is drawn inward and the diaphragm rises upward, driving air out of the lungs in a strong, steady stream. Not only is diaphragmic breathing the most efficient way to breathe, it also utilizes the diaphragm to perform another vital function for which it was designed: to assist the heart in pumping blood through the body, thereby taking a huge workload off the heart muscle and prolonging the life of the whole organism. Respiratory expert Dr. A. Salmanoff describes the cardio-vascular functions of the diaphragm as follows:

> It is the most powerful muscle in the body; it acts like a perfect force-pump, compressing the liver, the spleen, the intestines, and stimulating the whole abdominal and portal circulation. By compressing the lymphatic and blood vessels of the abdomen, the diaphragm aids the venous circulation from the abdomen toward the thorax. The number of movements of the diaphragm per minute is a quarter of those of the heart. But its haemodynamic power is much greater that that of cardiac contractions because the surface of the force-pump is much greater and because its propelling power is superior to that of the heart. We have only to visualize the surface of the diaphragm to accept the fact that it acts like another heart.

When the diaphragm descends into the abdominal cavity on inhalation, it exerts strong internal pressure on the vena cava, a major vein that drains stale blood from the abdominal organs and delivers it up to the heart and lungs to discharge carbon dioxide and replenish the blood with fresh oxygen. The descending diaphragmic pressure acts like a force-pump to drive stale blood from the internal organs through the vena cave up to the chest. This saves the heart an enormous amount of energy and effectively transforms the diaphragm into a "second heart" to help drive circulation.

Furthermore, when you consider the fact that the brain is irrigated by about 1,760 quarts of blood per day, and that the cerebral cortex contain thousands of yards of microcapillaries, you begin to realize how important it is to keep blood flowing freely through the brain. What a hard job that is for the heart, a job made even harder by working against the force of gravity. Deep abdominal breathing takes the bulk of this workload off the heart and transfers it down to the diaphragm, which helps pump blood up to the brain with each and every breath.

As the diaphragm descends down into the abdominal cavity, it increases internal abdominal pressure, providing a stimulating therapeutic massage to all the internal organs and glands, especially the kidneys, adrenal glands, and liver, which are seated directly beneath the diaphragm. Listed below are some of the additional health benefits enjoyed by those who practice deep diaphragmic breathing:

- For every extra millimeter of flex the diaphragm develops on inhalation, lung capacity increases by a volume of 250–300 ml. Studies in China have demonstrated that after six months of breathing practice, the average flex of the diaphragm increases by 4 mm, thereby overall increasing lung capacity by 1,000–2,000 ml per breath.
- A study conducted in India showed that after only fifteen minutes of deep diaphragmic breathing, the average volume of air inhaled per breath rose by 50 percent, while the average number of breaths per minute dropped from fifteen to five. This makes breathing by far more energy efficient and literally "saves breath."
- A major study on breathing conducted in China showed a big rise in red blood-cell count after only thirty minutes of regulated deep-breathing exercise. This greatly enhances the blood's capacity to hold and carry oxygen, which is a major advantage during detox.
- All digestive functions are immediately improved by a session of deep-breathing exercise, which stimulates secretions of bile, pepsin, and other digestive juices in the liver, stomach, and pancreas, and enhances peristaltic contractions throughout the digestive tract.
- Deep diaphragmic breathing activates the body's innate cleansing and healing responses by switching the nervous system into the restorative parasympathetic branch, thereby triggering the release of neurotransmitters and hormones that signal the body to detoxify and repair itself.

All of these benefits have obvious applications for the detox process and may be easily utilized at any time and in any place during the course of a detox program, to relieve discomfort, assist the detox and healing process, alkalize and oxygenate the blood, eliminate bad moods, relax body and mind, and keep the entire system in an optimum state of internal harmony and balance.

Deep diaphragmic breathing is performed in four distinct stages, and its therapeutic effects may be further amplified by the three maneuvers known in chi gung and yoga as the "Three Locks," which are applied during the retention stage. The four stages are as follows:

> **Inhalation:** Relax the diaphragm and let it expand slowly downward into the abdominal cavity, while drawing in a steady stream of air through flared nostrils and sending it down into the lower lungs. When the lower lungs are full, expand the rib cage and clavicles a bit to allow air in to "top off" the narrow upper portions of the lungs, then gently press the entire "bubble" of inhaled air down into the diaphragm, which causes the abdominal wall to bulge out.
>
> **Retention:** Apply the Three Locks to "lock up" the breath and increase the internal pressure within the abdomen and sacrum, retain the breath and hold the locks for three to ten seconds, no longer, then relax the locks and release the breath.
>
> **Exhalation:** Draw the abdominal wall inward and let the diaphragm rise upward into the chest to drive the breath out of the lungs in a long, slow, steady stream of air, either through the nose or through the mouth, depending on the exercise.
>
> **Pause:** Pause briefly after exhalation is complete to allow the abdominal wall and diaphragm to relax again and fall back into place, before commencing the next inhalation.

It is the retention stage that produces the strongest therapeutic benefits in four-stage diaphragmic breathing, especially when the effects are amplified with the Three Locks. Retentions of longer than ten seconds should never be attempted without prior training from a qualified teacher, but even short retentions of three to ten seconds, which may be safely practiced without supervision, provide profound therapeutic effects throughout the body.

Breath retention triggers what's known as the "dive response," or "cellular respiration," whereby heartbeats slow by half and blood pressure drops, while the cells start "breathing" spontaneously to produce energy by breaking down sugars and releasing oxygen to generate internal body heat. Seals use this mechanism when diving for fish in freezing cold seas, and infants instinctively apply it when submerged underwater, but adults lose it due to incorrect breathing habits. Practicing four-stage deep breathing with retention gradually restores this innate metabolic response.

Breathing deeply and briefly retaining the breath instantly calms the nervous system by switching it over to the parasympathetic branch and quickly lowers blood pressure by reducing the pulse. Activating cellular respiration prompts the cells to discharge toxins and produce energy. Breath retention increases the partial pressure of oxygen in the blood against the capillary walls, thereby enhancing the exchange of gas between the bloodstream and the cells. It is also the retention stage of breathing that signals the stomach to secrete pepsin and other digestive enzymes, and stimulates peristalsis in the intestinal tract. In addition, retention applied in conjunction with the three locks squeezes stale blood from the internal organs by increasing abdominal pressure and drives it up through the vena cava to the heart and lungs for replenishment. It also disperses stagnant energy from the organs through the meridian system.

To amplify internal pressure within the abdominal cavity and seal it up during the brief retention stage, you may apply the ancient Asian breath enhancement maneuvers known as the "Three Locks." Here's a quick review of how to do it:

Anal Lock

The bottom of the sacral cavity is supported by a web of muscle and sinew known as the "urogenital diaphragm," which controls the activities of the anus, rectum, bladder perineum, and urogenital canal. As the lungs fill and the diaphragm descends into the abdomen during inhalation, the pelvic floor below is pushed down by growing pressure from the diaphragm above, stretching the tissues of the urogenital diaphragm downward and reducing internal pressure on the abdominal organs and glands. The downward pressure on the urogenital diaphragm also causes internal energy to leak out through the anal and urogenital orifices.

To prevent this loss of internal pressure and energy, apply the anal lock as soon as inhalation is complete, by deliberately contracting the anal sphincter and extending the contraction to the urogenital orifice, as though you needed to pee and poop but couldn't find a toilet. This tightens all the tissues of the urogenital diaphragm and lifts up the entire pelvic floor. Known in yoga as *mula banda* and in chi gung as *ti gang* (literally "lifting the anus"), the anal lock effectively seals in and prevents the loss of internal pressure and energy from below, thereby helping sustain elevated diaphragmic pressure within the abdomen and sacrum and amplifying the therapeutic effects of breath retention. Contracting the anus and lifting the pelvic floor at the end of inhalation counteracts the downward push on the urogenital diaphragm and prevents the escape of internal energy and therapeutic pressure from the abdomen and sacrum.

Applying the anal lock flexes the myriad muscles and tendons, nerves and blood vessels of the sacrum, including those involved in urination, bowel movements, orgasm, menstruation, and prostate and ovary functions. All of these functions are stimulated and balanced by anal contractions because their tissues are all interwoven within the urogenital diaphragm. Practicing this maneuver also helps prevent and cure hemorrhoids, by flushing stagnant blood from the clogged capillaries of the anal sphincter and irrigating them with freshly oxygenated blood. In fact, if you carefully observe animals, such as cows and horses, dogs and cats, you will notice that they rhythmically contract and relax the anus a few times immediately after every defecation. This helps propel residual feces from the rectum at the end of a bowel movement, and replenishes the anal tissues with fresh circulation of blood and energy.

The anal lock should be held until the end of the retention stage, for three to ten seconds only, and released at the beginning of exhalation.

Abdominal Lock

The abdominal lock is applied immediately after the anal lock is set, by deliberately drawing the abdominal wall slightly inward toward the spine, thereby preventing the loss of internal pressure from the front. As the lungs fill up and the diaphragm descends, the abdominal wall balloons outward due to growing internal pressure within the abdominal cavity. Unless you pull the abdominal wall back in a bit at the end of inhalation, its outward expansion reduces internal pressure within the abdomen, and some of the therapeutic benefits of retention are lost. Applying the abdominal lock seals internal pressure in from the front, while the anal lock prevents it from escaping below. From above, internal pressure is firmly locked into the abdomen by the descending diaphragm, and the spine provides a strong retaining wall in back. The abdominal and anal locks thus complete the sealing in of elevated pressure within in the abdomen and sacrum, and the therapeutic benefits of this enhanced internal pressure on the organs and glands continues until the locks are relaxed and the breath released.

Neck Lock

The neck lock is not directly involved in maintaining enhanced pressure within the abdomen. Instead, it is designed to help press the breath down into the lower lungs and hold it there, and to prevent enhanced internal pressure in the abdomen from causing a sudden surge of blood to rush up into the brain during the retention phase. The neck lock also pulls on the spinal cord from above, giving it a stimulating stretch. To apply the neck lock, contract the muscles of the throat in front and close the glottis over the bronchial entrance inside, while also tucking in the chin a bit and slightly stretching up the back of the neck, without bending the neck forward. The neck lock shuts the entrance to the throat, making it much easier to press down and retain the breath, while also partially constricting the carotid arteries to prevent blood from flooding up into the brain. While contracting and closing the throat in front, the neck lock gives a slight stretch to the neck in back, opening the nerve and energy channels that enter the head from the spine and giving a therapeutic tug to the entire spinal cord. This stretch activates energy flow in the spinal channels and encourages it to rise up through the meridians from sacrum to brain, where it energizes all cerebral functions. Partial pressure on the carotid arteries also regulates the heart by slowing and deepening the pulse, greatly increasing cardiovascular efficiency.

Like the other two locks, the neck lock is held until the end of retention, then relaxed with the release of breath at the beginning of exhalation. When applying the neck lock, there is a tendency at first to hunch up the shoulders, which causes tension in the neck and upper back and obstructs free flow of nerve and energy pulses there, so check your posture after the neck lock is set and make sure your shoulders remain relaxed.

The Three Locks are applied only when practicing complete, four-stage deep breathing exercises in still sitting or still standing postures. When practicing moving forms of chi gung breathing exercise, such as Tai Chi or the Eight Pieces of Brocade, which involve continuous rhythmic movements of the body, natural two-stage breathing is used, without retention or pause. Each inhalation and exhalation follows and flows smoothly into one another in seamless succession, like the swinging pendulums of a clock. Four-stage breathing in still postures, and two-stage breathing timed to rhythmic bodily movements, each have their own respective therapeutic benefits. Four-stage deep breathing with retention is particularly effective for assimilating essential elements from air and discharging toxins from blood and tissues, and for stimulating cellular metabolism. Slow rhythmic body movements, synchronized with two-stage deep breathing, is best for giving a strong boost to circulation of blood and energy throughout the system, clearing blocked meridians, transforming stagnant energy, draining lymph channels, and activating all the "hinges" of the body.

Let's take a brief look at both styles.

BREATHING IN STILLNESS

Still breathing exercises may be practiced either sitting or standing. The traditional standing posture used for practicing Chinese breathing exer-

cises is called the "Horse" stance (figure 6). Feet should be placed parallel and shoulder-width apart on the floor or ground, with knees slightly
bent, pelvis tucked forward, shoulders relaxed and neck straight, arms
hanging loosely down with palms facing toward the rear. There should
be a straight line running from the crown of the head through the center of the body to a point midway between the navel and spine, then
down through the perineum to a point midway between the feet on the
ground. Body weight should rest a bit forward on the balls of the feet,
not back on the heels, with the body's center of balance located in the
middle of the lower abdomen, two inches below the navel. This point
lies in the second chakra and is known in Chinese as the *dan-tien,* or
"Elixir Field." This is the body's "sweet spot," the place where energy
collects when doing breathing exercises and the best place to focus attention while practicing deep breathing.

*Fig. 6. The basic Horse
Stance for chi gung practice.*

Fig. 7. Two basic sitting postures for still sitting chi gung and meditation:
A) Sitting flat with legs crossed; B) Sitting erect on a stool, feet on the floor.

Most people prefer to practice still breathing exercises in the sitting position, which has two basic forms (figure 7). One way is to sit with legs crossed on a cushion or mat placed on the floor, either in full- or half-lotus posture. The half-lotus posture, as depicted in the illustration, is much easier to hold for prolonged periods of practice and is therefore recommended for beginners. Alternatively, you may sit on the edge of a low stool or chair, with both feet planted firmly on the floor, parallel and shoulder-width. If sitting crossed-legged on the floor causes your legs to go numb and strains your lower back, choose the stool posture, which is very easy to maintain without straining any part of the body. In both forms, the hands should rest relaxed and open on the thighs, with palms up, just above the knees. This permits energy to flow freely through the powerful *lao gung* points located in the center of the palms.

Regardless which posture you prefer, it is very important to pay close attention to proper alignment of the spine. Otherwise much of the therapeutic benefit of the breathing exercise is lost. The spine must be held as straight as possible, with neck and sacrum aligned with the spinal column. To align the neck, tuck your chin slightly down toward the throat in front, while straightening up the back of the neck a bit, as in the neck lock but not quite as stretched as in that posture. To align the sacrum, tuck the pelvis forward to take some of the curve out of the lower spine. As noted above, you should be able to trace an imaginary line from the crown of the head down through the throat and chest to the *dan-tien* point in the center of the lower abdomen. This is the path of the Central Channel (also called the Thrusting Channel), through which the cosmic energies of the sky ("Heaven") and the elemental energies in the ground ("Earth") travel and mix with the organic energies of the human system ("Humanity").

Heaven, Earth, and Humanity *(tien, di, ren)* are known as the "Three Powers" in Taoist internal alchemy, and they represent the sum total of all the vital energies in the universe that contribute power to life on earth. Chinese breathing exercises are designed to tap into these infinite sources of primordial energy, and to harmonize and circulate them through the human system to protect health and prolong life. The spine, known as the

"Ladder to Heaven," links the earth energies that rise up from the ground with the cosmic energies that rain down from the sky and transforms them into frequencies and patterns that may be utilized by the human energy system. If the spine is blocked or kinked, or misaligned with the head and sacrum, the spinal energy channels cannot properly conduct and transform the various energies that the breathing exercises generate.

Three distinct types of energy travel through the spine, each within its own respective channels (as you will see in figure 8). The most obvious is nerve-signal energy, which travels through the spinal cord and links the brain to the peripheral parts of the body. During deep-breathing exercises, the calming parasympathetic branch of the nervous system is activated, which then links the brain directly with the endocrine glands that govern detoxification and immune responses. Another form of energy that travels along the spine is the energy that controls the various internal organs. This energy moves through major meridians located along the spine. The meridians then distribute the energy to the organs and other tissues of the body through a network of twelve main organ-energy channels and countless smaller branch channels. The third type of energy associated with the spine is the cosmic energy that enters the human system through the crown of the head and moves down through the chakra system to the sacrum. The chakras, known as "elixir fields" in Chinese, function as energy transformers to "step down" the subtle high-frequency energies that enter the human system from the sky, so that they may be utilized by the human body and mind. All of these various vital energies flow first through the main spinal channels, which then disperse them via branch channels to the organs and tissues. If the spine is misaligned, cramped, or blocked due to injuries or habitual poor posture, all three forms of energy are obstructed and become stagnant. Then the entire system grows weak and sluggish and becomes vulnerable to disease and degeneration.

In the yoga tradition of India, deep-breathing exercises are known as *pranayama* and are practiced in conjunction with various yoga postures called *asanas,* or sitting still with legs crossed. However, pranayama should only be practiced under the guidance of a qualified teacher, because some of the breathing techniques it employs are quite power-

Fig. 8. Channels, Chakras, and Nerve Plexus: A) The Central Channel of the meridian network and its major power points; B) The seven "energy wheels" of the chakra system; C) The spinal cord and the major nerve plexus of the central nervous system.

ful and complex and, if not performed precisely right and in correct sequence, can cause serious internal energy deviations.

In China, deep-breathing exercise is a branch of chi gung and is practiced in both still and moving modes. Chi gung, which literally means "energy work" or "breathing skill," is usually practiced in synchronized conjunction with slow body movements, but there are also still forms that may be practiced standing or sitting. Basic chi gung breathing exercises may be safely practiced by beginners from a book, without prior instruction from a teacher, as long as the basic guidelines on form and posture are followed, and breath retention never exceeds ten seconds. Detailed instructions for a variety of such exercises are introduced in several of the author's previous books, including important precautions and points of attention for each exercise. As a result, we'll limit our discussion in this book to one simple breathing exercise that anyone can easily practice anywhere and at any time, to facilitate internal cleansing, alkalize and oxygenate the bloodstream, calm the mind, soothe the nerves, and rebalance the entire energy system. This form of breathing is called *tu na*, literally "expel and collect," and it is both safe and easy to do.

Tu na breathing has been practiced in China for thousands of years as a simple and effective means of healing and preventive health care. It involves the four-stage breathing sequence, with the three locks applied during a brief retention. The idea is to first "expel" stagnant air from the lungs and stagnant energy from the meridians with a long, strong exhalation, and then "collect" fresh air and energy with a long, deep inhalation. During the retention stage, the bloodstream "collects" oxygen and negative-ion energy from air in the lungs. The cells, in turn, "collect" the oxygen and energy from the blood through the capillaries. Thus the whole system is completely recharged. To insure balance and stability, tu na should be practiced in one of the still sitting postures, not standing, at least until the body grows accustomed to the enhanced circulation of blood and energy. After that, tu na may be practiced standing in the "Horse" stance, as well.

Adopt a stable sitting posture, with spine erect and head aligned with sacrum, then flare open the nostrils and commence a long, slow inhalation, drawing the air down deeply into the lower lungs, then "topping off" the upper lungs and gently sinking the entire breath as far down into the diaphragm as possible. Immediately apply the anal, neck, and abdominal locks, relax the shoulders, and retain the breath for just three to five seconds. (Later, you may work up to longer retentions of five to ten seconds, if you wish.) Next, relax the locks and release the breath, exhaling in a long, steady stream while gradually drawing in the abdominal wall and letting the diaphragm rise up into the chest cavity to completely expel the breath. Pause briefly and allow the diaphragm and abdominal muscles to relax again, then start the next inhalation. To obtain effective therapeutic results, tu na should be practiced for at least fifteen minutes per session.

Exhalation may be done either through the nose or mouth, depending on which aspect of the exercise you wish to emphasize—elimination or assimilation. Exhaling through the nose places primary emphasis on the "collect" aspect, allowing the blood and tissues to rapidly assimilate and store fresh supplies of oxygen and energy. Exhaling through the mouth shifts the emphasis to the "expel" phase, increasing the discharge of carbon dioxide from the blood, expelling residual stale air from the lungs, and driving stagnant energy from the meridians. Both types of exhalation may be practiced at the same sitting. Exhaling through the mouth can be done in two different ways. One way is to purse the lips and blow the breath out in a long, steady stream through a narrow slit in the mouth, as though trying to move a candle flame a meter in front of your face without blowing it out; the other is to constrict the top of the throat by partially closing the glottis, then exhaling the breath slowly and strongly from the back of the mouth while making a low, hoarse "haw" sound.

Another form of this breathing exercise is to combine it with long, rhythmic extensions of the spine (as you will see in figure 9). To do this form, sit properly on the edge of a stool or chair, with feet planted firmly on the floor and hands placed palms down on the thighs above the knees. Inhale, applying the three locks, and briefly retain the breath while sitting with spine erect. Then relax the locks and jut the chin out in front, extending the spine as you slowly stretch forward and down in synchronicity with exhalation, timing it so that your body is extended fully forward at the end of the exhalation stage. Then relax the neck and let the head hang down naturally for a brief pause, before commencing the next inhalation. As you inhale again, return the spine back to the erect position by pushing the body up slowly, with your hands pressing on the thighs for support. Apply the three locks again, retain briefly, and start another round. This exercise flexes the entire spinal cord and all its supporting muscles and tendons and realigns the spinal vertebrae, stimulating all the major nerve networks and energy meridians located along the spine, and activating free flow of cerebrospinal fluids within the spinal shaft. The rhythmic arching and bowing of the spine also activates the seven chakras and stimulates secretions of vital hormones from the respectively related glands—pineal (crown chakra), pituitary

("Third Eye" chakra), thyroid (throat chakra), thymus (heart chakra), adrenals (solar plexus chakra), testicles/ovaries (lower abdomen chakra), and prostate/vaginal glands (root chakra). A good way to combine still sitting tu na with the moving spinal extension form is to start with a few minutes of the moving form to stretch and align the spine and stimulate the nerves and chakras, then finish with ten to fifteen minutes in the still sitting form, focusing on expelling and collecting air and energy.

Fig. 9. Tu na chi gung breathing with spinal-stretch movement: A) Starting posture, inhale; B) Extend chin and stretch forward, start exhalation; C) Full stretch forward, complete exhalation; D) Tuck chin in and arch spine up, breath, pause; E) Straighten back up, start inhalation; F) Return to start, complete inhalation.

BREATHING WITH BODY MOVEMENT

Deep diaphragmic breathing synchronized with slow, rhythmic body movements, performed in a state of physical relaxation and mental calm, has been practiced as a form of preventive and curative health therapy since ancient times in China. As the great Chinese alchemist and healer Ko Hung explained back in the fourth century AD, "The onset of illness is a sign that energy is not flowing. One must exercise in order to unblock the myriad meridians and facilitate the free flow of energy."

Synchronized breathing and body movement provides a powerful dynamic boost to the circulation of blood and energy throughout the body. Since these exercises are always practiced slowly, softly, and smoothly, with minimal muscular exertion, they do not cause a build-up of lactic acid in the tissues, as hard exercise does. Deep diaphragmic breathing enhances the free flow of blood and energy, driving them through their respective channels, while the long extensions of the limbs and gentle twists and turns of the torso guide this enhanced circulation out to the farthest extremities of the body and into the deepest tissues of the internal organs. This quickly clears the meridians of stagnant energy and purges the organs and other tissues of stale blood, suffusing every cell in the body with fresh supplies of both. TCM has always viewed the free flow of blood and energy as the primary foundations of health and viewed imbalances in either as the basic causes of disease. The famous physician Hua To, who lived a century before Ko Hung and who treated princes and peasants alike, stated this principle very succinctly, "When the blood pulses unobstructed through the veins, illness cannot take root."

Hua To developed a series of gentle rhythmic breathing exercises based upon the movements of animals in nature and prescribed them as curative therapy for a wide range of ailments, including arthritis, rheumatism, digestive difficulties, heart and circulatory problems, nervous system disorders, and many other conditions. Known as *dao yin* ("induce and guide"), these exercises induce the flow of blood and energy and guide them as they circulate through the system. Because these forms were based on the way animals naturally move, they were also called *wu chin hsi,* or the "Play of the Five Creatures." Cheng Yuan-lin, a contemporary of Hua To, commented on this form of therapy, saying, "Breathing practiced together with the movements resembling a bear, bird, and other animals helps move our energy, nourishes our bodies, and builds our spirits."

This type of therapeutic breathing with synchronized body movement is the basis of all moving forms of Chinese chi gung exercise, which brings body, breath, and mind into a unified state of harmony. In Chinese, the ideogram for *chi* may be used to denote "energy" as well as "breath" and "air" and reflects the view that vital energy, not oxygen, is the most essential component in air and that breath is the vehicle for bringing this essential energy into the body. Gung refers to any skill or work that takes a long time and lots of practice to perfect. Chi gung was originally developed about five thousand years ago as a sort of therapeutic dance to ward off rheumatism, energy stagnation, respiratory disorders, and other ailments caused by the excessively damp climate in the flood-prone plains of the Yellow River valley, where Chinese civilization first evolved. In a text entitled *Dance Verse,* written in the second century AD, scholar Fu Yi states, "Chi gung is an art that pleases the spirit, slows the aging process, and prolongs life."

The most widely practiced form of moving chi gung today is *Tai Chi Chuan,* the graceful, flowing form of martial art inspired when a Taoist sage observed a snake and crane locked in mortal battle. But Tai Chi is a complex form that requires special training from a qualified master and takes many long years of practice to reach a level of proficiency that delivers concrete therapeutic benefits. Very few people these days are willing to commit that much time and effort to practicing anything until they reach perfection of the form. Fortunately, much simpler chi gung forms exist, many of which may easily be learned from a book. These forms provide equally beneficial therapeutic benefits when practiced daily, but they take a lot less time and patience to learn to perform properly. These simpler forms include the "Eight Pieces of Brocade" set, the "Six Healing Sounds" set, the "Five Elements" set, and even easier single-step forms.

A brief review of some of the major health benefits provided by regular chi gung practice is in order here, so that readers understand why millions of Chinese people having been practicing it continuously for thousands of years, and why it is such a suitable system of therapeutic exercise for people today. About three hundred years ago, the Taoist adept Shen Chia-shu remarked, "Breathing and related exercises are one hundred times more effective as medical therapy than any drug. This knowledge is indispensable to man, and every physician should study it thoroughly." The leading edge of modern medical science is finally beginning to awaken to the truth of this statement, which has been verified with concrete scientific evidence. Here are some of the facts:

Blood and Marrow

Red blood cells, which deliver oxygen to the cells, and one type of white blood cell essential for immune response are produced in the marrow of bones. Healthy marrow produces 480,000,000 red blood cells per minute. In *The Root of Chinese Chi Kung,* contemporary chi gung master Dr. Yang Jwing-ming explains the significance of this as follows:

> According to Chinese medicine, your body deteriorates mainly because your blood loses its ability to feed and protect your body. Your bone marrow produces the red blood cells and one type of the white blood cells, but as you grow older, the marrow . . . produces fewer and fewer useful blood cells. . . . To keep marrow fresh and alive and functioning properly, chi must be plentiful and continuously supplied. Whenever there is a shortage of chi, the marrow will not function properly.

The best way to insure a continuous supply of fresh chi to the marrow is to practice chi gung on a regular basis. During a detox program, sufficient production of red blood cells is even more important than usual, because the bloodstream requires a very high red blood cell count to supply the additional amounts of oxygen the cells need during detox, and extra white blood cells are needed to keep immune response strong.

Brain and Central Nervous System

As we have already seen, deep breathing synchronized with slow body movements switches the autonomous nervous system over to the calming parasympathetic branch, which governs the body's natural self-cleansing and healing responses. During detox, it is essential to keep your nervous system at rest in this healing mode throughout the program, and there's no better way to do that than by practicing chi gung every day.

Electroencephalographic (EEG) devices have shown that chi gung energizes and activates the 90 percent of the brain that in most people lies perpetually dormant. We've all been told that on average we use less than 10 percent of the more than fifteen billion brain cells in our heads, but after a session of chi gung the entire brain is brought "online," whether you are consciously aware of it or not. This significantly improves all cerebral functions such as memory and learning, and in some cases, when diligently practiced, it also awakens some of the more extraordinary mental powers that lie dormant in our brains, such as telepathy, ESP, clairvoyance, and so forth. Even more significant, EEG scans of elderly adults in China who practice chi gung daily show a pattern and frequency of brain waves that are normally found only in young children, indicating that those who practice chi gung can restore their cerebral functions to those of youth and rejuvenate their minds. Chinese medical literature abounds with references to the *fan lao, huan tung* ("resist age, restore youth") benefits of chi gung practice, and these studies using modern EEG technology shed scientific light on this claim.

Chi gung not only charges the brain with energy, it also increases supplies of "vital essence" by stimulating secretions of important neurotransmitters such as serotonin, dopamine, and encephalin. This effect balances all brain functions, enhances mental clarity, and facilitates communications between the brain and peripheral nervous system.

Immune Response

We've already seen how chi gung enhances immune response by switching the nervous system to the parasympathetic healing mode and by stimulating production of red and white blood cells in the marrow. But it also boosts immunity in several other ways. Chi gung stimulates the thymus and other glands to secrete the full spectrum of immune factors, while inhibiting secretions of the adrenal stress hormones released by the "fight or flight" response, which have strong immunosuppressive effects. Chi gung also increases production of natural steroids, thereby relieving arthritis without the need to resort to the toxic synthetic steroids that most doctors prescribe for this condition.

One of the most significant recent discoveries about chi gung is the fact that it activates the PNI response, or "psychoneuroimmunology." PNI is one of the body's most powerful healing mechanisms, whereby specific neurotransmitters secreted in the brain communicate directly with the glands of the immune system to activate detox and healing responses throughout the body. In a May 1992 article that she wrote for *Omni,* the magazine's editor Kathy Keaton describes the response as follows:

> It has been discovered . . . that there are nerve fibers in the thymus, the immune system's master gland, as well as in the spleen, the lymph nodes, and the bone marrow—all vital parts of the immune system. . . . In other words, there's a growing body of evidence to suggest that the brain talks directly to the immune system via this electrochemical version of AT&T.

For the brain to release the neuropeptides that activate the body's glandular immune responses, the mind must remain calm, the body relaxed, and the nervous system switched over to the parasympathetic branch. Chi gung produces this balanced state of mental calm and physical relaxation quickly and efficiently, providing a convenient tool to activate the PNI healing response and open a direct line of healing biofeedback between the nervous and endocrine systems.

Heart and Circulatory System
As we've already noted above, correct breathing transforms the diaphragm into a virtual "second heart" to assist in the circulation of blood.

Studies in China show that twenty minutes of chi gung practice reduces the pulse by an average 15 percent, while increasing overall volume of blood circulated, and further, that this effect continues for several hours after the practice. This enhancement in circulatory power is due entirely to the way chi gung shifts the major burden of work in blood circulation from the heart over to the diaphragm. High blood pressure, which has become a major life-threatening condition throughout the world, can easily be controlled by daily chi gung practice, without the need for drugs. A study conducted on one hundred cases of chronic high blood pressure and hypertension at the Shanghai Research Institute for Hypertension demonstrated that after only five minutes of practice, blood-pressure levels in all of the patients began to drop dramatically, and after twenty minutes, their blood pressure went down to the same level it normally reached three hours after taking the blood-pressure drugs normally prescribed for this condition by modern Western medicine. Ninety-seven of these patients remained permanently free of high blood pressure and no longer needed to use the drugs, simply by continuing to practice chi gung at home every day, while the three who declined to continue their practice soon suffered relapses and had to go back on drug therapy.

Digestion

Indigestion has become such a common condition for people on modern Western diets that gastric distress is almost taken for granted now as an inevitable side-effect of eating. More than half of all Americans surveyed complain of chronic gastrointestinal discomfort, including gas, bloating, constipation, acid reflux, and stomachaches. Studies in China have shown that fifteen minutes of chi gung practice produces a major elevation in secretions of pepsin and other digestive enzymes in the stomach, and lysozyme in the salivary glands of the mouth. Chi gung balances pH in the stomach, thereby helping prevent "acid indigestion," and the downward movement of the diaphragm in chi gung breathing provides an invigorating massage to the liver, stomach, pancreas, and other digestive organs and glands within the abdomen, expelling gas and moving stagnant fluids and stimulating digestive functions.

pH Balance

Acidosis has become one of the great banes of modern lifestyles. Excessive acidity of blood and tissues is one of the primary preconditions for the onset of all disease and degenerative conditions; conversely, alkalization of blood and tissues is a primary strategy in healing and one of the main goals in any detox program. Chi gung quickly alkalizes the bloodstream, thereby restoring proper pH balance so that the blood can flush acid wastes from the cells and tissues. This helps detoxify the body and immediately raises resistance to disease. As Dr. Charles Gaspard Peschier and Dr. Michel remarked after conducting extensive studies on the benefits of deep breathing in France:

> Every organic or functional disorder leading to conditions of illness is susceptible to the influence, if not always the cure, of controlled breathing. Controlled breathing is the most outstanding method known to us for increasing organic resistance. . . . It confers on the balance of the acid/alkaline a regularity that is reestablished with every breath.

Antioxidant Effect

Free radicals are the main culprits in the premature aging and degeneration of the human body, and antioxidants, also known as "free-radical scavengers," are the body's primary line of defense against free-radical damage. Most health enthusiasts are already familiar with antioxidant supplements such as vitamins C and E, the minerals selenium and zinc, and various herbs but are probably not aware that deep breathing exercises can also greatly enhance the body's antioxidant activity. The most potent free-radical scavenger produced in the body is the enzyme superoxide dismutase (SOD). Laboratory analysis of blood samples taken from elderly practitioners of chi gung show that after a thirty-minute session of practice, the level of SOD in their blood rises to more than double the average found in those who do not practice. This finding is particularly significant for detox programs, because during detox, the body requires abundant and continuous supplies of SOD and other antioxidant enzymes to deal with all the free-radical activity from the toxins released in the tissues. Chi gung is therefore a quick and easy way to double the availability of SOD during a detox program—as well as in daily life.

For further details about the manifold benefits of chi gung for human health and longevity, and for detox in particular, the reader may refer to the author's previous title, *The Complete Guide to Chi Gung*. The points discussed above suffice to demonstrate how useful chi gung can be as a therapeutic tool for human health and healing. The many advantages of chi gung as a form of medical therapy include the fact that it costs nothing and is easy to administer; it is safe and effective and has no negative side effects when properly practiced; it can be practiced at any time and place without any special equipment; virtually anyone, including children and the elderly, can learn how to do it; it balances body as well as mind simultaneously to correct problems on both levels; and best of all, as Shen Chia-shu said, it is one hundred times more effective for medical therapy than any drug.

"YIN PARTICLES"

While we all know that we need to breathe air to supply our blood and tissues with life-sustaining oxygen, few people realize that air is more than just oxygen. What counts most in air quality is not its oxygen content but rather a particular form of energy that activates healthy air and gives it the dynamic vitality required to sustain life. The source of this essential, air-borne energy is highly active molecular particles called negative ions, each of which has a negative charge equivalent to that of one free electron. In Chinese, these units of negatively charged energy are called *yin li dze,* or "yin particles." In the Taoist principle of yin/yang polarity, yin is always the "negative" pole and yang is the "positive."

Negative-ion count is the most accurate measure of air quality in terms of its benefits for human health. Negative ions are produced in air by the action of wind and sun, especially at high altitudes, and by the movement of air over large bodies of water. That is why since time immemorial people have always felt so refreshed and rejuvenated after spending a day at the beach or trekking in high mountains: every breath you take in air that is rich in negative ions recharges your blood and cellular batteries with fresh supplies of purifying, energizing negative ions. All air pollutants, such as smoke, dust, and toxic chemicals, take the form of large, sluggish molecules with a positive charge. In urban areas, where the air is especially dense with pollutants, the heavy positive ions slow down and trap the vibrant negative ions in the air, reducing their activity, negating their energy, and robbing the air of its vitality and healing potential. Clean country air, for example, contains an average ratio of three negative ions to one positive, while polluted city air has about 500 positive molecules for every negative ion, a massive 1,500-fold drop in air quality. Negative ions are also removed from air by air-conditioning and central heating, severely degrading air quality in modern office and apartment buildings. The poor air quality is the reason people who work at desk jobs in air-conditioned offices with sealed windows feel more depleted and "wiped out" after a day of doing nothing but "pushing papers" and taking phone calls, than farmers and outdoor construction workers who work up a sweat doing hard physical labor in the sun and open air.

Let's take a look at the negative-ion count in the various types of air typically found on the earth today:

"Polluted Air," such as that in factories, airtight urban spaces, chemical plants, and heavy traffic, produces 320–3200 negative ions/cubic inch/sec. Breathing this sort of air causes illness, stress reactions, and toxemia of the blood and tissues.

"Unhealthy Air," such as that in inner cities, high-rise office buildings, and shopping malls, produces 3200–8000 negative ions/cubic inch/sec. Breathing this grade air can cause headaches, irritability, chronic fatigue, and various respiratory problems such as asthma.

"Average Air," such as that in suburbs and lowland farm areas, produces 8,000–16,000 negative ions/cubic inch/sec. This type of air does not cause any specific health problems, but it also has no positive benefits for health, other than providing basic oxygen requirements.

"Good Air," such as that by the ocean, in a big forest, or in low to medium mountain regions, produces 16,000–32,000 negative ion/cubic inch/sec. Breathing air of this quality has distinctive rejuvenating effects and energizes the whole system. It also helps purify the bloodstream.

"Healthy Air," such as that on high mountains, produces over 64,000 negative ions/cubic inch/sec. This is the purest, most therapeutically beneficial air on earth. It has potent detoxifying properties, invigorates the blood, recharges the human energy system, and accelerates new cell and tissue growth. It also stimulates the brain and activates dormant cerebral powers, which is why the yogins and hermits of ancient India, China, and Tibet often chose to live in remote caves among the wild and wind-swept peaks of Asia's highest mountain ranges. The ancient Chinese ideogram for "immortal sage" is *hsien,* which consists of the symbols for "man" and "mountain."

To remain healthy and strong, the human body needs to breathe air with a count of about 32,000 negative ions/cubic inch/sec. That high a count of negative ions of air is found at unpolluted seashores, deep in pristine forests, and high up in the mountains. Most people today, however, live nowhere near such places, which means that they are breathing air that not only is half as rich in oxygen as it was two hundred years ago but also is critically deficient in the essential energy of negative ions. The only viable way to compensate for the continuing degradation in air quality throughout the world today is to increase the efficiency of our breathing methods.

It is no accident that health resorts and spas have traditionally been located high up in the mountains, or else down along the shores of oceans and lakes. It was discovered by accumulative, extensive experience that the air in the mountains and by the sea has a potent vitality that rapidly cleanses the bloodstream, energizes the nervous system, and regenerates the body. That vitality comes from the high negative-ion count in the air at such locations.

One reason that negative ions are such an important factor in air, especially for purposes of detox and healing, is that they function as powerful antioxidants to scavenge free radicals in the blood and tissues. Considering how toxic most people are and how polluted the environment is, these days, this protective factor in air is more important than ever for those who wish to live long in good health. Besides scavenging free radicals, negative ions help eliminate all sorts of other toxins as well, by binding with their positive charge and allowing them to be carried away for excretion.

Air that is rich in negative ions continuously purges tissues of toxins and purifies the bloodstream with each and every breath. During detox, when the blood must carry an overload of toxic wastes from the tissues to the excretory organs for elimination, negative ions become an important ally, because they help to keep the bloodstream clean, thereby facilitating the blood's capacity to continuously flush toxins and acid wastes from the internal organs and tissues and deliver them to the excretory drains. Negative-ion energy from air also increases the electrical potential of each and every cell in the body, and collectively this boost amplifies the power and vibrancy of the entire human energy field. Not only does this amplification increase the body's overall resistance to disease, it also helps to shield the body from invasion by aberrant, external energies such as those produced by artificial electromagnetic fields, microwaves, atomic radiation, and other forms of "energy pollution."

The most convenient and effective way to increase your assimilation of negative ions is to practice deep breathing exercises in good quality air on a daily basis. The fact remains, however, that most people are unwilling to take the time and effort required to learn and practice chi gung. For such individuals, modern technology has come up with some electronic devices that effectively recharge the air in a room, office, or automobile with high concentrations of negative ions, so that the people may assimilate abundant amounts of this essential energy, even while lounging in a hammock or armchair.

One such device is the negative-ion generator, which emits a constant stream of negative ions into the air from electrically charged metallic pins. These devices, which come in a variety of sizes and output capacities, may be placed in any office, bedroom, work space, or other human habitat to compensate for negative-ion deficiency in the air. Many modern office buildings and high-rise hotels and apartment blocks in Japan are routinely equipped with negative-ion generators to purify and energize the air that people must breathe inside, and perhaps this helps account, at least in part, for the fact that the Japanese people continue to lead the world in longevity. Special units are also designed for use in automobiles, as are compact battery-operated units that may be taken anywhere, including on airplanes.

The commercial airline industry has for years resisted the call to install negative-ion generators on all flights, apparently because doing so would acknowledge the basic problem with the air on airplanes that has existed all along. This problem became even worse once we entered the jet age, when the commercial airline industry decided to stop drawing fresh air into aircraft to save the costs of pressurizing and heating it at such high altitudes. Instead, the air on all commercial airliners is now recycled throughout the duration of all flights, forcing passengers to breathe and rebreathe the same stale, germ-ridden air exhaled by other passengers. On long flights, this situation can pose serious health hazards for unsuspecting passengers, especially those with weak immune systems.

The need for negative-ion generators in aircraft was first discovered during the early days of the space program, when it was noted that early astronauts such as John Glenn could not remain aloft in space for more than one day without experiencing debilitating fatigue and mental confusion. It was the Russians who first recognized that the source of the problem was negative-ion deficiency, and they solved it by installing negative-ion generators in their spacecraft, which immediately enabled their cosmonauts to endure much longer space flights. Today, airline passengers throughout the world are complaining of circulatory problems, jet lag, virulent diseases contracted in flight, breathing difficulties, and other health problems, all of which are due primarily to the critical deficiency of negative ions in the air within aircraft. A negative-ion generator of sufficient output to infuse a large room with life-sustaining negative ions draws less power than that required by a 60-watt light bulb, so expense is certainly no excuse for not installing these devices on all airplanes. Nevertheless, until the airline industry is compelled by public demand to make the air in aircraft safe and suitable for human consumption by installing negative-ion generators (or offering passengers portable units at the beginning of all flights, as they offer earphones for in-flight entertainment), your best bet to protect yourself from the dangers of the dead, contaminated air that you're forced to breathe on airline flights is to bring along your own portable, battery-operated negative-ion generator. Such units are now available.

During a detox program, it is very helpful to keep a negative-ion generator going in your bedroom while sleeping at night. Not only does this neutralize and precipitate all dust, smoke, and other pollutants in the air of the room in which you sleep, it also provides strong, continuous antioxidant activity in your blood and tissues while you're sleeping, so that the detox process may continue efficiently and without interruption even while you're asleep. In addition, it protects you from bacterial infections: the natural decay rate for bacteria in ordinary air today is about 23 percent, but when air is charged with negative ions, the bacterial decay rate rises more than threefold to 78 percent. In light of how many patients contract deadly bacterial infections in hospitals today, installing negative-ion generators in all hospital rooms would save a lot of lives at negligible expense.

"ACTIVATED AIR"

A new device has recently appeared on the market in Australia that generates a stream of air with a negative-ion count of eighty million ions/cubic inch/sec. Known as an "Activated Air System" and manufactured by "GEOMED Biomedicine," this new technology is showing great promise as a swift, powerful, and totally safe therapeutic tool for treating a wide range of ailments and degenerative conditions that are caused by blood and tissue toxicity. This is one of the most effective electronic detox technologies on the market today.

The GEOMED Activated Air System works by producing a steady stream of highly ionized air containing the same natural ratios of oxygen and nitrogen as ordinary air. Ionized oxygen greatly improves the blood's capacity to cleanse and nourish the tissues. However, nitrogen is equally as important for detox purposes, because it functions as a bonding molecule for the discharge of various waste products such as uric acid and ammonia. The GEOMED generates both ionized oxygen and nitrogen, thereby producing air that has extremely potent detoxifying and rejuvenating properties.

Inhaling this activated ionized air for a period of just thirty minutes produces an immediate, measurable increase in the body's overall metabolic rate and a huge boost to immune response, particularly antioxidant activity. These effects greatly amplify and accelerate the detox process and facilitate healing and regeneration on the cellular level. Those interested in ordering or obtaining further information about the GEOMED Activated Air System, may contact the appropriate supplier listed at the back of this book.

"THE NOSE KNOWS!"

While the lungs are designed to assimilate oxygen and discharge carbon dioxide through breathing, the more subtle energy elements in air, such as negative ions and the medicinal energies in the volatile vapors released into the air by aromatherapy, are absorbed primarily by special receptors located in the lining of the nasal passages and sinus cavities. To keep their nasal receptors clean and sensitive, the yogins of ancient India developed the Neti nasal douche, to allow the essential energies carried in the air to be freely assimilated. These receptors, when clean and functioning properly, transmit the energy of negative ions and volatile aromatic vapors directly into the energy meridians, blood vessels, and nerves of the head, from where they are distributed to the brain and body.

Aromatic vapors released into the air from essential oils and flowers by evaporation carry the essential energies of those plants and transport their potent therapeutic properties directly into the human system via the nasal and sinus receptors. Medieval Arab physicians frequently noted the fact that when cholera, smallpox, and other contagious plagues periodically swept through the Middle East, perfumers and incense makers, who work daily with the potent aromatic essence of plants, rarely succumbed to these deadly diseases. Their imperviousness to disease was due to the fact that they were protected by the potent medicinal properties of the natural aromatic plants from which they extracted essential scents to make perfume and incense all day long. Today, the same phenomenon is observed in professional florists, who work amidst the fragrant energies of fresh flowers and consequently rarely catch colds, the flu, and other contagious ailments that routinely infect others.

It should be noted that only scents derived from natural plant sources provide medicinal benefits and may therefore be effectively used for aromatherapy. This includes various flowers, seeds, roots, barks, leaves, and other plant parts that contain volatile aromatic elements. Synthetic scents have a "smell," but they don't have any bioactive energies with therapeutic properties, and any well trained nose can instantly detect the difference between natural and synthetic scents, not so much by their actual smell but by the subtle effects of their vibrant energy. Those distinctive effects are produced by the ionized energies released into the air from the essential oils of aromatic plants by the process of evaporation. In Taoist terminology, synthetic substances are devoid of the natural "essence" (jing) required to produce the bio-active "energy" (chi) found in the ionized vapors of medicinal plants. The French medical scientist Dr. J. Valent, writing in the journal L'Hopital in 1960, explains how aromatherapy works:

Carried by the bloodstream, the ionized plant aroma impregnates every corner of the body, powerfully revitalizes the polarized and discharged cells, replenishes electronic shortages by recharging the bio-electromagnetic batteries, and disperses cellular residue by

dissolving the viscous and diseased substances of body fluids. It oxidizes poisonous metabolic waste products, increases energy balance,
frees the mechanism of organic oxidation and of self-regulation, and
reaches the lungs and kidneys, whence it is excreted or exhaled without a trace.

Here we see how useful aromatherapy can be when applied to the
detox process. The ionized essential energy assimilated from the inhaled
vapors of medicinal plants penetrates the deepest tissues of the body
and reaches into each and every cell, where, as Dr. Valent says, it disperses cellular residue by dissolving the viscous and diseased substances
of body fluids and oxidizes poisonous metabolic waste products, send-
ing them all out to the lungs and kidneys for excretion. The practical
applications of aromatherapy for detox are obvious. By keeping an aromatherapy vaporizer operating in the rooms in which you sleep at night
and spend the most time by day, you saturate the air you breathe with
the potent ionized energies of medicinal plants, which in turn enter your
body with each breath, assisting and accelerating the detoxification and
healing process.

During the day, you should select essential oils that are known for
their strong blood and tissue-cleansing properties, such as sage, rosemary, and juniper. At night, while sleeping, it is best to use aromas with
calming nervine properties, such as lavender, frankincense, or sandal-
wood to help you sleep well. These also have detoxifying properties,
but they are gentler than those used by day, so they won't interfere with
sleep.

"SILENCE IS GOLDEN"

We've all heard this slogan before, but what does it actually mean? Let's
hear what Master Chang San-feng, the Taoist sage credited with developing Tai Chi Chuan six hundred years ago, had to say about this con-
cept. He advised, "Forget about words and your energy won't scatter."
The Taoist adept and commentator, Liu I-ming, writing about two hun-

dred years ago, said basically the same thing: "When the mouth speaks, energy scatters." And in the Tibetan Buddhist tradition, the word for "speech" is often used to denote "energy," because speech expends and dissipates a tremendous amount of breath and energy. The only sort of speech that focuses rather than scatters energy is mantra, prayer, and harmonious song.

Today, with all the manifold pressures and chronic stress of modern life, many people seem to have acquired a "motor-mouth" syndrome. They feel compelled to sustain a constant stream of small talk, gossip, and marathon monologues, regardless of whether anyone else is really listening or responding to their words or not. Indeed, some people are so addicted to "blowing off steam" this way that they talk to themselves constantly when there's no one else around to listen. This book is not the place to speculate on the psychological and emotional implications of the modern motor-mouth syndrome, but it is certainly appropriate to point out the fact that constant chatter drains away vital energy and depletes your "bio-batteries." Since energy is the fundamental fuel required to detox, repair, and rebalance the human body, especially during an intensive detox program, it doesn't make much sense to needlessly waste this vital resource by spewing it out of your mouth in a fountain of words. It's far better to remain silent and focus your energy inward for healing purposes.

It is, therefore, advisable to speak no more than necessary during a detox program and remain as silent as possible, to conserve your limited supplies of vital energy for internal cleansing. Try to resist spending a lot of time on the telephone talking to friends, or making long-distance calls to check on your business affairs. All of that activity can wait until the program is over. Also try not to spend all afternoon scattering your energy to the wind by gossiping with other guests at spas and health resorts; that chatter definitely slows down the detox process and prevents the nervous system from remaining at rest in the healing mode. Instead, have a massage or steam bath, take a stroll in the forest or along the beach, or practice chi gung. Speak only when necessary to communicate something important, and say it softly, with a minimum waste of energy. By "saving your breath" this way, you'll also be reserving your energy for internal cleansing and healing. That extra supply of energy is "as good as gold" in terms of its value to human health and healing.

And that's why "silence is golden," because it conserves your energy assets so that your body can draw upon them in times of need to protect your health and prolong your life.

5
DETOX DIET AND SUPPLEMENTS

What you don't eat is actually more important than what you do eat during a detox program. In fact, the best detox diet of all is to eat nothing. The basic dietary strategy for detox is to totally eliminate all acid-forming foods and beverages and to consume only small amounts of a few simple alkalizing items that provide the basic mix of essential nutrients required by the body when it is in detox mode. By keeping the diet as simple and sparse as possible, digestive wastes are reduced to a bare minimum, and the enormous amount of energy and the vast number of enzymes that our bodies normally burn up to meet the constant, complex digestive demands of our daily diets are diverted instead to detox duty. The less food you eat and the more water you drink, the faster and more efficiently your body detoxifies and repairs itself.

On the other hand, some nutrients actively assist the detox process, so whatever you choose to eat during a detox program should be selected to provide precisely those elements. The most important nutritional elements the body needs to purify the bloodstream and detoxify the tissues are enzymes, minerals, trace elements, and vitamins. Animal protein, fat, refined sugar, and starch, which constitute about 90 percent of the calories most people in the Western world consume these days, not only are useless for detox purposes, but also actually block the cleansing process as well as produce large amounts of acid wastes and putrefactive sludge. These items, therefore, must strictly be eliminated from a detox diet.

Short of fasting, which remains by far the best way to detoxify the body, the dietary approach to detox includes four basic strategies. First and foremost is to abstain entirely from eating or drinking anything that acidifies the blood and tissues. The next step is to design a detox diet based on just a few simple, unrefined plant-source foods that alkalize the blood and tissues while also providing the basic nutrients the body needs to support the detox process from start to finish. Third is to select a variety of special supplements made entirely from natural sources to assist and accelerate the detox process by providing pure, concentrated forms of essential nutrients and alkalizing agents. Fourth is to reduce calorie intake as much as possible, to decrease production of digestive and metabolic wastes and conserve energy and enzymes for detox rather than digestive purposes.

ACID ABSTINENCE

"The longest journey begins with a single step." The first step in the direction of detox is to abstain completely from eating or drinking anything that produces an acid reaction in the digestive tract and leaves acid residues in the blood and tissues. This step should be taken a week or more before you start your full detox program. Some processed foods, such as refined sugar and starch, as well as many chemical food additives, have addictive properties similar to drugs when consumed in large amounts over long periods of time, and it is much easier on the body to withdraw these items from the diet gradually, rather than stopping suddenly. Leaping abruptly from a highly acidic state of toxemia into an alkaline state of intensive detox can produce unpleasant withdrawal symptoms. By starting to abstain from all acid-forming food and drink a week or more before implementing the main parts of your detox program, you give your body a chance to adjust incrementally to the rigors of the alkalization and detoxification process.

First and foremost, you should eliminate all animal-source food products from your diet during detox, including meat, eggs, and dairy products. All animal products are extremely acidifying to the digestive tract and bloodstream, and they also produce highly putrefactive protein wastes in the bowels. Cancer cells thrive on animal proteins and multiply rapidly in the highly acidic environment they create in the body, while worms and parasites flourish in the toxic sludge they leave glued to the bowel wall. By eliminating all acid-forming animal products from your diet and taking additional measures to alkalize your blood and tissues, you starve any cancer cells that may be developing in the body and rob them of the acidic environment they require to multiply and form tumors. In light of the pandemic spread of cancer throughout all segments of society today, this preventive strategy against cancer is a primary goal of any detox program.

Animal-based foods require a tremendous amount of energy and enzyme power to digest and process, far more than plant-based foods. If you eat meat and dairy products while trying to detoxify your blood and tissues, there is simply no way your body can muster the extra reserves of energy and enzymes it needs to cleanse and repair itself. Rather than using these reserves for detox functions such as dissolving developing tumors, dismantling damaged cells, and destroying dangerous microbes, your body will be forced by your diet to divert most of its energy and enzyme power to digestive duty to process the complex proteins and heavy fats in animal foods, and to deal with the putrid acid wastes they produce in the digestive tract. This high-energy drain defeats the very purpose of detox and should be strictly avoided.

Another category of food that should be deleted completely from the diet during detox is refined starch, especially white flour products such as bread, pasta, and pastries. These items are highly acid-forming and burn up a tremendous amount of energy and enzymes to process. Moreover, since they provide absolutely nothing of nutritional value to the detox process, they should be totally cut from the detox diet. All highly refined food products that enter the human body stripped naked of their essential nutrients must borrow the missing nutrients from the body's reserves to complete their nutritional profiles so that they may be properly digested and metabolized in the body. Consequently, eating highly refined, processed foods actually robs the body of the essential nutrients it needs to support the detox process.

The most hazardous dietary item of all in terms of its acid-forming, nutrient-robbing properties is refined white sugar. Refined sugar, or "sucrose," acidifies the bloodstream faster and more severely than any other food on earth, and by far the worst offender in this category is the sugary sweet, fizzy "Acid Bomb" known as the soft drink. One 12-ounce serving of Coke, Pepsi, or a similar soft drink delivers straight to the bloodstream a sugar fix equivalent to about 9 teaspoons of refined white sugar. That sugar spike instantly acidifies the bloodstream to the extreme point that, without an immediate emergency response from the body, it would kill you in a matter of minutes. To counteract the sudden radical rise in blood acidity that a glass of sweet, carbonated soda causes and to reestablish a viable balance in blood pH before you drop dead, you'd have to quickly drink thirty-two glasses of alkaline water. Of course, nobody drinks thirty-two glasses of alkaline water after each serving of a soft drink. Instead, to prevent death by acidosis, the body reacts swiftly by drawing huge amounts of organic calcium from the bones and teeth and pouring it into the bloodstream to neutralize the excess acids and to restore alkaline balance quickly. Calcium is the body's most potent alkalizing agent and one of the most essential elements required for detox. If you consume soft drinks and other refined sweets during a detox program, not only will they continuously acidify your blood and tissues when you're supposed to be alkalizing them instead, they'll also drain away all your vital calcium reserves, and force your body to leach additional calcium from your bones and teeth to combat the constant influx of acids. This defensive response to excess acidosis in the bloodstream has become one of the main causes of osteoporosis, particularly in America, where people consume an astounding average of fifty-three teaspoons of refined white sugar per day, much of it in the form of carbonated soft drinks.

It is not just the sugar in soft drinks that makes them so dangerously acidifying to the blood and other bodily fluids. The carbonation in soft drinks is produced by forcing carbon dioxide gas into the sweet liquid and sealing it under pressure, so that when the can or bottle is opened, the gas is released as fizzy bubbles. As we already know, carbon dioxide is a waste product of human metabolism and a primary contributing factor to blood acidosis. To make matters even worse, the active ingredient in most of these fizzy, sweet soft drinks is phosphoric acid, which has an extremely acid pH value of 2.8. Since human blood must maintain a slightly alkaline pH of 7.35 at all times—and even small fluctuations can cause severe reactions—dropping an "Acid Bomb" of sugar plus carbon dioxide plus phosphoric acid into your stomach causes a constant, rapid drain on your body's calcium resources. If you drink this stuff while trying to detox, its strong acid-forming properties will prevent your blood and tissues from ever reaching the degree of alkalinity required for the body's detox and healing mechanisms to switch on and function. Instead, your blood and tissues will remain in a constant state of acidosis. Rather than cleansing and repairing itself, your body will be forced to fight a running biochemical battle just to keep your blood pH from dropping to critically dangerous levels.

ALKALINE À LA CARTE

The basic purpose of a detox diet is to provide a highly alkalizing, totally nonacidifying source of nutrition that supports the detox process while producing as little waste as possible in the body and requiring the least amount of energy to digest. Everything consumed during detox should specifically assist in alkalizing the body, purifying the bloodstream, and detoxifying the tissues, while also helping to eliminate acid wastes and toxic residues through the excretory organs. All of the manifold symptoms of blood and tissue toxicity, such as chronic headaches and body pain, joint and tissue inflammation, bloating and swelling, indigestion and constipation, liver congestion and nervous tension respond quickly to a well-planned detox diet, which not only provides symptomatic relief but also helps eliminate the root cause of all these conditions, which is toxemia.

The twin pillars of the detox diet are fresh fruits and fresh vegetables. These foods must not only be fresh but also be organically grown and free of chemical pesticides, genetically modified varieties, and irradiation. Any fruit or vegetable that has been genetically modified, irradiated, or grown with chemical pesticides and fertilizers is useless for detox purposes. Such food is not fit for daily human consumption, either. On the other hand, fresh, organic produce is a pure and potent source of alkalizing elements and antioxidant factors, as well as a source of essential nutrients, all of which assist the detox and healing process. Fruits have primarily cleansing and purging properties, while vegetables are mainly curative and regenerative. Both are highly alkalizing, produce very little waste, and don't require much energy and or many enzymes to digest. Together, fruit and vegetables provide the full spectrum of nutritional and therapeutic elements required to detoxify and repair the body.

Fresh fruits are such a pure and simple form of food that most of them require no digestion whatsoever in the stomach. Instead, they move quickly into the duodenum, where they dissolve and release their nutrients for quick assimilation into the bloodstream within half an hour of ingestion. If there is any other food digesting in the stomach when fresh fruit is eaten, however, the fruit must back up and wait until the other food has been processed before it can move on through to the duodenum. During this delay, the ever-present bacteria in the stomach feast on the fruit, metabolizing its nutrients and causing the fruit and everything else in the stomach to ferment rather than digest, producing toxic acid wastes and intestinal gas and upsetting the entire digestive tract. Fruit that would normally alkalize, nourish, and cleanse the body thus becomes a source of acidosis, toxicity, and indigestion instead. Therefore, the basic rule regarding fruit is, "Eat it alone or leave it alone." Some vegetables, especially when eaten raw, can take up to three hours to digest due to their high cellulose content, and therefore fruits and vegetables should always be consumed separately from each other. In a detox diet, for example, vegetables may be included with the main meals at breakfast, lunch, and dinner, and fruits may be eaten as snacks in between meals.

First, let's take a look at the vegetable section of the detox menu. The best choices in vegetables are those that actively cleanse and heal the body, alkalize the blood and tissues, and deliver optimum nutrition at minimum digestive cost. Such vegetables include sweet potatoes, yams, squash, pumpkin, carrot, beet, cabbage, celery, parsley, and all dark leafy greens. These items are rich in organic carotenes, which rank among the most powerful dietary healing factors. Such vegetables also include other elements that are specifically beneficial in supporting the excretory functions of the liver, lungs, kidneys, and bowels. Garlic, ginger, and onion also have potent cleansing and curative properties and may therefore be included in the detox diet to spice up the taste of otherwise bland vegetables.

Vegetables may be prepared three ways for consumption during detox: as a clear broth of boiled vegetables; as fresh-cut vegetables cooked by steaming, stewing, or stir-frying; and as freshly extracted raw vegetable juice. Note that raw vegetable salads are not recommended during detox. The cell walls of raw vegetables, especially those with high cellulose content such as lettuce, celery, and carrots, are very tough and require a long time and a lot of enzyme power to digest before their nutrients can be released. Not only does this waste a lot of precious energy on digestion but it also delays delivery of nutrients and other healing factors into the bloodstream, thereby slowing down detox. For detox purposes, raw vegetables should only be consumed as freshly extracted juices in which the cell walls of the vegetables have been crushed to release all the nutrients and healing factors in a fluid form that swiftly enters the bloodstream without requiring much digestion.

Clear Broth

Clear vegetable broth is a good choice for people with stomach ulcers or weak digestive systems because the stomach and bowels need not process the bulky solids and waste products of whole vegetables. While the cooking process destroys the enzymes and some of the vitamins, all the essential minerals and trace elements are retained and easily assimilated, and these are the most important nutrients for detox purposes. Since clear vegetable broth requires no digestion in the stomach, it may be sipped in small amounts throughout the day or taken along with other cooked vegetables at meals. You may also stir a spoonful of organic miso paste into a cup of hot vegetable broth to increase its nutritional and therapeutic value, as well as to aid in digestion. A recommended combination of vegetables for preparing clear broth is given in the section on "Recipes and Formulas" (see page 304).

Cooked Vegetables

Vegetables may be cooked by steaming, stewing, or stir-frying. The only seasonings that should be added to the vegetables are a bit of sea salt, some chopped ginger root, and a clove or two of garlic or some chopped onion, if desired. Sea salt provides the full spectrum of minerals and trace elements to complement the primary nutrients in the vegetables and to assist in their digestion and assimilation. Ginger root is a strong alkalizer and also assists digestion, while garlic has potent antibacterial and tissue-cleansing properties and is one of the few dietary sources of the trace element selenium, which the body requires to produce its most powerful antioxidant enzyme. Onions also contain a variety of useful elements for purifying the blood and detoxifying the tissues.

Because *The Tao of Detox* is not a cookbook, we'll simply review the basic methods of preparing vegetables for use in a detox diet rather than discuss detailed recipes. We will leave the cooking style to your own culinary imagination.

Steaming

You can steam pumpkins, sweet potatoes, carrots, squash, and beets together in the same steamer. Simply cut them into large chunks, including the skin, and steam for twenty to thirty minutes. Leaf vegetables only require a few minutes to steam. If you wish to season the vegetables with sea salt, ginger, and/or garlic, add those items during the last minute of cooking.

Stewing

Cut all vegetables into bite-sized pieces and place them in a large cooking pot. Add sea salt, ginger, and garlic, if desired. Add enough water to completely cover the vegetables. Then bring to a boil, cover with a lid and simmer slowly over low heat for thirty to forty-five minutes. Stir occasionally. Add extra water if the mixture gets too dry. A good combination includes pumpkin, sweet potato, carrot, cabbage, and celery, with some chopped parsley and spinach thrown in during the last five minutes of cooking. Pumpkin has mild laxative and diuretic properties, which helps support the excretory functions of the bowels and kidneys during detox.

Stir-frying

This method is definitely the best way to cook fresh vegetables to preserve their fresh flavors and crisp textures, as well as their nutritional value. The high heat softens the cell walls of the cellulose and cooks the vegetables just enough to make them easy to digest, while the short cooking time prevents their crispy textures from wilting and their bright colors from fading. When stir-frying vegetables, chopped ginger and garlic may be added to the pan together with the vegetables, but the salt should be added only at the very end of the cooking process. Root vegetables such as carrots, yams, and beets are not very suitable for stir-frying, but squash, pumpkin, and celery as well as all green leafy vegetables lend themselves very well to stir-fry cooking. It is best to use only olive oil for stir-frying, because it provides the most beneficial forms of essential fatty acids and does not produce an abundance of free radicals at high cooking temperatures, as most other oils do. Good choices for stir-fried vegetables in the detox diet include spinach, kale, mustard greens, cabbage, bok choi, bamboo shoots, and watercress. Watercress supplies abundant amounts of organic sulfur, calcium, and magnesium and has particularly potent blood-purifying properties. If your kidneys and bladder are ailing and need a cleansing alkaline flush-out, try stir-frying some tender fresh asparagus with ginger, garlic, and sea salt. Asparagus is one of the most powerful natural alkalizers in the vegetable kingdom. It flushes so much acid waste from the blood and kidneys so quickly that you can smell the ammonia in your urine within half an hour after eating asparagus. If you prefer, asparagus may also be steamed for two or three minutes, rather than stir-fried.

Raw Vegetable Juice

To extract juice from fresh raw vegetables, use a proper vegetable extractor that can press the juice from the vegetable cells under high pressure, extracting the essential fluid content and discarding the fibrous pulp. The great advantage of raw juice is that it retains all the potent, active enzymes from the vegetables, which are destroyed by heat in the cooking process. Raw juice also preserves all of the vitamins and other essential nutrients in vegetables and delivers them into the stomach in a ready-to-assimilate fluid form that requires no digestion. A glass of raw vegetable juice is the perfect complementary beverage for a detox meal of cooked vegetables; the juice provides the active enzymes and vitamins missing from the cooked vegetables, and the cooked vegetables provide the fiber removed from the juice.

Vegetable juices may be taken individually or blended in various combinations to provide specific therapeutic benefits to particular organs, glands, and other tissues by virtue of their natural pharmacodynamic affinity for specific parts of the body. Many good books are available these days on raw-juice therapy, and many health spas now feature special "juice bars" where guests can enjoy their "Happy Hour" over a carrot and beet cocktail rather than a beer or whisky. A few tried-and-true vegetable juices for detox are briefly introduced below:

Carrot

This is perhaps the single most valuable vegetable juice for detox purposes. It cleanses the liver of stale bile and the coagulated toxic residues that accumulate there year after year as a result of eating chemically contaminated foods and wrong food combinations. Carrot juice provides abundant supplies of organic sulfur and chlorine for tissue cleansing purposes, calcium and magnesium to support the detox process, and natural carotenes, which provide strong antioxidant activity. Carrot is also the best base juice for blending special combinations with other juices.

Beet

Beet juice is a potent cleanser of the liver and lower bowel. It also nourishes red blood cells, increases their capacity to carry oxygen, and helps regulate menstrual cycles in women. Beet juice is quite strong and therefore only 2–4 ounces, combined with 6–8 ounces of carrot and/or other juices, should be taken per serving, and no more than 8 ounces (1 cup) should be used per day.

Celery

Celery juice is an excellent source of organic sodium chloride, which has strong cleansing and alkalizing properties and helps cool down the whole system. It is also a rich source of magnesium, which is required to produce alkaline enzymes for detox purposes. Celery juice is an effective remedy for disorders of the nervous system, including insomnia and nervous tension. Celery's nervine properties help keep body and mind relaxed and at ease during detox. A glass of fresh celery juice in the morning is a very good way to soothe a hangover after a night of drinking, which is something that hopefully won't happen during a detox program. This remedy, however, can come in handy in daily life, should such a situation arise.

Parsley

Parsley, like asparagus, is a powerful alkalizer with strong affinity for the kidneys and bladder. In addition to its potent kidney- and bladder-cleansing properties, parsley juice soothes and reduces inflammation in the urogenital canal and detoxifies the liver. Parsley is a rich source of organic calcium and magnesium and it helps purify the blood. In combination with carrot juice, parsley nourishes the eyes and improves vision. Parsley juice is strong medicine and should be taken only in combination with other juices, such as carrot juice. Don't use more than 3 ounces a day.

Wheat-Grass Juice

If you have access to freshly extracted wheat-grass juice, or if you're equipped to prepare it at home, include 2–3 ounces a day in your detox diet, combined with carrot and other juices. Wheat-grass juice is the ideal detox food. It provides fresh organic chlorophyll to purify the bloodstream and build strong blood; it alkalizes the blood and tissues; it contains the full range of essential amino acids, minerals, and vitamins required for cellular regeneration; and it is brimming with active enzymes.

Breuss Vegetable Juice

This juice recipe is used in the cancer treatment developed by Dr. Rudolf Breuss, an Austrian naturopath whose program has helped over forty-thousand people cure themselves of cancer. It also serves as an excellent therapeutic blend for general detox purposes. To make enough juice for one day, put the following vegetables through a good juice extractor, then strain the liquid through a fine sieve or cheesecloth to remove all sediment. Combine 10 ounces of beets; 3½ ounces of carrots; 3½ ounces of celery root, 2½ ounces of potatoes, and one ounce of white turnips (Chinese radish). You may drink a glass of this juice as part of a detox meal, or sip it slowly, an ounce at a time, throughout the day as part of your detox diet. Breuss Vegetable Juice is also produced in bottled form by the Biotta Company of Switzerland. Made only from organic, chemical-free vegetables that have been cold-pressed to preserve all the vital nutrients, enzymes, and other healing factors, this exceptional product is a pure, living vegetable juice that retains the therapeutic benefits and nutritional value of fresh, raw juice. Juice is a very convenient way to take your vegetables during detox. In fact, two glasses per day of Breuss Vegetable Juice, either homemade or bottled from Biotta, is sufficient to provide all the nutritional support and alkalizing factors required during a detox program.

Fruits

Fresh fruits are the other mainstay of the detox diet, but not all fruits are suitable for detox purposes. The best choices for internal cleansing are citrus fruits and semisweet fruits from temperate climates such as apples, pears, watermelons, black cherries, and black grapes. Tropical fruits such as mangos, pineapples, bananas, and litchi have a very high content of fruit sugars and tend to overheat the system; the only exception is papaya, which facilitates detox and is particularly cleansing to the digestive tract owing to its rich content of active protease (protein-digesting) enzymes, which dissolve partially digested proteins and mucoid matter in the intestines. All fruits included in the detox diet should be organically grown and totally free of pesticides and other chemical sprays. In addition, only fresh fruits should be eaten. Do not substitute dried fruits. As a result of the dehydration process, dried fruits contain much denser concentrations of fruit sugars and far fewer enzymes than fresh fruits. Therefore the body must spend its own energy and enzymes to process dried fruit. Fresh fruits, which are over 95 percent water and contain their own active enzymes, virtually digest themselves.

Three ways are recommended for eating fruit during detox. One way is to extract the juice and strain out most of the pulp. This process renders a very pure, highly alkalizing nectar that is easy to absorb and that reaches the bloodstream quickly. A second way is to use a blender to make a "fruit smoothie," but without adding any milk, yogurt, soy milk, honey, or any other ingredients. Use only fresh fruit and pure water. This produces a drink in which the juice is blended together with the pureed pulp. It provides an excellent source of hydrated fiber for the digestive tract. The third way is simply to eat the fruit whole, with or without the peel. The peel of fruits such as apples, pears, and grapes contain many valuable nutrients and healing factors, but they must be very well chewed in the mouth before swallowing to extract those nutrients, and the fruit must be certified organic to avoid poisoning yourself with the chemical sprays used on most commercial crops.

Many people are confused regarding the role of citrus fruits in maintaining proper pH balance in the stomach and bloodstream. Citrus fruit juices are very cleansing to the stomach and digestive tract and help dissolve impacted mucus and putrefactive wastes, but if you measure the pH value of any citrus juice with litmus paper, you'll find that it falls decisively into the acid range. The pH value of a food outside the stomach, however, does not determine whether it has "acid-forming" or "alkaline-forming" effects within the stomach. What counts is how a particular food *reacts* with the digestive juices and other foods in the stomach after it is eaten, and whether it acidifies or alkalizes the bloodstream after it has been digested. In the case of citrus fruits, if they are eaten on an empty stomach and allowed to pass unobstructed into the duodenum, they become highly alkalizing and very beneficial for internal cleansing and detox. However, if you drink a glass of orange or grapefruit juice with a meal of toast, eggs, pancakes, and/or cereal—as millions of people do every day when eating a modern Western-style breakfast—the citrus juice, unable to pass into the duodenum, sits on top of the other food and quickly ferments, preventing the proper digestion of everything else in the stomach and turning it all into a frothing, fermentive stew that causes gas, forms acid wastes, and increases tissue toxicity. To gain maximum benefit from citrus fruits' cleansing and alkalizing properties, and to avoid their acid-forming reactions with other foods, they should always be eaten separately from any other foods, including all other types of fruit.

As with all items in the detox diet, the fewer your choices in fruit, and the more simply you combine them, the better they will work to purify your blood, detoxify your tissues, and cleanse your digestive tract. Here are a few suggestions:

Apples

Apples aid digestion and cleanse the intestinal tract. They may be eaten whole or juiced. Apple cores are very rich in pectin, which acts as a potent intestinal detoxificant. Raw apple juice usually reduces the fever and tissue inflammation that sometimes occur during detox as heavy toxins are dislodged and released into the bloodstream for excretion. Another raw apple product that may be used for detox purposes is organic apple cider vinegar. Unlike all other vinegars, which contain acetic acid and are therefore acid-forming, apple cider vinegar contains malic acid, which is alkalizing to the body. Two tablespoons of apple cider vinegar with one teaspoon of raw honey stirred into a glass of warm water may be taken once or twice a day, before meals, to cleanse the stomach and balance pH throughout the digestive system. This is particularly beneficial for those who suffer from gastritis.

Pears

Pears are loaded with alkalizing elements and have a natural affinity for the kidneys, where they provide a gentle diuretic effect, cleansing the kidneys, and dissolving crystallized acid residue before it can form kidney stones.

Grapes

The best type of grapes for detox purposes are black grapes. The juice of raw black grapes is known among vegans as "vegetarian milk" because of its capacity to sustain nursing infants deprived of mother's milk, without using dairy milk. Black grapes are particularly effective for treating constipation and gastritis, detoxifying the liver and kidneys, and purifying the blood. In Russia, entire clinics are devoted exclusively to what is called "The Grape Cure." In the clinics, patients are fed nothing but raw black grapes for up to a full month or more. This regimen has been effectively used to cure various forms of cancer, heart disease, hepatitis, nervous system disorders, and many other serious conditions that conventional medicine often views as "incurable." Glucose, which is also known as "blood sugar" and is the main form of sugar found in grapes, is the body's primary metabolic fuel and is especially important for brain functions. Since grapes directly provide the bloodstream with the precise form of fuel required by the cells, they help curb the craving for rich foods that often manifests when you're trying to restrict your diet to just a few simple items. The skins and seeds of grapes are also rich in nutrients and cleansing factors, but they must be chewed very well to release these elements for assimilation. If you don't have the patience to chew the skins and seeds of whole grapes, you may puree them whole in a blender, which does the chewing job for you. Like all other fruits, grapes should be eaten at least one or two hours apart from vegetables and other foods. If you choose to eat nothing else but grapes for your detox diet, you may eat as many of them as you wish, from morning till night.

Citrus

Oranges, grapefruits, and lemons are wonderful alkalizers and cleansers when consumed alone, either whole or juiced. They help dissolve mucus and phlegm throughout the system, alkalize the blood and bodily fluids, and decongest the liver. Fresh grapefruit is extraordinarily rich in salicylic acid, which dissolves crystallized calcium deposits in the joints, thereby relieving arthritis. In conjunction with long-term reforms in daily diet after a few detox programs, arthritis can be gradually and permanently cured with grapefruit therapy. Citrus juice also has strong antiseptic and antifungal properties, which can be important during detox. Never add sugar or any other sweetener to fresh citrus juice because any additive will cause it to ferment in the stomach and become highly acid-forming, rather than alkalizing. As explained earlier, always consume citrus fruits and juices separately from other foods, and on an empty stomach.

Watermelon

Watermelon is an excellent internal organ cleanser, especially for the kidneys and bladder. When eaten whole, it should be cut up into bite-sized chunks and chewed slowly, bite by bite, throughout the day. Alternatively, it may be pureed in a blender, including the white rind, which contains potent kidney-cleansing factors. Watermelon is one of the most alkalizing of fruits. In addition, owing to its natural affinity for the kidneys, it helps dissolve and prevent the formation of kidney stones.

Papaya

Papaya's abundant supplies of protease enzymes makes it particularly effective as a digestive aid and a detoxifying agent for bowels that are clogged with putrefactive protein wastes from excessive consumption of meat, eggs, and dairy products. Papaya also stimulates secretions of digestive juices in the stomach and duodenum, and when there's nothing else in the stomach, these digestive enzymes travel down to dissolve mucus and break down putrid waste matter in the intestines.

GRAINS AND NUTS

Almost all major grain foods are acid-forming and require significant energy and enzymes to digest. Therefore in the detox diet, grains should either be eliminated entirely, or else strictly limited. The only major grain food that is alkaline-forming is millet, so it is the best choice when grains are included in the detox diet. If millet is unavailable, the next best options, in order of preference, are spelt, barley, rye, buckwheat, or brown rice. All wheat products should be eliminated completely. Wheat not only is one of the most acid-forming grains but also is the cause of allergic reactions in many people. Both these reactions become particularly severe during detox.

Only whole, organically grown grains should be included in the detox diet. Absolutely no flour products, such as bread, pasta, and pastry, should be allowed. The grain should be washed well and presoaked in pure water for at least six hours, or overnight, then boiled for a few hours with plenty of water and a teaspoon of sea salt until it forms a thin gruel or porridge. In Chinese, this sort of watery boiled grain is called *hsi-fan,* literally "diluted rice," or "congee." During cooking, if the porridge becomes too thick, stir in another cup or two of water. Millet makes an excellent porridge, and so do barley and brown rice. An even better choice for porridge is a tasty medicinal grain called "Job's Tears" *(Coix lacryma-jobi),* or *yi-yi-ren* in Chinese, which has diuretic properties, decongests the lungs, eliminates phlegm, and removes excess dampness from the joints and tissues. A simple recipe for Job's Tears and Brown Rice Porridge is given in the "Recipes & Formulas" section (appendix 1, page 305).

Thin porridge made from whole grain is relatively easy to digest and provides a variety of essential nutrients, including B vitamins, minerals, and amino acids. Porridge also adds fibrous bulk to the diet to facilitate bowel movements and provides carbohydrates for metabolic energy. As noted above, it is generally best to abstain from grain during detox and save the digestive energy and enzymes for internal cleansing purposes instead. In some cases, however, such as when doing a liver and nerve detox, it is good to include a limited amount of whole-grains porridge as a source of B vitamins, amino acids, and other factors of specific benefit to liver and nerve tissue.

All grains become alkaline-forming when sprouted. Sprouting transforms them into complete living foods bursting with essential nutrients, active enzymes, and energy. So freshly sprouted grains may always be included with the main meals in a detox diet.

Raw nuts and seeds are an excellent source of vegetable protein, essential fatty acids, vitamins, and minerals, but to digest them and extract their nutritional benefits, raw nuts and seeds must be presoaked overnight in pure water before you eat them. All nuts and seeds have a special "antidigestive" factor built into them, specifically designed by nature to prevent them from rotting (i.e., digesting themselves). That factor allows nuts and seeds to be kept unrefrigerated for a long time without decaying. However, if you eat them like that, this natural preservative factor also prevents your stomach from properly digesting them, and consequently they ferment instead, producing gas and acid wastes. When raw nuts and seeds are presoaked overnight, the water eliminates the antidigestive factor and signals the nut or seed to "wake up," just as it would if the nut or seed were planted in the ground and watered. While soaking in water overnight, nuts and seeds come to life and release their rich reserves of nutrients and other health factors. When you eat them like this, they become very easy to digest, and all of their abundant nutritional potential becomes available for assimilation.

Like grains, however, most nuts and seeds are acid-forming in the body and should therefore not be eaten during detox. Fortunately, the only exception is the most beneficial nut of all, the almighty almond, which is not only alkalizing to the human system but also ranks as one of the very best foods in nature for human health and longevity. Almonds are one of the purest, most potent sources of the essential amino acids and fatty acids that form the "bricks and mortar" of cell and tissue construction. Almonds also provide abundant amounts of other vital nutrient cofactors, particularly calcium and magnesium—the "Dynamic Duo" of mineral elements for detox. The famous clairvoyant healer, Edgar Cayce, who successfully diagnosed and cured thousands of severely sick people, often said that anyone who eats a few raw almonds every day will never develop cancer.

To prepare almonds for eating, use only raw, preferably organically grown whole almonds that have been shelled but not blanched. Place them in a bowl, cover with pure water, and set aside to soak overnight. Next morning, drain off the water, and the almonds are ready to eat. Peel off the brown skins, which are very easy to remove after the nuts have been soaked, because any contaminants to which the nuts have been exposed will be trapped in the skin and are eliminated by peeling them. Soaked almonds remain fresh and ready to eat all day; any left-overs should be kept in the refrigerator and may still be eaten the next day. Soaked almonds are so satisfying to the appetite, so easy to digest, and so rich in nutritional value, that including them as a staple in the detox diet makes it relatively easy to abstain from heavy, acid-forming foods such as meat, dairy products, bread, and pasta that most people normally eat as staples in their daily diets. By depending on almonds during detox, you may even grow so fond of their fine flavor and crunchy texture that you'll start substituting almonds for some of the heavier, acid-forming foods in your daily diet.

DETOX BEVERAGES

What you drink is as much a part of your diet as what you eat, and in a detox diet, water and other liquid nourishment are particularly important. To continuously flush toxins out the kidneys and replenish all bodily fluids with pure water, you must drink *at least* six to eight glasses (1½ to 2 quarts) of pure, preferably alkaline and ionized, water each and every day throughout the duration of a detox program. This much water is absolutely essential for success. A glass of fruit or vegetable juice or a cup of herbal tea does not count as a glass of water just because you are drinking a fluid that contains water. Juices and teas function in an entirely different way than pure water does in the human body. Only water that is consumed "straight" can purify the blood, detoxify the tissues, rehydrate the cells, and replenish bodily fluids. Water should be consumed separately from food, not with meals, and the first two glasses should be taken immediately upon arising in the morning, before eating anything, to flush mucus and food residues from the stomach and digestive tract. Drink another glass or two between breakfast and lunch, and again between lunch and dinner, and the last one between dinner and bedtime.

Another important beverage during detox is herbal tea, which is especially supportive for various aspects of the detoxification and purification process. The teas enhance the functions of the organs and glands involved in the relief of the symptomatic discomforts of detox. Almost all herbal teas are alkalizing and have therapeutic benefits for detox. They may therefore be sipped freely throughout the day. Depending on which organs and tissues require the most attention during a detox program, you may select specific herbal teas that have what TCM refers to as "natural affinity" *(gui jing)* for those particular organs and tissues, such as using dandelion and milk thistle to detoxify the liver, horsetail and nettle to clean the kidneys, valerian and passion flower to soothe the nerves, and so forth. A variety of herbal teas and other herbal formulas, which may be used as supplements to help detoxify specific organs and tissues and relieve the discomforts of detox, are presented in chapter 8, "Herbal Detox." You may include a selection of these in any detox program, according to your personal requirements.

Sage tea is generally beneficial for all detox and internal-cleansing purposes and may be included in all detox programs. Sage tea also plays a central role in the "Breuss Cancer Cure." An old Roman proverb asks, "Why die, when there is sage in the garden?" Sage has been known since ancient times for its potent cleansing and healing properties and has been used for centuries as an effective preventive medicine against disease and degeneration. It contains factors that nourish all of the glands as well as the spinal cord, thereby helping the body to produce the hormones and neurochemicals involved in the cleansing, healing, and regeneration of the whole system. A large thermos full of hot Sage Tea may be prepared first thing each morning and taken as desired throughout the day and evening. The recipe for this excellent herbal detox tea is given in "Recipes & Formulas" (in appendix 1, page 306).

DETOX SUPPLEMENTS

To fortify the detox diet with extra cleansing and healing power, various nutritional supplements may be included to selectively assist different dimensions of the detox process, and to target specific organs and tissues for extra attention. Only supplements made from natural food concentrates and pure plant or mineral extracts should be included in the detox diet. Anything synthesized from chemicals or other artificial ingredients should be strictly avoided.

Supplements serve three basic purposes in the detox diet. They help alkalize the blood and tissues, thereby maintaining the internal "climate" of alkalinity required for cleansing and healing responses to function properly. They provide additional supplies of antioxidants, chlorophyll, carotenes, and other essential detoxifying elements. And they supply extra reserves of vital detox nutrients, especially the all-important vitamin and mineral factors that are so centrally involved in the myriad metabolic enzyme reactions that occur during detox. A few of the most useful detox supplements are briefly introduced below:

Minerals

Include some form of full-spectrum, easily assimilated mineral supplement in all detox programs. The best choice for this purpose is sea water, which may be taken straight from clean ocean waters or made from a concentrated fluid extract of pure marine minerals. Another good source is homemade bittern of Celtic or Himalayan Glacial sea salt, or ⅓ teaspoon of either of these sea salts dissolved in a glass of pure water. Sea water and sea salt contain the full range of minerals and trace elements required by the body, and in precisely the proper proportions. In fact, the mineral composition and pH value of human blood and natural sea water are virtually identical.

In addition to full-spectrum mineral supplementation, the body also requires extra amounts of calcium and magnesium during detox. Calcium is the body's primary alkalizing agent. Calcium is also needed for balanced functioning of all the major organ systems, including the nervous system. It is involved in every major metabolic reaction and is essential for new cell growth and tissue regeneration. An excellent source of this macromineral is coral calcium, which is exceptionally alkalizing and relatively easy to assimilate. Simply dissolve the powder in pure water and take it two or three times daily, with or without food.

Magnesium is a key component in a wide range of alkaline enzymes that the body must produce to conduct the detox process, and it is also a vital factor for balancing heart and nervous-system functions. Calcium and magnesium work together as the "Dynamic Duo" of detox. It is important to obtain sufficient quantities of both for either one to be completely effective. The easiest form of magnesium to assimilate is magnesium chloride, as found in the sea. An excellent source is the magnesium-rich bittern extracted from Celtic sea salt, which you can easily prepare at home as described in chapter 2. Alternatively, you may use pure magnesium chloride in fluid form ("magnesium oil"), or concentrated marine mineral extracts derived from pure sea water, which is available at many health food stores or by mail order.

Green Food

Green food refers to any purified food concentrate made from the freshly extracted juice of young cereal grasses, such as wheat, rye, and barley, or extracted from water plants and green algae, which grow on the surface of large, unpolluted lakes. These foods products are called green due to their high concentration of pure organic chlorophyll, which is one of nature's most potent blood purifiers and tissue cleansers and is essential for any detox program. It is an interesting and significant fact of nature that, with the sole exception of a single molecule, the chlorophyll in plants and the hemoglobin in human blood have precisely the same biochemical composition. The only difference is that in the place in which hemoglobin has a molecule of iron, chlorophyll has a molecule of magnesium.

Hemoglobin is the factor in blood that is responsible for carrying oxygen. Without sufficient hemoglobin, the blood's capacity to carry oxygen diminishes rapidly, reducing its power to detoxify and nourish the tissues. Chlorophyll builds strong hemoglobin and swiftly purifies the bloodstream, thereby supporting the entire detox process by enhancing the blood's capacity to hold oxygen and deliver it to the tissues. As Dr. Bernard Jensen, one of the leading authorities on detox therapy, states, "Chlorophyll can speed up the rate of cleansing the bowel, bloodstream, and liver." Since cleansing the bowel, bloodstream, and liver represents about 75 percent of the work in detox, chlorophyll is the sovereign element for getting the detox job done swiftly and effectively.

Green food also contains the full range of essential amino acids required for reproducing cells and repairing tissues, as well all the essential vitamins, minerals, and enzymes that the body needs to cleanse and heal itself. Green food supplies all of these elements in their purest, most bio-available forms. As a nutritionally complete food as well as a rich source of blood and tissue cleansing factors, green food may be used as the sole form of nutrition during a detox program, without the need for any other type of food. Since green foods are pure, highly concentrated extracts of living plants, they're loaded with active enzymes and they therefore can be digested without requiring any additional energy or enzymes from your body. Their nutrients are rapidly released for immediate assimilation into the bloodstream and swift delivery to the cells and tissues, which means that they produce virtually no acid wastes in the body—an obvious advantage during detox—while still delivering the full range of essential nutrients in the purest, most readily utilized form possible in any food.

Although all forms of wheat *grain* are forbidden when one is detoxing, the juice of young cereal *grasses,* such as wheat and barley, is one of the most widely used green foods for detox purposes. Such juice may be taken either freshly extracted (which requires a special machine) or in the form of dried powder pressed into tablets. One of the best wheatgrass supplements on the market today is called "Green Life." It is made in the United States by the V. E. Irons Company as part of its line of "Vit-ra-tox" internal-cleansing products. Green Life is made from the dried, cold-extracted juices of organically grown cereal grasses, including wheat, barley, oats, and rye, and is available either as loose powder or pressed tablets. It also contains powdered extract of whole beet juice to detoxify the liver and bowels, sea kelp to rebuild the blood, and papaya enzymes to dissolve putrefactive proteins and impacted dried mucoid matter in the intestinal tract. This product contains all the elements required by the body to detoxify and purify itself, including 50,000 IU of natural beta carotene per 3½-ounce portion, almost double the amount found in fresh carrots. In addition, it contains about 25 percent pure vegetable protein, including a properly balanced blend of twenty natural amino acids, which help build new cells and repair damaged tissues.

Another excellent green-food supplement is "Barley Green," produced by AIM International in the USA. This supplement comes in a light green powder that may be stirred into juice or water, or swallowed dry by the spoonful and washed down with juice or water. Extracted from pure barley grass, the powder is densely packed with chlorophyll, nutrients, and active enzymes in highly concentrated form.

Spirulina, blue-green algae, and chlorella are examples of green foods made from the simple, single-celled aquatic plants that grow on the surfaces of large, unpolluted lakes located in pristine mountains and forest regions. These organisms are among the oldest forms of life on earth, having first appeared about two billion years ago, when plant life still ruled the planet. Their nutritional profile includes an amazing 2 ounces of pure vegetable protein and .075 ounces of pure organic chlorophyll per 3½ ounce serving.

Like green foods derived from cereal grasses, spirulina and other micro-algae also provide all the essential B vitamins required for detox and healing, including the highest known vegetable source of vitamin B12, which is very difficult to obtain from any other nonanimal food source. B vitamins are particularly important for repairing and rebalancing the liver, brain, and nervous system. Since the normal dietary sources of these vitamins are grains and animal products, which are highly acid-forming and should be avoided during detox, green foods provide a convenient alternative source of these essential nutritional factors in a pure, potent form that alkalizes rather than acidifies the body.

Blackstrap Molasses

Natural, unsulfured molasses is one of the richest and most easily assimilated sources of essential minerals in balanced, organic form. The roots of sugar cane can grow as deep as 5½ to 6½ yards into the ground, allowing them to tap into the abundant reserves of minerals that lie beneath depleted topsoils and that are out of reach of other, shallower crops. Since mineralization of blood and tissues is one of the primary strategies in all detox programs, molasses is a convenient and effective supplement for this purpose, especially for people with long-term mineral deficiency. Molasses is also one of the best natural sources of both organic iron and copper, which is an essential cofactor for the utilization of iron in the body. This composition makes molasses an excellent supplement for building strong blood, and a good tonic for those suffering from anemia. In addition, molasses provides lots of calcium and magnesium, both of which the body needs extra supplies of during detox.

Alkaline Vitamin C

Alkaline vitamin C, or "C-salts," is a nonacidic form of vitamin C bound to various alkaline mineral salts. C-salts can be used in large dosages without the acidifying effects produced by the more common, less expensive acetic acid form of vitamin C. Vitamin C is both a potent antioxidant and an important nutrient. Because of vitamin C's indispensable metabolic role in the detox process, it is wise to include a supplemental source of alkaline vitamin C in all detox programs. Calcium ascorbate and sodium ascorbate are the two most widely used C-salts, and both are available in tablets or pure powdered form; the latter may be stirred into water or juice throughout the day. One-tenth ounce to .175 ounces per day of alkaline vitamin C is a suitable dosage for most detox purposes, although C may also be taken in much larger amounts for additional antioxidant activity.

Liquid Bentonite

Also known as "clay water," bentonite is a superfine, colloidal form of volcanic ash consisting of micromolecules that are five hundred times smaller than water molecules, each of which carries a strong negative charge. These molecules saturate the blood and bodily fluids, penetrating places where even water cannot go. They act like millions of micro-magnets to attract and neutralize positively charged toxic molecules lodged deep in tissues and fluids throughout the body. The neutralized toxins are then carried away in the bloodstream for excretion. A single molecule of bentonite can adsorb two hundred times its own weight in toxic wastes, and its cleansing action is entirely mechanical, producing no chemical reactions whatsoever in the body. One of the best grades of liquid bentonite on the market is the "Vit-ra-tox" label, which may be ordered by mail from the address provided in the "Suppliers" section. One tablespoon of bentonite stirred into a glass of water and taken two to three times per day, separately from food, is an adequate dosage for most detox programs, although it may be taken in double those amounts in extreme cases of blood and tissue toxicity. If you're also using psyllium, take the bentonite as a "chaser" immediately after the psyllium.

Psyllium Seed

The ground seed and husk of psyllium *(plantago ovato blond)*, known in India as "Flea Seed," is by far the most effective available natural fiber-bulking supplement for clearing clogged bowels of impacted feces, dry mucoid plaque, and putrefactive food residues. No better remedy exists for chronic constipation and sluggish bowels than ground psyllium. Like liquid bentonite, psyllium functions entirely on a mechanical basis, without causing any chemical reactions whatsoever. One teaspoon of ground psyllium shaken well with about ten ounces of water and drunk down quickly on an empty stomach forms a dense, mucilaginous bolus that sweeps like a broom throughout the entire digestive tract, loosening and eliminating pockets of impacted putrefactive waste and mucoid sludge from the deep folds of the colon. Psyllium facilitates regular bowel movements, dredges the colon of dangerous toxic residues that have festered there for years, and accelerates the entire detox process. One or two doses per day on an empty stomach is sufficient when using psyllium as a supplement in the detox diet. When fasting, however, four doses per day should be taken to provide a constant cleansing action within the bowels. Always remember to drink an extra glass of water immediately after taking a dose of psyllium, and if you're also using bentonite, add it to the second glass of water. The ground psyllium seed powder produced by "Vit-ra-tox" as part of its line of detox supplements is called "Intestinal Cleanser" and is one of the best on the market today. Another excellent variety of this important detox supplement is "Herbal Fiber Blend," produced under the AIM label.

This product is a balanced blend of eighteen cleansing herbs combined in a base of ground psyllium. The herbs eliminate intestinal parasites, stimulate excretory functions, detoxify the internal organs, and rebalance the entire digestive system.

Cayenne

Cayenne is one of the most effective healing herbs on earth, and it has strong cleansing properties that greatly assist the detox process. Cayenne gives a big boost to blood circulation and balances heart functions, thereby insuring sufficient supplies of oxygen and nutrients to all tissues. In addition, cayenne stimulates the entire endocrine system, strengthens immune response, clears liver congestion, activates peristalsis and lower bowel functions, and energizes the whole digestive system. Believe it or not, cayenne is also one of the best remedies for stomach ulcers. It cleanses and disinfects the ulcers and promotes their rapid healing. On top of all that, cayenne is highly alkalizing, which makes it a perfect detox supplement, especially for those with circulatory and heart problems, stomach ulcers, and/or stagnant digestive systems. One or two capsules taken once or twice a day with a glass of warm water is an effective therapeutic dosage for detox purposes. Cayenne is most effective taken on an empty stomach, but it may also be taken with meals to buffer the heat it produces in the stomach. You can quickly quell the heat of cayenne taken between meals by eating an apple with it.

Lemon

Fresh lemon is the only food in the world that is anionic, which means it carries a negative molecular charge. This does not apply to any other citrus fruit such as lime or grapefruit, but only to fresh lemon, the juice of which must be consumed freshly extracted to retain its detoxifying anionic properties. The negative charge, combined with lemon's strong alkalizing effects, makes fresh lemon juice one of the most powerful detoxifying supplements of all. It may be used to assist any type of detox program. Fresh lemon juice should always be taken on an empty stomach, mixed into a glass of pure water, without the addition of any sweeteners. Fresh lemon juice assists the production of bile in the liver, and without adequate bile production, it is impossible to properly digest food and assimilate nutrients. An excellent way to use fresh lemon juice as a detox supplement is to blend it with ground whole flax seed, alkaline vitamin C powder, and selected herbs to make a "Lemon-Flax Shake." This drink may be taken twice daily, between meals, throughout the duration of a detox program. The recipe is provided in the "Recipes and Formulas" section, appendix 1, page 312.

DAILY DETOX MENUS

The dietary guidelines given in this chapter, including the sample menus presented below, are specifically designed for detox purposes, not for daily life. Since one tries to remain calm and quiet during detox, resting in a state of uninterrupted relaxation and avoiding all stress and strain that might activate the "fight or flight" response, while also refraining from strenuous muscular exertion that produces lactic acid in the tissues, the body requires far fewer calories during detox than it does in daily life. Moreover, detox requires a diet that produces minimal acid wastes and consumes minimal digestive energy, while delivering maximum nutrition and providing precisely the elements the body needs to detoxify and cleanse itself. Such a diet does not meet the requirements of daily life for an active person, because it does not provide sufficient calories to generate the energy required for an active lifestyle, nor does it contain the proper mixture of food elements the body needs for daily life. Therefore, the detox diet outlined in this chapter should only be used for the specific purpose of deliberately detoxifying the body, preferably in conjunction with other detox modalities introduced in this book, for periods of three days up to three weeks. After that, if you wish to reform your personal daily diet in ways that protect your health and prolong your life by producing minimum toxicity and providing maximum nutrition, you may adopt some of the dietary suggestions offered in the chapter "Retox Diet and Supplements" in part 2 of this book.

As a general guideline to assist the reader in composing his or her own daily menus for detox programs of three days to three weeks duration, six sample detox menus are presented for reference below. These menus are geared to various different appetites, tastes, and detox requirements, and each one focuses primary therapeutic attention on particular organs and tissues that need the most work. Feel free to mix and match the recommended foods and supplements in whatever ways best suit your own personal tastes and individual therapeutic needs, as long as you do not include any items or combinations that are counterproductive to detox and healing.

Generally speaking, the more fluid and less solid, the more raw and less cooked, the more nutrient-dense and fewer calorie-rich items you include in your detox diet, the more detoxifying that diet becomes and the more effectively it heals your body. It is important to remember that in the detox diet, "less is more." The less you eat, the more you detox. In fact, the best detox diet of all is fasting, as we shall see in the following chapter. Therefore, please do not feel obliged to strictly follow the suggestions below when designing your own personal detox programs. Instead, use them as general dietary guidelines to help you compose menus that satisfy your own therapeutic requirements without overly offending your basic tastes in food. Once you've decided on a particular detox menu, it is best not to stray too far from it for the duration of your program. The simpler and more consistent you make the diet, the better it will work for you.

A few basic items should be included in all the detox menus suggested below. Most important of all is to drink at least six to eight glasses (1⅓ to 1¾ quarts) of pure alkaline water each and every day, as follows: two 8-ounce glasses immediately upon arising in the morning; one to two glasses between breakfast and lunch; two to three glasses between lunch and dinner; and one glass between dinner and bedtime. Sage tea is recommended for general cleansing and healing purposes in all these detox menus, in addition to various other herbal teas for specific conditions. Some form of full-spectrum mineral supplement, such as marine minerals or Celtic sea salt, is recommended in all menus, as well as some type of "green food," such as wheat- or barley-grass juice, spirulina or chlorella. Other supplements may be included to enhance various aspects of the detox process according to your own individual requirements.

MENU NUMBER 1

Therapeutic Focus: General Tissue Detox

Breakfast:
Steamed Pumpkin with Shredded Ginger and Celtic Sea Salt
Vegetable Juice: 1 generous cup fresh Breuss Vegetable Juice or bottled "Biotta" brand
8–12 presoaked raw Almonds

Mid-Morning Snack:
Fresh Apples and/or Black Grapes

Lunch:
Half a Fresh Avocado with Chopped Garlic, Celtic Sea Salt, and Olive Oil
Vegetable Juice: 1 generous cup fresh Breuss Vegetable Juice or "Biotta" brand

Mid-Afternoon Snack:
Fresh Papaya or Watermelon Juice

Dinner:
Spinach or Watercress Stir-fried with Ginger and Garlic
Millet or Job's Tears & Brown Rice Porridge

Evening Snack:
Fresh Apples and/or Black Grapes

Herb Tea:
Sage Tea

Supplements:
Green Food, 3 times per day with meals
Marine Minerals and Coral Calcium, 1–2 times per day, with meals
Psyllium Seed, 1–2 times per day, on an empty stomach

Summary: Avocado may be eaten as it is, rather than as juice, because the flesh does not contain tough cellulose; it is a rich source of essential fatty acids, vegetable protein, and other nutrients and provides abundant fuel for metabolic energy. If arthritis is a problem, use freshly squeezed grapefruit juice rather than other fruits for the three snacks. Grapefruit is one of the best sources available for organic salicylic acid, which dissolves inorganic calcium deposits from the joints.

MENU NUMBER 2

Therapeutic Focus: Bowels and Digestive Tract

Breakfast:
Stewed Vegetables: Carrot, Pumpkin, Turnip, Squash
Clear Vegetable Broth with Miso Paste
12–15 presoaked raw Almonds

Mid-Morning Snack:
Fresh Papaya, Apples

Lunch:
12–15 presoaked raw Almonds
Vegetable Juice: ¾ cup carrot, ¼ cup beet

Afternoon Snack:
Fresh Papaya, Apples

Dinner:
Steamed Okra with Chopped Garlic, Ginger, and Sea Salt
Half a fresh Avocado with Garlic, Sea Salt, and Olive Oil
Clear Vegetable Broth with Miso Paste

Evening Snack:
Black Grapes

Herb Tea:
Sage Tea

Supplements:
Psyllium seed, 2 times per day, on an empty stomach
Liquid Bentonite, 2 times per day, immediately after Psyllium
Cayenne, 1 cap, 2 times per day, with lunch and dinner
Green Food, 3 times per day, with meals
Aloe Vera Juice, fresh or bottled, 1–2 times per day

Summary: Cooked vegetables and whole, raw fruits provide plenty of natural fiber to help dredge wastes from the bowels, and okra is particularly effective for cleansing the colon and facilitating bowel movements. Miso provides a rich source of active enzymes to assist in the digestion of putrefactive wastes lodged in the bowels. Psyllium supplies additional pure vegetable fiber to loosen and eliminate impacted mucoid wastes, while bentonite adsorbs toxic particles released from the lining of the digestive tract by the psyllium. Cayenne cleanses and heals ulcers in the stomach and intestinal tract, and aloe vera juice is one of nature's most effective digestive tract cleansers, as well as an excellent remedy for constipation and colitis.

MENU NUMBER 3

Therapeutic Focus: Heart and Circulatory System

Breakfast:
Half a fresh Avocado with Olive Oil
Vegetable Juice: ¾ cup carrot, 1¼ ounces spinach, 1¼ ounces celery
8–12 presoaked raw Almonds

Mid-Morning Snack:
Fresh Orange Juice

Lunch:
Spinach or Watercress Stir-fried with Garlic
Steamed Pumpkin with Ginger

Mid-Afternoon Snack:
Fresh Orange Juice or Black Grapes

Dinner:
Millet or Barley or Job's Tears & Brown Rice Porridge
Stir-fried Leafy Greens with Garlic
Vegetable Juice: 1¼ cup carrot

Evening Snack:
Apples and/or Black Grapes

Herb Tea:
Sage Tea; Hawthorne Berry Tea

Supplements:
Marine Minerals and Coral Calcium, 1 time per day, before breakfast
Cayenne, 1 cap, 2 times per day, with lunch and dinner
CoQ_{10}, 60 mg daily, after breakfast
Green Food, 2 times per day, with breakfast and dinner
Hawthorn Berry Extract, 1–2 times per day, in warm water, between meals

Summary: Garlic helps cleanse the blood vessels and remove plaque, while cayenne is the single most beneficial herb for regulating heart function, balancing pulse, and stimulating blood circulation. Marine minerals provide the essential trace elements required by the heart and bloodstream to regulate blood pressure, green food purifies the bloodstream and increases the blood's capacity to carry oxygen, and raw almonds are a rich source of organic calcium and magnesium. Hawthorn Berry fortifies the heart muscle and coronary vessels and helps stabilize heartbeat, and CoQ_{10} has been shown to help correct imbalances in heart function.

MENU NUMBER 4

Therapeutic Focus: Brain and Nervous System

Breakfast: 12–15 presoaked raw Almonds
Clear Vegetable Broth
Steamed Pumpkin with Ginger and Sea Salt

Mid-Morning Snack: Black Cherries and/or Black Grapes

Lunch: Millet or Barley or Job's Tears & Brown Rice Porridge
Spinach or Watercress or Kale Stir-fried with Garlic and
Sea Salt
Vegetable Juice: ¾ cup carrot, ¼ cup celery

Mid-Afternoon Snack: Fresh Apples and/or Pears
Black Cherries and/or Black Grapes

Dinner: Millet or Barley or Job's Tears & Brown Rice Porridge
Stewed Vegetables
Vegetable Juice: ¼ cup carrot, ⅛ cup celery

Evening Snack: Apples and/or Pears

Herb Tea: Sage Tea; Chamomile Tea; Passion Flower & Lemon
Balm Tea

Supplements: Nervine Herbal Formulas (see chapter 8), 2 times per
day, between meals
Cilantro (Coriander) Extract, 2–3 times per day,
between meals
Gingko Biloba, 2 times per day, after breakfast and
lunch
Marine Minerals, 2 times per day, before breakfast and
dinner

Summary: Concentrated extract of cilantro is a potent detoxifier of brain cells and nerve tissue, and it is especially effective for removing heavy-metal toxins. Gingko biloba provides powerful antioxidant activity in the brain and nerves and also increases microcirculation in the brain. The body requires B vitamins to detoxify and repair nerve and brain tissue, and these vitamins are provided by the porridge, almonds, and green food. Celery juice contains elements that calm the nervous system and relieve insomnia. Marine minerals and sea salt provide the full spectrum of essential minerals and trace elements that the brain and nervous system need to function properly, and the nervine herbal teas and extracts keep the nervous system relaxed, prevent anxiety from developing during the detox process, and promote sound sleep.

MENU NUMBER 5

Therapeutic Focus: Kidneys and Bladder

Breakfast: Vegetable Juice: ⅞ cup carrot, ⅛ cup beet, 1⅓ tablespoons parsley
8–12 presoaked raw Almonds
Clear Vegetable Broth with Miso Paste

Mid-Morning Snack: Fresh Watermelon, cut into small bite-sized pieces and eaten slowly
Lunch: Vegetable Juice: 1 cup and 1 tablespoon fresh Breuss Vegetable Juice or bottled "Biotta" brand
Watercress Stir-fried with Garlic

Mid-Afternoon Snack: Fresh Watermelon, small pieces eaten slowly

Dinner: Steamed or Poached Fresh Asparagus with Garlic and Sea Salt
Millet Porridge
Vegetable Juice: ¼ cup carrot, 1 tablespoon beet, 2 teaspoons parsley

Evening Snack: Black Cherries or Black Grapes

Herb Tea: Sage Tea; Breuss Kidney Tea

Supplements: Green Food, 2 times per day, with breakfast and dinner
Marine Minerals or Celtic Sea Salt Bittern, 2 times per day, before breakfast and dinner

Summary: Asparagus has strong cleansing effects on the kidneys and bladder, flushing out acid wastes so fast that you can smell the ammonia in urine shortly after eating asparagus. Parsley purifies and protects kidney tissues, which is especially important when the kidneys are working overtime to excrete toxic wastes. It is important to drink plenty of water when cleansing the kidneys, and better to eat more fluid foods and fewer solid foods. Eating fresh watermelon slowly produces a steady stream of cleansing elements that flow through the kidneys and bladder, detoxifying and soothing inflammation in those tissues.

MENU NUMBER 6

Therapeutic Focus: Liver and Blood

Breakfast:	Steamed Pumpkin with Ginger and Sea Salt Vegetable Juice: ¾ cup carrot, 2 tablespoons beet 8–12 presoaked raw Almonds
Mid-Morning Snack:	Black Grapes
Lunch: Veg. Juice:	Fresh Tomato, ¾ cup Job's Tears & Brown Rice 　　Porridge Steamed Pumpkin (leftover from breakfast)
Mid-Afternoon Snack:	Black Grapes
Dinner:	Spinach or Watercress Stir-fried with Garlic and Sea 　　Salt
Veg. Juice:	¾ cup carrot, 2 tablespoons beet Job's Tears & Brown Rice Porridge
Evening Snack:	Black Grapes
Herb Tea:	Sage Tea; Milk Thistle & Dandelion Tea; Licorice 　　Root & Chrysanthemum Tea
Supplements:	Bentonite, 2 times per day between meals Green Food, 3 times per day, with meals Milk Thistle Extract or Silimarin Tablets Herbal Liver Formulas (see chapter 8)

Summary: Pumpkin, dark leafy greens, carrots, and green food are packed with organic carotenes, which are essential for detoxifying and repairing the liver. Beet juice, milk thistle, and dandelion all help detoxify and rebuild liver tissue. Since the liver filters the blood, a toxic liver means a toxic bloodstream and vice-versa, so both must be cleansed together. Black grapes help clean both the bloodstream and the liver, especially if the skins and seeds are chewed very well and eaten together with the pulp. The chlorophyll in green food purifies blood and increases its capacity to carry oxygen, while bentonite molecules actively adsorb any toxins floating in the bloodstream and transport them to the kidneys for excretion. Licorice and chrysanthemum tea detoxify and cool both the blood and the liver, and other herbal formulas may be included to amplify this effect.

6

THE "FAST LANE": FASTING AND COLONIC IRRIGATION

Fasting is a perfect example of the hidden powers of nature that awaken when the ancient Taoist principle of *wu-wei,* "not-doing" or "noninterference," is put into practice. "By doing nothing," notes the *Tao Teh Ching,* "the sage accomplishes everything." In dietary terms, "doing nothing" means eating nothing and letting nature take its course, and this abstinence awakens the body's most powerful cleansing and healing responses.

Fasting is nature's way of curing disease, restoring health, and prolonging life. As all zookeepers and pet owners know, animals of every species instinctively refuse to eat when they are sick, and the same rule applies to animals in the wilderness. Long ago, humans also shared this natural, self-healing instinct, and even today, primitive tribes in remote regions of Africa, Asia, and the Amazon still have special "sick houses" located on the outskirts of their villages, where the sick rest quietly and comfortably, without eating any food, for as long as it takes to recover their health.

Today, however, therapeutic fasting is dismissed by mainstream modern medicine as "primitive." As a prominent surgeon in New York once told this writer, "Fasting went out with the horse-and-buggy!" Nevertheless, owing to the pioneering work of a few courageous health professionals during the latter half of the twentieth century, the Western world has rediscovered the profound healing powers of fasting, and practitioners of alternative medicine are now applying it with success for conditions in which all other treatments fail. Moreover, recent scientific research, backed by extensive clinical studies, has established conclusive proof that periodic fasting and calorie restriction are the one and only proven way to significantly extend lifespan.

On May 28, 1986, the Associated Press reported the following U.S. scientific study on aging, in which laboratory rats were periodically put on forced fasts:

> When the diets of laboratory rats are severely restricted, they live far longer than do otherwise identical animals that are allowed to eat as much as they want. In fact, researchers say such food limits are the only way they know of significantly extending these rodents' normal lifespans.

More recently, Dr. Roy Walford, who was a member of the team that lived for two years in the experimental "Biosphere" project in the United States, conducted even more exhaustive research on the link between calorie restriction and lifespan, using a variety of different species for his studies, including rats and dogs. In his book *Beyond the 120 Year Diet,* he presents evidence that clearly demonstrates that calorie restriction prolongs the lifespan of all species tested by a factor of 50–80 percent. In human terms, that would mean a lifespan of 120–150 years.

While long-term human studies on the effects of fasting on longevity have not yet been concluded, individual examples of several contemporary practitioners of therapeutic fasting are highly inspiring and very encouraging. Dr. Norman Walker, for example, who advocated periodic fasting and daily consumption of raw juices and practiced what he preached, lived to the ripe age of 116, remaining active until the very end. Paul Bragg, who fasted for ten days fours times a year for most of his life, lived almost as long as Dr. Walker, and he too stayed healthy and productive until his final days. V. E. Irons, who cured himself of an "incurable" crippling disease by fasting, then went on to develop an extremely efficient do-it-yourself fasting and internal colonic cleansing system, would no doubt have lived a "normal" human lifespan of 120, if fate had not intervened with a car accident at the age of 98. Each of these individuals, and others like them, rediscovered through their own experience what all animals and primitive tribesmen still know: that fasting is nature's way of cleansing and healing the body and regenerating the life force.

Abstaining from food permits the body's innate detox mechanisms to function at full capacity and allows immune responses to operate in high gear. When fasting, all of the energy and enzyme power that the body must normally use to digest and process food is diverted instead to digesting toxic debris and acid wastes, while the digestive system itself remains dormant and produces no new wastes in the body. Fasting also triggers the production of human growth hormone in the pituitary gland and releases it into the bloodstream, where it circulates throughout the body to repair damaged tissues, regenerate vital functions, and rejuvenate the whole system. Normally, the production of growth hormone diminishes rapidly after humans reach adulthood, and the ever-dwindling supply of this powerful regenerative hormone is one of the primary causes of aging and the onset of chronic degenerative conditions. By stimulating secretion of human growth hormone, fasting not only helps cure disease and repair the body, it also slows down the aging process, restores flagging vitality, and prolongs life.

THE CURE OF THE SAGES

Fasting is not new. Hindu yogis, Buddhist monks, and Taoist hermits have been fasting for thousands of years to enhance their vitality and extend their lifespans. A few years ago in India, an elderly meditation master set a world record by fasting nonstop for two hundred days, during which time he took nothing whatsoever but plain water. Plato, Aristotle, and other Greek philosophers whose thought laid the foundations of Western civilization fasted regularly to improve their physical health and sharpen their mental powers, and Pythagoras required all of his senior students to fast for forty days as a means of purifying their bodies and minds prior to receiving his highest teachings. Practitioners of traditional medicine in ancient China also understood the direct link between human disease and the toxic filth that accumulates in the bowels as a result of unnatural eating habits. The Sung Dynasty physician Chang Tsung-cheng observed, "If the stomach and bowels are blocked, then blood and energy stagnate," while the famous Chinese doctor, Chai Yu-hua, wrote, "Purging the bowels eliminates the source of poison, thereby permitting blood and energy to regenerate naturally. By cleaning the bowels we repair the body."

The Bible mentions fasting seventy-four times, and Jesus himself fasted frequently, sometimes for as long as forty days. When the Dead Sea Scrolls were unearthed in Palestine in the early twentieth century, a most remarkable document written in Aramaic and dating from the third century CE came to light. Translated into English in 1937 by Edmond Szekely under the title *The Essene Gospel of Peace,* this ancient text recounts in detail some of the most important healing work performed by Jesus among the people of Palestine, and much of it sounds very similar to what Dr. Bernard Jensen writes about fasting and colonic irrigation in his book *Tissue Cleansing Through Bowel Management.* Unfortunately, none of this information ever found its way into the Bible, despite the fact that this gospel was recorded several hundred years earlier than other gospels that appear in the Bible. Perhaps the early editors of the Bible found the topic of colonic irrigation to be of too delicate a nature for inclusion in the Christian scriptures, but since this ancient historical document contains teachings of vital significance to the health of the Western world today, let's take a quick look at some key passages and listen to what Jesus, in *The Essene Gospel of Peace,* said to his followers on the subject of detox and human health:

Renew yourselves and fast. . . . Seek the fresh air of the forest and of the fields, and there in the midst of them shall you find the angel of air. . . . Then breathe long and deeply, that the angel of air may be brought within you. I tell you truly, the angle of air shall cast out of your body all uncleannesses which defiled it without and within.

. . . After the angel of air, seek the angel of water. . . . Think not that it is sufficient that the angel of water embrace you outwards only. I tell you truly, the uncleanness within is greater by much than the uncleanness without. . . . Seek, therefore, a large trailing gourd, having a stalk the length of a man; take out its inwards and fill it with water from the river which the sun has warmed. Hang it upon the branch of a tree, and kneel upon the ground . . . and suffer the end of the stalk of the trailing gourd to enter your hinder parts, that the water may flow through all your bowels. . . . Then let the water run out from your body, that it may carry away from within it all the unclean and evil-smelling things. . . . And you shall see with your eyes and smell with your nose all the abominations and uncleannesses which defiled the temple of your body. . . . Renew your baptizing with water every day of your fast, till the day when you see that the water which flows out of you is as pure as the river's foam.

This method of cleansing and healing the body by means of colonic irrigation using a trailing gourd and warm river water was commonly practiced among the ancient Essenes, with whom Jesus lived and studied during his early, formative years, and it constitutes one of his most beneficial teachings for the welfare of humanity. Unfortunately, since all mention of this period in Jesus's life was deliberately excluded from the Christian scriptures, this aspect of his work remains virtually unknown among Christians today, although it was common knowledge to Jesus's own disciples. The sages of the ancient world were well aware of the inseparable link between the state of the body and the state of the mind, for they knew that toxic blood and tissues form a breeding ground not only for disease and degeneration of the human body but also for the darkening and degradation of the human spirit. They knew the law that modern physicians and philosophers alike have forgotten: that whatever pollutes the body also pollutes the mind. That's why so many sacred scriptures of the ancient world prescribe fasting and detox as the first preliminary steps on the path of spiritual cultivation.

Today, the mutual dependence of physical and spiritual health has been largely forgotten, and few people see the causal connection between the massive pollution of the planet and degradation of the human body, and the rampant crime, chronic violence, and spiritual malaise that marks human life in contemporary times. According to the psychophysiological prescription of the ancient sages who gave birth to Western civilization, cleaning up the planet and detoxifying the human body are the best medicine of all for restoring peace on earth and reviving the health and spiritual integrity of humanity, and scientific evidence validating the truth of this ancient teaching is beginning to emerge. In 1972, for example, the Moscow Research Institute of Psychiatry reported results of a clinical study in which fasting and tissue detox were successfully used, without recourse to any drugs whatsoever, to cure over seven thousand patients suffering from a variety of serious mental disorders that neither psychiatry nor drug therapy had helped in any way. This methodology has since become known as the "Hunger Cure" and is still practiced in Russia.

Even a cursory glance at the current state of human affairs throughout the world today reveals two indisputable facts: one is that people everywhere and in all walks of life are getting sicker and more toxic than ever before in human history; and the other is that human behavior is growing more angry and violent, and world affairs are becoming more cruel and barbaric, day by day. Maybe it is already too late to take the slow lane of detox by gradual dietary reform. Perhaps our only remaining hope is to take the plunge and leap directly into the "fast lane" of detox by the "angels" of air and water alone.

THE "FAST LANE"

Tissue toxicity is a deadly serious condition, especially today, when so many carcinogens and other toxic chemicals contaminate our food and water and pollute the air we breathe. To give the reader an idea of just how serious the situation is, and what can be done about it, here's a graphic excerpt from the book *Detox Diet and Wellness Lifestyle,* by Dr. Grady Deal, who operates a detox clinic in Hawaii:

You may be unaware that the colon remains chronically impacted with accumulated feces and mucus backed all the way up to the small intestine. . . . In effect, your intestinal plumbing. . . backs up like a full and overflowing septic tank. The blood vessels and lymph vessels in the colon pick up the toxins and carry them to all parts of the body. . . . The bloodstream becomes increasingly filled to overflowing with disease organisms . . . and toxins, where they circulate around the body, causing inflammation, water retention, weight gain, irritation, corrosion, damage, and disease. Feces and toxins abnormally recirculated in the bloodstream as a result of chronic constipation explains why the eliminative organs of the skin and lungs have a strangely familiar unpleasant odor . . . in the form of smelly sweat . . . and bad breath that smells like feces. . . . As a protective measure to get the disease-causing toxins out of circulation, the body removes these poisons from the bloodstream and stores them in cells and tissues, out of the way . . . causing what Dr. Norman Walker calls tissue constipation, meaning the tissues are burdened with excess toxins which then cause cellular and tissue inflammation, congestion, eruptions, and disease. In general, excess toxins are continually stored in the cells [and] tissues . . . as long as the person is taking in that particular offending unhealthy food, allergen, drug, etc. When that specific food or substance is completely eliminated from the diet, only then do the cells eliminate that particular toxin from the cells back into the bloodstream and lymph on its way to the eliminative organs and out of the body. Once back in the bloodstream and lymph, the toxin does its dirty work of inflaming and irritating the body until it is eliminated and out of the body. This aggravation or worsening of symptoms is called a healing crisis. People detoxifying from a toxin may get worse before they get better and they tend to crave the very food or habit which made them toxic initially.

Fasting is the fastest and most effective way to deal with this sort of blood and tissue toxicity, and to rid the body of the toxic residues and putrefactive wastes in the colon that continuously poison the blood-stream, clog the cells, and sap vitality. Until these toxins are eliminated, there's simply no way that the body can repair and rebalance itself. Although there are milder methods of detox than fasting, they all take much longer and work less effectively, and none can match the deep healing power and life-prolonging benefits of fasting.

To gain those benefits, one must be willing to tolerate the unpleasant symptoms of the so-called "healing crisis" that fasting always triggers after the third day. The healing crisis opens the gate to the state of radiant health and longevity that only fasting can create, and the discomfort of detox is the price one pays to pass through that gateway. The choice is yours: either you flush those poisons out of your system, or else you live with the consequences of retaining them for the rest of your life. As this author notes in *The Tao of Health, Sex, and Longevity:*

> Unless you live an ascetic life far from civilization and avoid all dietary folly, your blood and other tissues are bound to accumulate toxins and gradually lose their functional vitality. If you don't purge yourself of these toxins on a regular basis, toxemia gets worse and worse, until the body cannot stand it any longer and either purges itself spontaneously in the form of diarrhea, acne, pimples, boils, "liver spots," foul perspiration, body odor, bad breath, and so forth, or else it simply gives up the battle and succumbs to cancer, tuberculosis, and other fatal conditions.

MEGAFASTS, MINIFASTS, AND SEMIFASTS

Many different types of therapeutic fasting programs exist, with varying degrees of intensity and duration. The most intensive detox and swiftest healing results are produced by completely foodless fasts in which nothing but water and a few internal cleansing supplements such as psyllium and bentonite are used. Semi-fasts using water and supplements, plus one type of vegetable or fruit juice to provide energy and nutrition are easier to tolerate, and they, too, provide excellent cleansing and healing results. The so-called "Grape Cure," in which nothing but black grapes are eaten for period of one week to a full month, also qualifies as a sort of "semifast," one that is particularly effective for purifying the bloodstream, detoxifying the liver, and correcting serious gastrointestinal disorders.

To be effective for detoxifying the blood and tissues, a therapeutic fast must continue for a minimum of three full days, which is how long it takes for the body's internal cleansing and healing mechanisms to shift into full gear. Three days is not long enough, however, to totally purify the bloodstream and detoxify the internal organs, nor is it long enough to experience the so-called "healing crisis" that normally occurs sometime between the third and fifth day of a fast. The healing crisis marks the point in a fast when tissue detox has reached its peak, and symptoms of the body's most serious conditions come out of hiding and begin to manifest. For example, in someone with arthritis, the healing crisis occurs when the deepest deposits of toxic residues are dislodged and drawn out of the joints, causing pain in the joints and connective tissues. For someone suffering from heavy liver toxicity, the healing crisis comes as the most poisonous substances are dissolved and eliminated from the tissues of the liver, bringing out all the unpleasant symptoms of liver toxemia, such as overwhelming fatigue and listlessness, anger and irritability, yellow eyes and skin, foul breath and body odor, and throbbing pain in the liver. The good news is that this "crisis" marks the midpoint from which the rest of the fast is all "downhill." It means that the worst part of the detox stage of the fast has passed, and that the healing stage is beginning. Hitting bottom at the midpoint is why that phase is called a "healing" crisis. Unless you continue a fast long enough to "hit the wall" and pass through the stormy gate of the healing crisis to reach the sunny side of radiant health, you will not succeed in fully correcting the root causes of your ills. Three days is certainly sufficient, however, to achieve a major cleansing of the bowels and bloodstream, and to rebalance the internal organs and partially detoxify the tissues.

The ideal duration for a therapeutic detox fast is seven to ten days, because it takes precisely seven days to completely purify the bloodstream and cleanse the lymphatic system of all residual wastes. When the blood and lymph have been totally purified, it means the whole body and all its parts are free of toxicity, because pure blood and clean lymph automatically cleanse the body and eliminate toxins from the tissues on a day-to-day basis. If you reform your eating habits and change your diet after a detox fast, your blood and lymph will be able to keep your tissues clean far longer and more efficiently than they would if you continued polluting yourself with wrong eating habits and wrong food choices. Eating properly also means you won't need to fast as often to rid yourself of accumulated putrefactive wastes and metabolic toxins. Generally speaking, one seven-to-ten-day detox fast each year, while taking care to control your diet in between, is usually sufficient to protect you from serious diseases such as cancer and arteriosclerosis, prevent the onset of common degenerative conditions such as arthritis and senility, and pave the path to a long and healthy life. Almost anyone is capable of completing a seven-day fast, but for those who have never tried it and worry about going that long without food, a few three-day minifasts may be tried first, as a sort of "warm-up." A minifast is a good way to gain confidence and gradually work up to a full, seven-day fast.

The remarkable Breuss Cancer Cure decribed earlier in this text is the longest therapeutic detox fast known to this writer. It involves a forty-two-day (six-week) fast during which only one cup of Breuss Vegetable Juice (fresh or bottled) is taken per day, sipped slowly by the teaspoonful, in addition to Sage Tea and one or two other herbal teas, depending upon the organs and tissues that need primary attention. While this fast may sound extreme, bear in mind that cancer is an extremely serious condition that can easily kill the patient, and that conventional therapies applied to cancer today, such as chemotherapy and radiation, are far more "extreme" in terms of the damage they do to the body than even the longest fast. In fact, mainstream cancer therapy often kills the patient faster than the cancer itself. On the other hand, no one has yet died as a result of trying the Breuss Cancer Cure, and to date there have been over forty thousand documented cases of successful cures from various forms of cancer, some of them already in advanced stages of development. Strangely, most people with cancer would rather submit to instant chemo or radiation therapy, despite the terrible side effects and dubious results, than endure a forty-two-day detox fast that has a proven track record as a real cure. It is hard to say whether patients' reluctance to try the fasting cure is due to lack of confidence in the method, or to an actual fear of fasting.

The Breuss Cancer Cure is not only effective for treating cancer. As noted earlier, cancer is the final stage of tissue toxicity, and chronic tissue toxicity is the root cause of cancer. Therefore, shorter versions of the Breuss fasting program may be used as a means of periodic cleansing and general tissue detox, serving as a very effective preventive therapy against the development of cancer. Unless you already have cancer and wish to use this method as a cure, it is not necessary to follow the Breuss fasting program for the full forty-two days. One to three weeks suffices to effectively detoxify the whole body.

Minifasts are those of fewer than three days. While these brief fasts are not effective for serious detox purposes, they are an excellent form of maintenance between longer therapeutic fasts. For example, some people fast for one full day every week, taking nothing but pure water or one variety of alkalizing fruit or vegetable juice. This gives the digestive system a weekly rest and allows the body a brief break from "active duty" to readjust and rebalance itself. Another way is to fast for a period of two or three days each month, which has similar benefits to a weekly one-day fast. While minifasts do not provide the dramatic cleansing results of longer fasts, they are still quite effective as a form of regular preventive medicine against a wide range of diseases and degenerative conditions, especially if you do longer detox fasts from time to time. As the Greek writer Plutarch suggested, "Instead of medicine, fast for a day."

FASTING SUPPLEMENTS

Water is the primary cleansing agent involved in therapeutic fasting; it is very important to drink at least 1¾ quarts a day of purified alkaline water throughout the duration of any fast, even if you're using raw juices as well. In addition to water, a variety of very effective fasting supplements may also be utilized to amplify and accelerate blood purification and tissue detox, and to promote rapid healing during the course of a fast. Below is a review of previously described standard tools of the trade for therapeutic fasts:

Psyllium

Psyllium is the single most important supplement for cleaning and clearing the digestive tract, particularly the lower bowels. Psyllium's mucilaginous bulking properties also help curb hunger by making the stomach and intestines feel "full."

Bentonite

Colloidal bentonite acts like a "magnetic mop" to neutralize and carry away toxins loosened from the bowel walls by the psyllium fiber. Five hundred times smaller than water molecules, the negatively charged micromolecules of bentonite enter the bloodstream and cellular fluids. Once there, they latch onto positively charged toxins that are up to two hundred times heavier than they are and carry those toxins through the bloodstream to the kidneys for excretion.

Green Food

Green food is by far the best nutritional supplement to use during a therapeutic fast. One of the richest and purest sources of blood-cleansing chlorophyll and life-sustaining nutrients, green foods are easy to assimilate and do not require complex digestion. They also provide sufficient metabolic energy to help counteract the food cravings that often arise while fasting.

Lemon Juice

During a fast, fresh lemon juice may be used to assist the detox process with its swift alkalizing and cleansing properties. As the only anionic (negative-ion charged) food source, it provides potent antioxidant activity and energizes the detox process. Lemon juice has a natural affinity for the liver and stimulates bile production, thereby helping to detoxify and repair the liver. An ounce or two of fresh lemon juice may be added to the water when shaking up a dose of psyllium powder, to improve the taste of the psyllium and enhance its cleansing properties.

Lactobacteria

These are the so-called "friendly flora" of the bowels, and they constitute one of the most important elements required for proper digestion of food, assimilation of nutrients, and processing of digestive wastes. In healthy bowels, friendly bacteria should constitute about 80 percent of total bacteria population, with putrefactive bacteria accounting for the remaining 20 percent. In toxic bowels, such as those in over 95 percent of the people on the planet today, the ratio is reversed, with putrefactive bacteria occupying 80 percent or more of the bowel terrain, and the "good guys" hanging on for dear life in ever dwindling numbers. A primary goal of any therapeutic fast is to completely dredge the bowels of *all* bacterial colonies, and to eliminate the septic filth in which they breed. After that, the entire intestinal tract must be replenished with fresh colonies of friendly lactobacteria. Psyllium and bentonite do the job of dredging out the old stuff very well, but you definitely need to take dietary measures to introduce new colonies of beneficial lactobacteria into the bowels after each fast, before the "bad guys" sneak back in and take over again.

One way to replenish the bowels with friendly bacteria is to take a good lactobacteria supplement such as acidopholus, bifudus, and other similar cultures used to make yogurt. These come in powdered and capsule form, but you must be careful to purchase a reliable brand that retains its potency on the shelf. Most brands on the market today contain virtually no living cultures. Another option is to eat fresh goat milk yogurt for about a week immediately after a fast, but yogurt is not as effective as a high-potency, powdered supplement, because milk products produce mucus in the bowels, and it is best not to consume mucus-forming foods until after you've firmly established a new colony of friendly flora in your colon.

There's also a third way, one that you can easily prepare at home in your own kitchen. Popularly known as Rejuvelac, fermented cabbage juice is one of the purest and most abundant sources of "rejuvenating lactobacteria" for the human digestive tract, and it does not require the use of any dairy products. After making the first batch, which takes about three days, each subsequent batch ferments quickly overnight by adding a few ounces of the previous batch as a starter to prepare the next one. You may therefore keep the culture going day by day for as long as you wish, simply by chopping some cabbage, adding water and some starter from the last batch, and setting it aside to ferment for a day. A recipe for making your own Rejuvelac at home is listed in appendix 1, page 312 "Recipes and Formulas."

Regardless of whether you use dairy-based lactobacteria or cabbage Rejuvelac, you should start taking it shortly before eating your first food when breaking a fast, and continue using it twice a day for at least ten days to insure that a new colony of friendly bacteria establishes itself firmly in your bowels. Thereafter, repeat this replenishing regimen several times each year, even without a fast, to assist the friendly bacterial allies in your bowels to flourish and keep putrefactive bacteria under control.

TAKING THE PLUNGE

While fasting for seven days completely purifies the bloodstream, cleanses the lymphatic system, and detoxifies the tissues, fasting by itself will not remove the five-to-fifteen pounds of tough, toxic, mucoid matter that becomes deeply impacted in the bowels from years of wrong eating habits and wrong food choices that begin in childhood. The only way to rid your bowels of this rubbery toxic sludge is to dredge it out with a series of colonic irrigations done in conjunction with a therapeutic fast.

A hundred years ago, when pneumonia was still the leading cause of death in the United States, Dr. J. H. Tilden of Denver, Colorado, cured thousands of people of this deadly disease, without ever losing a single patient, simply by treating them with fasting and colonic irrigation and nothing else, then putting them on a strict diet of fresh raw foods consisting mostly of fruit and vegetables. After decades of dependence on antibiotics, pneumonia has grown resistant to drug therapy and has once again become a major killer throughout the world. As with most infectious diseases, the real cure for pneumonia is not a new drug; it is an ancient naturopathic method that long predates allopathic medicine but has lain buried and unnoticed for centuries in the archives of medical literature. That method is fasting and colonic cleansing.

One man who went to the library in search of a better cure back in 1935 and thereby rediscovered the curative powers of fasting and colonic irrigation, was V. E. Irons, an ordinary American businessman who, at the age of forty, had been diagnosed with a crippling arthritic spinal ailment called "ankylosing spondylosis." His doctors told him that it was incurable and that he would soon be confined to a wheelchair. Refusing to accept their verdict, Irons began to study the medical literature recorded by such early luminaries of naturopathic medicine in the United States as Dr. Tilden, Dr. Kellogg, and others. Irons then decided to take matters into his own hands by treating his condition with a series of therapeutic fasts and self-administered colonics. Says he:

> Within two months I had no more pain from displacement and within fourteen months practically no spurs. All done with cleansing, fasting, and natural foods—no drugs!

His experience, and the complete cure it effected, impressed him so deeply that he devoted the rest of his long life to research and development of this natural way to detoxify and heal the human body. In the process, he created a line of products that enables anyone to practice this powerful self-healing therapy safely and effectively at home. During the 1950s, V. E. Irons was briefly imprisoned in a federal penitentiary in the United States for publicly stating his revolutionary views on human health and healing and for refusing to recant them under legal pressure from the American medical establishment. Fifty years later, in an ironic turn of events that must have amused Irons, President Reagan heaped public praise on Irons for his excellent work in health and healing and presented him with a national award for his contributions to the science of longevity. Irons remained healthy and active throughout the ninety-eight years of his life, starting a second family at the age of seventy-two and fathering his last child at the age of eighty.

During the course of his life, Irons perfected a system of self-detoxification based on fasting and colonic cleansing that this writer regards as one of the most important contributions to modern medicine and world health in the twentieth century. In addition to his line of "Vit-ra-tox" internal cleansing supplements, Irons played a key role in the invention and development of the "Colema Board" (figure 10)—the bowel's "best friend" and an indispensable tool for doing colonics yourself at home. Operated entirely by gravity, the Colema Board allows virtually anyone to safely administer their own colonic irrigations in the privacy of their own bathrooms. As Irons notes in an interview, it's so easy that even a child can do it:

> My seven-year-old son Robert frequently takes home colonics—all by himself. I'm 87 and I take them all the time. So, if you're any-where between the ages of 7 and 87, you should have no problems. . . . It is completely safe.

And yet, while people today don't hesitate to discuss the most intimate details of their—and others'—personal sex lives, the moment the word "colon" or "bowel" crops up in a conversation, everyone winces uncomfortably and looks away, quickly changing the subject. Suggest that their bowels are bursting at the seams with mounds of foul, putrefactive filth and that it might be a good idea for them to flush it all out with a series of colonics, and most people leap to their feet and start looking for the nearest exit. Here's what Irons has to say about such "colonic cry-babies" in an interview he gave in 1982:

> If people can't take a simple home colonic to clean out their clogged, constipated, putrid colons, then tell them to start looking for an old

rocking chair and cane. . . . If these people are afraid of all the "horrors" that may happen to them when they stick a tiny plastic tube one "micro-inch" up their fanny, there is just not much hope for them. . . . Many people will easily talk about the most intimate sexual experiences—but by golly, they will revolt at the first thought of discussing the colon.

Some people claim that fasting and raw-juice therapy alone can remove the hardened mucoid plaque from the colon wall, but they are mistaken. Irons replies to this claim by saying, "Forget it! It won't work. . . . You must use the Colema Board together with the intestinal cleansers, if you really want to cleanse your colon properly. If you don't, the thick mucus coating on the intestinal wall will never come off. It will stay there till you die."

It is important to remember that this tough, toxic layer of putrefied mucus and partially digested protein was put there by you, not by mother nature, as a result of your own unnatural eating habits and food choices. Your body's natural cleansing mechanisms are not designed to deal with this unnatural mess; it requires special methods to eliminate it. Those methods are fasting and colonic cleansing, and anyone with the pluck to take the plunge always gets spectacular results and never regrets the decision to do it. Listen to Irons describe what happens when you do

Fig. 10. The "Colema Board": The bowel's best friend.

colonic irrigations in conjunction with a therapeutic fast, based on some of the cases he personally handled:

> You'll get fabulous results. Some of the worst smelling material known to man comes out when people do the program right. . . . One woman passed more than a quart of black, vomitus, putrid material for three days in a row. One man passed a whole lot of material that looked like afterbirth. One man I know recently passed fourteen pounds of rotting material—all in one treatment. . . . Just about everyone should get a lot of black, hardened mucus on about the fourth or fifth day, if he takes two five-gallon colonics a day. . . . Most of this mucus is as black as charcoal and so tough you can't even cut it with a knife. In many cases, the mucus is as tough as the rubber tubing of a bicycle tire. . . . The longest we have had is twenty-seven feet, in one piece. Sometimes it will come out as a pile weighing as much as eleven pounds and continuing to come out for several days to a week.

Despite the clear and present evidence, most people these days react with disbelief when told by a naturopath that their worst chronic ailments are caused by the seepage of poisons into the bloodstream from clogged, toxic bowels, and that they need a series of colonic irrigations to clear their bowels and cure themselves. These people often reply defensively, "Who, me?" The answer to that question is a resounding, "Yes, you!" Thirty years ago, in a rare moment of candor, public health authorities in the USA acknowledged that "over 90 percent" of all Americans are running around with seriously clogged colons, such as those depicted in figure 11. If, at the turn of the twentieth century, Dr. Harvey Kellogg said he had never found a single normal colon, it boggles the mind to imagine what a century of junk food, synthetic additives, chemically contaminated beef and dairy products, frozen pizzas, and now genetically modified foods have done to the contemporary Western colon. As Irons puts it, "Regardless of your financial standing, regardless of your past health history, regardless of your age or sex, you do have this hardened mucus in your colon, and you will be amazed by what comes out of you."

The only way to find out what comes out of you and to get rid of it once and for all is to climb aboard the "Colema Express" for a seven-day adventure of fasting and colonic irrigation.

SEVEN DAYS ABOARD THE COLEMA EXPRESS

The seven-day fast and internal cleansing program using "Vit-ra-tox" supplements and the Colema Board is V. E. Irons's great gift to the science of health and longevity. Today, Irons's family in California continues to produce and distribute this fine line of products and to provide printed information regarding the program to anyone who requests it. Those interested in obtaining further information or ordering the products may do so by contacting the address given in the "Suppliers" section.

To give the reader an idea of what to expect on a seven-day cleansing

Fig. 11. Clogged Plumbing: The colon is the most "out of shape" organ today. A) Healthy colon as depicted in anatomy books; B) X-Ray profiles of typical human colons today.

fast using detox supplements and colonics, here's a day-by-day description, based on personal experience, of a week on the "Colema Express"—the fast lane to health, longevity, and a squeaky clean colon:

Day 1

It is best to skip dinner the night before starting a therapeutic fast, or just eat fresh fruit, and to take two or three "Vit-ra-tox" herbal laxatives before bed, so that you begin the first day of the fast by completely evacuating the bowels of all residual feces. First thing in the morning, start taking the psyllium and bentonite cleansers, followed an hour or two later by the Greenlife and other nutritional supplements, according to the schedule outlined in the program brochure, and take one or two five-gallon colonics per day. The first day is very easy and causes no discomfort, because the body's detox mechanisms have not yet reached high gear, and the tissues have not yet begun to discharge their most deeply impacted toxins into the bloodstream.

Day 2

Continue taking the supplements and colonics. By midafternoon, you will probably begin to feel a bit weak and wobbly, tired and listless. This is *not* due to starvation or lack of nutrition. How you feel is due entirely to the onset of the detox process, which switches on about thirty-six hours after you stop eating food. Digestive enzymes normally engaged in the endless task of digesting food in the stomach now enter the bloodstream instead and patrol the body on "search and destroy" missions, dismantling damaged and cancerous cells, killing bacteria and viruses, and dissolving toxic deposits in the joints, organs, and other tissues. All of these toxic wastes are then dumped into the bloodstream for excretion. For the first few days, the toxins come pouring out of the tissues much faster than the kidneys and skin can excrete them, leaving a backlog of toxic residues floating in the bloodstream. These toxins circulate around the body and through the brain while waiting to be eliminated, like aircraft circling an airfield while waiting their turn to land. They can cause headaches, body pain, fatigue, and irritability. You may, perhaps, derive a small measure of comfort from the knowledge that the worse you feel, the better the program is working for you to detoxify and heal your body. Also be assured that the discomfort will pass in a few more days. There is no shortcut to bypass the symptomatic discomforts of detox, although you may lessen them with herbal teas, hot mineral baths, massage, and other methods. There's always a certain degree of "no pain, no gain" dynamics when it comes to detox. But with fasting, the gain is so much greater and lasts so much longer than the temporary discomfort it causes that it seems a negligible price to pay for the benefits.

Day 3

The detox process continues to accelerate and intensify today, making you feel even more tired and uncomfortable. If you feel particularly low, you may take a few extra doses of bentonite, which helps to neutralize the toxic overload in the bloodstream. You may also take some extra Greenlife to increase the blood's capacity to carry oxygen and provide additional fuel for metabolic energy. This is the day that you start to approach the threshold of the healing crisis, which marks the peak intensity of the detox phase and the beginning of the healing process. It is no coincidence that this day is when first-time fasters start to waver and toy with the idea of terminating the fast. Do *not* surrender to that temptation! You've already come this far, and you'll regret it if you deprive yourself of the final rewards of the fast by quitting now.

Day 4

For most people, this is the most difficult day, especially if they are highly toxic, because this is the day that the healing crisis usually occurs. The body excretes a foul odor and clammy sweat, the breath stinks of rotting sewage, and the tongue becomes coated with white and yellow slime. All of this reaction is the toxic waste from the deepest tissues of the body coming to the surface for elimination, and the body's rancid reactions are always a sign of a successful detox. Don't give up now! This is the halfway mark, and if you can make it through to the end of the day, the rest is all downhill, and you will easily finish the program.

Day 5

Depending upon how toxic you were to begin with, the healing crisis will either pass today, or continue with ever diminishing intensity until the next morning. Either way, you will start feeling better today. Since the heaviest toxins are now out of your body, you will have a lot more energy to spare for ordinary functions. You'll start to notice a lightness in your limbs, a supple flexibility in your joints, and a rapidly growing clarity and joy in your mind. You will realize from the way you feel on this day, without a shadow of doubt, that you are in the midst of the most profound cleansing and healing experience of your life, and that what you are doing is the best possible way to repair your body, preserve your health, and prolong your lifespan. That insight alone usually suffices to carry you through to the end of the program.

Day 6

Energy returns rapidly now, and the blood and tissues are almost completely purified. Your body has already begun to replace damaged cells, rebuild blood, and repair organs and tissues, and as a result you feel yourself growing stronger by the hour, even though you have not eaten any food for nearly a week. You should continue taking one or two colonics per day, because the biggest amounts of the most deeply impacted mucoid matter and putrefactive waste are flushed out of the colon on the last two or three days of the fast, after the superficial layers of sludge have been removed. As Irons says, and as anyone else who has ever done this program has observed, "You will be amazed by what comes out of you," especially in the last few days, despite not having eaten anything for nearly a week.

Day 7

By now, you should feel healthier and more energized and well balanced than you can ever remember feeling, and you probably won't have much hunger for food. You well might feel as though you could easily fast for a few more days, and indeed you could, if you wished. Recalling the heavy heaps of putrid waste matter that poured out of your bowels and realizing how much better you feel after ridding your body of this toxic load, you will probably resolve to change your diet and eating habits to avoid polluting your bowels, blood, and bodily tissues again with wrong food choices, indigestible food combinations, and foods loaded with chemical contaminants.

Don't forget to take a good lactobacteria supplement for a week or two after any fast, and be sure to break your fast gradually and carefully by eating only fresh fruits and vegetables for a day or two. Then slowly returning to a normal daily diet of wholesome natural foods properly prepared and correctly combined.

Try taking the "Colema Express." You may not like the ride very much, but you'll love the results.

7

"THE ANGEL OF SUNLIGHT": HELIOTHERAPY

Ancient Chinese medical texts describe sunlight as a form of "nourishment for the brain," and the prescription they give to correct conditions caused by deficiency of this vital "nutrient" is to "administer sunbeams" to the patient's eyes and skin. These texts clearly state that "sunlight benefits the brain by stimulating production of vital essence." In the brain, "vital essence" refers to pituitary hormones and essential neurotransmitters.

Many ancient cultures understood the vital link between health and sunlight, and they knew that sunlight could be applied as a form of medicine to purify, heal, and rebalance the human system. In *The Essene Gospel of Peace,* after teaching his followers how to cleanse their bodies internally with water, Jesus advises them as follows:

> Seek the angel of sunlight. Put off your shoes and your clothing and suffer the angel of sunlight to embrace all your body . . . that the angel of sunlight may be brought within you. And the angel of sunlight shall cast out of your body all evil-smelling and unclean things that defiled it without and within.

Modern medical science has unraveled the mystery of the mechanism whereby "the angel of sunlight" casts out "unclean things" from the human body. They call it the "oculo-endocrine system," and the new branch of science spawned by this discovery is known as "photobiology." The essential factor in sunlight that "nourishes the brain" is the invisible band of long-wave ultraviolet (UV) light that enters the eye along with the visible frequencies of light. UV light has both long-wave and short-wave forms; it is only excessive exposure to the short-wave variety that damages the eyes and skin. Long-wave UV light, however, is an absolutely essential factor for sustaining human health; it can also be applied as a tool for detox and healing.

Here's how the oculo-endocrine system works: when natural, full-spectrum sunlight enters the eyes, the visible bands of light excite the cells in the retina known as "rods" and "cones" to produce the colors and forms of ordinary vision. The invisible, long-wave UV frequencies, which hit the retina together with the visible bands, activate a special layer of cells in the retina called "epithelial cells," which are designed by nature precisely for the purpose of receiving these invisible frequencies of ultraviolet light within the eyes. Long-wave UV stimulation to the epithelial cells in the retina produces a powerful neural pulse that is carried along the optic nerve and delivered directly to the pituitary and pineal glands, where these signals stimulate the production of essential hormones that regulate the entire endocrine system and thereby determine the strength and speed of the body's natural immune responses.

The pituitary plays a particularly important role in the ocular-endocrine system, especially for immune response. Known as the body's "master gland," the pituitary secretes hormones that regulate and balance all the other glands in the endocrine system. Without sufficient stimulation from long-wave UV light via the retina and optic nerve, the pituitary is deprived of its most essential form of "nourishment" and the entire oculo-endocrine system malfunctions, resulting in impaired immune response. With all the smog, smoke, dust, chemicals, and other pollution in the air today, the strength and quality of sunlight reaching the earth has been seriously reduced, resulting in widespread "UV deficiency" and contributing to the overall deterioration in human immune response. The Smithsonian Institute reports a 15 percent reduction in the overall intensity of sunlight reaching the earth over the past seventy-five years, with an even greater drop of 27 percent in the UV part of the spectrum. This is causing problems for human health that are quite similar to the immuno-suppressive effects produced by polluted sources of food, water, and air.

The biggest problem caused by sunlight deficiency is weak immune response and low resistance, which not only reduces defense against disease and degeneration, but also erodes the body's ability to detoxify and repair itself. The effects of "light pollution" on human health in big cities and heavily industrialized regions are similar to those of pollutants in food, water, and air: critical deficiency of the essential elements and energies required to sustain strong immunity and resistance. This problem is further aggravated by the sedentary, indoor lifestyles of contemporary times, which keep most people out of the sun all day long and usually keep a layer of glass between their eyes and sunlight whenever they do venture briefly into the light of day.

All glass blocks out beneficial, long-wave UV frequencies in sunlight. That means your oculo-endocrine system receives no nourishment and stimulation when you're sitting behind the windshield of a car, looking through a window in your home or office, riding in a bus or train, or walking in broad sunlight wearing any kind of eye glasses. Only plastic windowpanes and lenses allow beneficial UV waves to pass through and enter the eyes. Herein lies another contributing factor in the modern syndrome of chronic fatigue, ill health, and mental malaise experienced by people who spend their entire working lives seated at desks in glass office towers, and most of their leisure time seated indoors at home watching television in artificially lit homes. The net result of such light-deficient lifestyles is an acquired immune deficiency caused by chronic "solar malnutrition" and the consequent malfunction of the oculo-endocrine system.

Let's look at a few concrete examples that illustrate this problem. During the Hong Kong Flu epidemic that swept through North America in the winter of 1968–1969, entire factories and department stores in

Sarasota County, Florida, were forced to close down due to the high incidence of flu among their employees. At one large factory, however, where plastic windowpanes and full-spectrum indoor lighting had recently been installed, not a single employee fell ill during the entire duration of the epidemic. Similar results have since been observed in other places where full-spectrum light sources have been installed.

Another good example of how crucial the oculo-endocrine system is to human health is the situation in public schools in the United States and other industrialized nations. Severe hyperactivity, chronic violence, inability to concentrate, and other behavioral problems have become so severe among young school children that many of them are now dosed daily with powerful sedatives, tranquilizers, and amphetamines, which in turn lead to even more severe life-long health problems, such as drug addiction and liver damage. When ordinary fluorescent lights, which have an extremely irritating effect on the oculo-endocrine system, were replaced with full-spectrum lighting and glass window panes were replaced with plastic in all classrooms in several selected school districts, however, these behavioral problems virtually vanished within a few weeks of the change in lighting, and many "problem children" suddenly transformed to become model students. Similar positive results were observed in every classroom tested. Incredibly, this research has been deliberately ignored and suppressed, owing to its implications for conventional indoor lighting systems everywhere.

A third example is the "winter blues" syndrome that has been observed for so long in countries such as Sweden and Canada, where long winters and short days produce a critical deficiency in beneficial UV stimulation during that time of year. By midwinter, these countries experienced a significant rise in death due to disease as well as suicide, and the reason turned out to be "starvation" of the pituitary gland due to insufficient exposure to full-spectrum sunlight. Today, these countries have "light clinics" where people can go for their daily dose of long-wave UV light energy, and many homes, offices, and public places use full-spectrum indoor lighting to compensate for the decrease in natural outdoor sources during the depths of winter.

"SKIN DEEP"

Skin is the second important receptor for assimilating essential nourishment and energy from solar radiation. In 1967, a group of Russian scientists reported the results of extensive research in this field as follows:

> If human skin is not exposed to solar radiation (direct or scattered) for long periods of time, disturbances will occur in the physiological equilibrium of the human system. The result will be functional disorders of the nervous system and a Vitamin-D deficiency, a weakening of the body's defenses, and an aggravation of chronic diseases.

The main mechanism whereby sunlight provides essential "nutrition" to the human body through exposure to skin is vitamin D production. Sunlight stimulates the tissues below the skin to produce vitamin D, which is an essential cofactor for the assimilation and utilization of calcium in the body. Without the presence of vitamin D, there's no way that the body can absorb even the purest, most potent sources of calcium, and without adequate supplies of calcium, there's no way the body can detoxify and repair itself. Solar deficiency is therefore a primary contributing factor to chronic calcium deficiency, and this in turn is one of the main reasons that modern man and woman, especially in urban areas, have such weak teeth and bones.

It is a fact of modern lifestyle that most people in the Western world do not get adequate exposure to clear, full-spectrum sunlight at the proper time of day. Those who occasionally do go out in the sun usually do so like the proverbial "mad dogs and Englishmen," tanning their hides in the noonday sun solely for cosmetic purposes. The pursuit of a suntan for the sake of browning the skin is an abuse of sunlight that is tantamount to gluttony in food. The proper daily "dosage" for sunlight is about thirty minutes, more or less, and this should be administered only before 10:30 AM or after 3:30 PM As Dr. Theodore Baroody states in his book *Alkalize or Die*, "At least ½ to one hour of direct sunlight a day is requisite for the body's system to produce proper hormonal levels and assist alkaline-acid balances. . . . Between 11:00 A.M. and 3:00 P.M., the sun is too direct and produces an acid effect in the body through its radiations."

So here again we see how insufficient exposure to beneficial sunlight, as well as excessive exposure to damaging sunlight, contribute to the current crisis in human health. Not only does this problem produce critical imbalances in the oculo-endocrine system, it also has an acid-forming influence on the blood and other bodily fluids, which makes it a major contributing factor to chronic acidosis and tissue toxemia.

HELIOTHERAPY FOR DETOX AND HEALING

The therapeutic power of sunlight is another reason that health resorts and healing spas have traditionally been located by the sea or high up in the mountains. Like the high negative-ion count in mountain and seaside air, the clear bright sunlight in such locations provides strong support for the many immune responses involved in detox and healing. By stimulating the pituitary gland via the oculo-endocrine system, sunlight assures an adequate daily supply of the essential hormones required to repair and rebalance the body. In addition, by prompting production of vitamin D, the essential cofactor required by the body to assimilate and utilize calcium, sunlight also assures the abundant supplies of calcium needed for detox and healing.

While it is definitely a big advantage to do a detox program at a time and a place with lots of sunshine, you don't need to spend a fortune at a fancy spa to find good sunlight for a week or two. You can avoid the expense of staying in health resorts and spas by designing your own detox program and doing it in a sunny time and place of your own choosing. If there is no sunny season where you live, or you cannot find sufficient peace and privacy at home, you may travel instead to the nearest mountains or seashore, rent an inexpensive room or cottage for a week or two, and do it yourself. You don't need luxury and fancy frills for a detox program; what you need is peace of mind, plenty of personal privacy, clean air, pure water, and clear, bright sunlight.

The best times of day for heliotherapy, or "therapeutic sun-bathing," are before 10:30 in the morning and after 3:30 in the afternoon, when the sun rides low in the sky and doesn't damage skin or eyes. Twenty to thirty minutes of exposure per session, and one or two sessions per day, are sufficient to achieve the desired therapeutic benefits. Total daily exposure should not exceed one hour. The more skin you expose while sun-bathing, the greater the therapeutic benefits. This exposure principle also applies to the eyes; don't wear sunglasses during heliotherapy, because they block out the beneficial, long-wave UV frequencies in sunlight—the solar factors that activate the ocular-endocrine system and elevate immune response.

Unfortunately, it's not always possible to find a sunny time and place to do a detox program, especially if it's midwinter in the northern latitudes and your finances are limited. Nevertheless, when the condition of your health demands that you detoxify your system without delay, you may bring the healing power of natural sunlight into your own home by installing full-spectrum light bulbs and lighting systems, all of which are now widely available. Like food, water, and air, modern technology has analyzed the active ingredients in sunlight and developed "solar supplements" to compensate for the degradation in the quality of natural sources of these essential elements for life. Much of this new light technology is based on the work of time-lapse photographer John Ott, who accidentally discovered the healing powers of sunlight when he stepped on his sunglasses and broke them while working on an outdoor project to film the growth cycles of plants. Too busy to buy new glasses, he worked without them. A few weeks later, Ott noticed that the painful arthritis he'd suffered for many years was swiftly disappearing. Subsequent research revealed that the UV light that his sunglasses had formerly blocked from entering his eyes had relieved his arthritis by stimulating his pituitary to secrete the hormones necessary to signal the adrenal glands to produce the natural steroids that constitute the body's own built-in remedy for this condition.

Today there is a wide range of full-spectrum lighting available on the market, including the "Ott Light" and the "Ott Bulb," which produce indoor light containing the complete spectrum of natural light frequencies, both visible and invisible, found in clear bright sunlight. These light fixtures may be used in any home or office. People can even take their own full-spectrum lightbulbs to a health resort or beach cottage and use them to light their rooms there. In the absence of adequate sources of whole, natural sunlight outdoors, full-spectrum indoor lighting provides all the essential frequencies of sunlight required to stimulate the oculo-endocrine system, thereby sustaining strong immune response and promoting production of vitamin-D for calcium assimilation. Full-spectrum lighting is an excellent form of preventive medicine in daily life as well. By lighting your home and your place of work with "whole light," you provide yourself with an additional line of defense against disease and degeneration, and help to counteract the immuno-suppressive effects of harmful artificial light frequencies such as those produced by television screens and fluorescent lights.

Another form of indoor heliotherapy that has recently been developed is the infrared sauna. Unlike ordinary saunas, which heat the bodily tissues and induce perspiration by sheer force of heat, infrared saunas heat the deepest organs and tissues of the body by virtue of the radiant penetrating energy of the infrared band of natural light. This radiant, infrared energy heats the internal tissues without overheating the skin and respiratory system, as ordinary saunas do. As it penetrates into the deeper, denser tissues below the skin, the infrared heat softens deposits of crystallized toxins and acid wastes in joints, nerves, and connective tissues, allowing them to be dissolved, diluted, and carried away for excretion via blood, lymph, and sweat. This kind of heat is particularly effective for eliminating heavy metals from the tissues. Holistic healing centers and health spas are beginning to include infrared saunas among their therapeutic facilities. Smaller units are also available for home installation.

"LET THERE BE LIGHT"

In previous chapters, we've already discussed how essential factors in food, water, and air may be utilized as effective tools for detox. Now sunlight may also be added to your growing arsenal of weapons to do battle with tissue toxicity, strengthen immune defenses, and protect your health. Similarly, just as good food, pure water, and clean air may be easily integrated into your daily life as long-term defenses against disease, degeneration, and premature death, so full-spectrum light may also be relied upon as a daily source of life-supporting elements and energies. While getting adequate daily exposure of eyes and skin to natural sunlight outdoors is no doubt the best way to achieve this balance, in reality, most people are either far too busy to take the time to do this on a daily basis, their schedules simply won't permit it, or else they live in places where the amount of sunshine is limited.

If your living situation does not allow for the right balance of sunlight, then you have two alternatives. If you live in a sun-starved area such as a big city or in a far northern latitude where the winters are long and the days short, you may follow the "let there be light" principle in your own home and office/shop/studio by using full-spectrum indoor lighting systems. Alternatively, if you live in a sunny region, you may harvest sufficient long-wave UV radiation from the sun each day by quickly doing a simple set of eye exercises early in the morning or late in the afternoon. To do this, stand facing the sun anytime between sunrise and 8:30 AM or between 4:30 PM and sunset. Without staring directly at the sun, roll your eyes in circles around the sun, so that sunlight bathes the entire surface of the retina. Roll the eyes ten to twenty times in each direction. Then close your eyes facing the sun and blink rapidly ten times, shut them again for a minute and blink rapidly another ten times. That's it. Your pituitary gland has now received its daily dose of whole, unrefined sunlight, and your endocrine system has received its solar tune up for the day.

Another way to feed your brain with the essential energy of sunlight is by practicing "sun gazing," a method developed by the yogis of ancient India. This practice should only be done within the first half hour after sunrise, or before sunset, and you are advised to practice this method on a daily basis. On the first day, gaze directly at the sun on the horizon, eyes wide open, for ten seconds, then increase the time to twenty seconds on the second day, thirty seconds on the third day, and so forth, adding ten seconds each consecutive day. For best results, stand barefoot on bare ground, not on concrete or grass, to establish a strong link between the energy currents of sky and earth. Practitioners of this method incrementally increase their exposure until they are gazing at the sun for up to fifteen minutes or more, and most of them report profound healing benefits for a wide variety of chronic conditions as well as an overall boost in vitality.

The "angel of sunlight" is always there, shining in the sky, freely available to one and all. Sunlight is one of the most powerful healers on earth. All you need to do is let it bathe your skin and shine into your eyes, and it will bestow on you the "glow of good health."

8

THE ELIMINATORS: HERBAL DETOX

Traditional herbal pharmacopoeia contain hundreds of medicinal herbs that effectively eliminate toxic substances and flush out residual metabolic wastes from the blood and tissues. They also help repair toxic damage to the organs and restore functional balance to the whole system. The great advantage of using natural herbs rather than chemical drugs to repair and rebalance the body is that each herb may be specifically selected to target particular organs and tissues with very precise and intensive detox therapy, without causing hazardous side effects in other parts of the body, as most chemical drugs do. Such therapeutic precision can only be achieved with medicines derived directly from nature by virtue of sympathetic resonance between their essential energies and similar organic energy frequencies in the body. Each and every herb has what TCM calls a "natural affinity" *(gui jing)* for specific tissues and organ-energy systems in the body. After many millennia of continuous clinical practice, traditional herbalists have determined the specific natural affinities and therapeutic actions of thousands of medicinal herbs. All of this knowledge has been carefully recorded and preserved for posterity in traditional herbal manuals that are still in use today, and such knowledge may easily be applied at home to produce swifter, deeper, more effective results in any detox program.

Herbal supplements may be used to accelerate and amplify detox and healing in programs based on detox diets, as well as in fasting programs. When using herbs for detox support in therapeutic fasting programs, it is best to prepare them as whole herbal teas, which have gentler, fewer aggressive effects than concentrated herbal extracts. When fasting, the body becomes far more sensitive to the effects of all external supplements. Therefore, a mild herbal tea delivers the same therapeutic potency to someone who's fasting as a concentrated extract of the same herb would to someone on a detox diet, but without the intensity of condensed extracts. When used as supplements in a detox diet, herbs may be taken in all forms, from the mildest teas to the strongest tinctures, powders, and tablets.

In traditional Chinese medicine, all herbs are categorized in two ways: according to their natural affinities for specific organs and tissues, which determines where in the body their therapeutic energies go; and according to the nature of their bio-active energies, which determines their therapeutic effects. The latter classification is based on the ancient Chinese theory of the Five Elemental Energies *(wu hsing),* which in food and medicine manifests as the Five Essential Flavors *(wu wei).* Most detox herbs in TCM belong to the "bitter" category of medicines, and this also holds true in traditional Western herbalogy. No doubt this characteristic is the origin of the term "bitter medicine," for prior to the advent of chemical drugs and artificially flavored foods, most diseases were treated with cleansing bitter herbs and foods, and medicinal herbal "bitters" were a common household item in homes throughout the world. Today, not only have insipid chemical pills replaced bitter herbal potions in medicine, but also widespread addiction to sugar has led to a "sweet tooth" syndrome that has virtually eliminated bitter flavors from modern Western diets. And yet, according to the principles of traditional herbalogy, bitter flavors are nature's antidote for toxemia, and bitter herbs and foods carry energies into the body that purify the bloodstream, detoxify the tissues, and initiate healing responses.

Let's take a look at the major organs systems involved in the detox process, and see how medicinal herbs may be utilized to cleanse their tissues and rebalance their functions, while also protecting them from toxic damage during the detox process.

LIVER: CLEANING THE FILTER

In TCM, the liver is described as the "Chief of Staff" of the internal organs. It holds responsibility for filtering toxins from the blood, breaking down complex proteins, fats, and carbohydrates, and providing the bloodstream with a constant infusion of nutrients for delivery to the various tissues of the body. External signs of internal liver toxicity include yellow eyes and blurry vision, brittle fingernails and cracked toenails, and the negative emotions of anger, depression, and irritability. During detox, the liver must store an overload of toxic wastes discharged from the tissues, while the bloodstream gradually moves them out to the various excretory organs for elimination. Therefore, people with a history of liver toxicity, especially from excessive use of alcohol and drugs, or from chemical contamination, should include a few herbal liver cleansers among the supplements they select as supports for a detox program.

The most effective herbs for detoxifying the liver are milk thistle and dandelion root, which may be taken as whole herbal teas, capsules of the ground powdered herbs, or liquid extracts. Milk thistle has particularly potent liver cleansing properties. Its primary active ingredient is silymarin, a compound that has stronger antioxidant properties in the liver than vitamins E, C, or beta carotene. Silymarin may be taken directly in tablet or capsule form, 100 mg three times a day, as liver support during detox. In addition to detoxifying the liver, milk thistle stimulates production of the proteins required to build new cells and repair damaged tissues in the liver. A formula for Liver Detox Tea, in which milk thistle and dandelion are combined with four other herbal liver cleansers, is given in the "Recipes and Formulas" section, appendix 1, page 306. Dragon River Herbals (see "Suppliers" section) produces a formula called "Rejuvenate" Liver Regenerator, which is a pure, high-potency blend of extracts of dandelion, milk thistle, red clover, burdock, and cleavers in concentrated liquid form. This formula is an excellent supplement to use for detoxifying and repairing the liver in conjunction with a detox diet of one-to-three weeks duration.

A quick and easy way to give the liver a deep, intensive cleanse is to do the "liver flush." This may be done once a day for a period of three-to-ten days, preferably in the morning, as a means of flushing extra toxins from the liver during a detox diet program, but the liver flush is not a suitable method to use while fasting. The liver flush prompts an intensive cleansing purge in the liver, and it's particularly beneficial in cases of long-term chronic liver toxicity. For best results, supplement the liver flush by drinking plenty of Liver Detox Tea. Here's how to do it:

Mix one cup of your choice of freshly squeezed citrus juices, such as orange and grapefruit, but be sure to include some fresh lemon juice. Add enough pure water to dilute it to taste. Add the juice of 2 cloves garlic and ½ tsp of freshly grated ginger juice (grate the ginger, then squeeze the pulp through cloth). Mix in 1 tablespoon high-grade virgin olive oil and ½ teaspoon cayenne, shake it all together in a glass jar with lid until well blended, and then drink it down. Follow with one or two cups of Liver Detox Tea, sipped slowly.

Although the liver flush includes two food items (lemon juice and olive oil), these are therapeutic foods with affinity for the liver, and they work synergistically with the three active herbal ingredients—garlic, ginger, and cayenne. Performed regularly once or twice a year, this is an excellent regimen for general liver maintenance and preventive protection against disease and degeneration in the liver.

Chinese herbal medicine, which is renowned for the efficacy of its formulas for treating liver damage, offers some special high-potency liver detox formulas that may be used in cases of severe liver toxicity due to drug, alcohol, or chemical poisoning. The formulas may also be used to treat the various forms of hepatitis. These powerful formulas have strong effects, and they should only be used within the context of an overall detox diet program, preferably with the assistance of a health professional. In a previous title, *A Handbook of Chinese Healing Herbs*, the author presents a classic Chinese formula for healing severe liver damage that has demonstrated repeated efficacy in clinical practice. Known as "Major Bupleurum with Artemisia Decoction," this formula is given in the "Recipes and Formulas" section, appendix 1, page 308, along with a few guidelines on diet and other factors that should be followed when using this formula.

BLOOD AND LYMPH: THE PIPELINES

In TCM, the condition of the bloodstream is regarded as a primary indicator of health and disease, and a decisive factor in healing. Blood is responsible for delivering oxygen and nutrients to the cells, and carrying away carbon dioxide and other metabolic wastes for excretion. In Chinese medicine, great emphasis is given to purifying the bloodstream as an essential preliminary step in curing any ailment. The lymph deals with the coarsest toxins and most highly acidic wastes in the body, and it plays an especially important role during detox, when the bloodstream becomes overloaded with toxic residues discharged from the tissues. Unlike blood, lymph does not have its own pump to move it through the system, as the heart pumps blood. Instead, lymph depends on the force of gravity and regular movements of the body for its mobility, which is why the lymphatic system becomes so vulnerable to stagnation in sedentary people.

Herbs that purify the blood and lymph are known as "alteratives," because they alter the state of these vital bodily fluids from toxic to pure. The most widely used blood alteratives in Western herbalogy include Echinacea, yerba mansa, chaparral, red clover, burdock, and yarrow. These may be taken singly or in various combinations, either as whole teas, or concentrated tablets and extracts. A tasty tea used in TCM to detoxify and "cool" the bloodstream is made by steeping dried chrysanthemum blossoms and licorice root for fifteen to twenty minutes in boiling hot water. This tea may be sipped throughout the day and night during any detox program to help keep the bloodstream clean and prevent overheating of the blood due to toxic overload. Cayenne also helps cleanse the bloodstream during detox, by giving a strong boost to circulation and thereby accelerating delivery of toxins to the excretory organs for elimination.

An alternative formula that cleanses both the blood and the lymph may be prepared by combining equal portions of concentrated liquid extracts of Echinacea, red root, baptisia root, thuja leaf, stillingia root, blue flag root, and prickly ash bark. Take twenty to thirty drops of this blend in warm water, three-to-five times a day, between meals. This treatment may be started during a detox program, then continued for up to three more months, especially when deep-tissue cleansing is required, or if the immune system is weak.

The most important herbs for cleansing lymph are red root, Echinacea, ocotillo, red clover, cleavers, mullein, figwort, prickly ash, and poke weed. As with blood alteratives, these may be taken singly or in various combinations, as teas, tablets, or tinctures. Remember, however, that during a therapeutic detox fast, these herbs should only be used in the form of steeped or simmered teas, not concentrated extracts. A formula for Lymphatic Detox Tea is given in appendix 1, page 310 of the "Recipes and Formulas" section.

KIDNEYS AND BLADDER: THE DRAINAGE SYSTEM

In TCM, the kidney system is referred to as the "Minister of Power," and its energy is so essential that it is also known as the "Root of Life." One reason that the kidney system is so important to overall health and vitality is that the adrenal glands are attached to the top of the kidneys. Therefore, whenever the kidneys become toxic or weak, the adrenal glands falter as well, weakening immune response as well as sexual potency. According to TCM, kidney-energy also regulates the condition of bone and marrow, which produces red and white blood cells. Therefore, when kidney energy is deficient, blood becomes weak and immune response is impaired. The kidneys themselves are responsible for filtering the fluid wastes of metabolism from the bloodstream, and the bladder is the primary outlet for eliminating these acid wastes from the body. For those with deficient kidney function and adrenal insufficiency, take some form of herbal kidney support during a detox program, to protect the kidneys and bladder from toxic damage and assist them in excreting wastes quickly from the body.

An excellent formula for cleansing the kidneys and bladder and balancing kidney functions is Breuss Kidney Tea, which may be used in detox diets as well as during therapeutic fasts. You should start drinking this tea on the first day of a detox program, and continue taking it three times a day for exactly three weeks, even if your detox program is only for a few days. You may also use this herbal tea for three consecutive weeks, once or twice a year, in conjunction with your regular daily diet, as an effective means of periodic kidney cleansing and preventive protection against kidney disease. The formula for Breuss Kidney Tea is listed in "Recipes and Formulas," appendix 1, page 307. Another formula that is particularly effective for cleansing the urinary tract and bladder is listed in appendix 1, page 309.

Parsley tea, which can easily be prepared in the kitchen from fresh or dried parsley leaf, has a strong affinity for the kidneys and is an excellent kidney cleanser. Parsley also soothes the kidney tissues when they become inflamed from passing too many toxins too fast during intensive detox. Since fresh parsley is readily available in most markets and many home gardens, keep some on hand in the kitchen, in case you need to give your kidneys a refreshing flush during detox. To prepare a potent herbal kidney cleanser that contains parsley as well as herbs that strengthen the entire urinary system, combine equal portions of finely ground powders of dried gravel root, juniper berries, hydrangea, uva ursi, parsley, marshmallow, bladderpod, ginger, and burdock root. Take 1 level teaspoon of this powder three times a day, between meals, either in capsules or stirred into a cup of hot water. Powdered herbs generally have stronger, longer-lasting therapeutic effects than whole teas, but should not be used while fasting.

BOWELS: DREDGING THE SEWER

Known in TCM as the "Minister of Transport," the colon transforms digestive wastes from liquid into solid form, recovering and recycling most of the water and moving the solids onward to the rectum for elimination. When the colon gets clogged with putrefactive wastes, toxic residues are diverted to the lungs and skin for excretion, causing lung congestion, bronchial infections, and festering skin eruptions. Of all the organs in the human body today, the lower bowel is by far the most congested with toxic waste, and dredging these poisonous wastes from the colon should be a primary goal of any detox program. Unless the colon is thoroughly cleansed, no matter how well you clean your blood, liver, and other tissues, they will all soon become polluted again by toxins seeping into the bloodstream from the colon.

In TCM, rhubarb is the sovereign remedy for constipation, and it may be used singly or in combination with other bowel-cleansing herbs. A classic Chinese formula using rhubarb, listed in *A Handbook of Chinese Healing Herbs* as "Moisten Bowel Decoction," is given in the "Recipes and Formulas" section, appendix 1, page 310. The "Vit-ra-tox" line of internal cleansing supplements includes an excellent herbal laxative in convenient tablet form, containing cascara sagrada, aloe curacao, and licorice. This formula assists the elimination of impacted mucoid matter and putrefactive bacterial wastes in the colon, softens and clears solid obstructions that clog the bowels, and stimulates vigorous peristalsis in the large intestine. It may be ordered by mail directly from the source listed in "Suppliers."

A very effective way to deal with chronic constipation and clear clogged bowels during a detox program is to use powdered psyllium seed blended with various powdered herbs that have colon-cleansing properties. "Herbal Fiber Blend," made by AIM, has already been mentioned as an excellent example of this supplement. You may also prepare your own blend of psyllium and bowel detox herbs by combining one cup of ground psyllium with one level teaspoon each of the following powdered herbs: licorice root, slippery elm, cascara sagrada, and black walnut hulls. Mix the powders together with the psyllium until well blended, and use it the same way as plain psyllium.

If you have fresh aloe vera growing in your garden, or know someone who does, you can make a potent intestinal and lower-bowel cleanser by extracting the fresh juice. Simply cut a large leaf of aloe and scrape away the spiked edges, but do not peel. Cut it into chunks, place them in a blender, and puree. Squeeze the puree through a fine gauze cloth to extract the pure fluid, and discard the pulp. Drink one-to-two teaspoons, more or less, stirred in a glass of water on an empty stomach, first thing in the morning and again at bedtime. If the purging effects are too strong, cut down the dosage; if they're not strong enough, increase it a bit. Fresh aloe juice may be used as a lower-bowel-cleansing supplement in conjunction with a detox diet, or taken occasionally as needed for a week or two to stimulate sluggish bowels, deal with chronic constipation, or simply give the colon a periodic purge.

During a detox program, people with long-term bowel toxicity and other digestive disorders will sometimes experience an excess production of gas in the intestinal tract. This is caused by the activity of putrefactive bacteria as they are rousted from the bowels, by fermentation of dislodged toxic wastes, and by other biochemical reactions triggered in the digestive system by detox. If gas becomes a problem, you may use herbs with "carminative" properties to reduce gas reactions in the intestinal tract and relieve the flatulence it causes. A formula for carminative herbal tea to control gas is listed in appendix 1, page 312 in "Recipes and Formulas."

LUNGS AND BRONCHIA: CLEARING THE AIR VENT

The lungs are known as the "Prime Minister" of the internal organs, assisting the "King" heart with the task of circulating blood through the body, and regulating pulse and blood pressure by virtue of diaphragmic breathing. In addition to governing respiration and metabolism by supplying oxygen to the cells, the lungs also excrete carbon dioxide and other gaseous wastes from the body. The condition of the lungs is reflected externally in the skin: blemishes and other skin problems are often a manifestation of impaired lung function, and when both the lungs and the bowels are congested and clogged with mucus, toxic wastes are forced out of the body through the skin, causing further skin damage. If a person has recently quit a long-term smoking habit, a detox program will usually trigger a major expulsion of phlegm from the lungs and bronchia, as the body cleanses and repairs the lung tissues. This process may be assisted with the use of herbal "expectorants," which help dissolve phlegm and propel it out of the lungs and bronchial tubes. "Antitussive" herbs may be added to lung formulas to help control coughing and relieve sore throats, and "demulcent" herbs can be included to soothe the inflammation of the mucus membranes, which sometimes occurs as the lungs purge themselves of toxins, microbes, and air pollutants.

Lungwort and pleurisy root are two of the most powerful herbs for decongesting and healing the lungs. Dragon River Herbal makes a very good herbal lung formula called "Breath of Life," as a concentrated liquid extract, using lungwort, pleurisy root, osha root, horehound, and other herbs with specific affinity for the lungs. In addition to detoxifying and decongesting the lungs and clearing the bronchial tubes, this formula also strengthens weak lungs, tones bronchial tissues, and helps restore impaired lung functions.

In TCM, a tasty tea for clearing phlegm from the lungs may be prepared by boiling fresh ginger and dried licorice root in water for ten minutes, then straining out the liquid and adding a bit of honey to taste. This blend helps decongest the lungs and assists expectoration of phlegm from the bronchia. If persistent coughing is a problem during detox, you may use bee propolis in tincture form to soothe itchy throat, control coughing, and protect tender bronchial tissues from microbial infection. Simply stir ½ teaspoon of propolis tincture into a few ounces of hot water, add some honey to taste, and sip very slowly, so that it dribbles continuously down the throat.

One of the best forms of herbal therapy for detoxifying, decongesting, and restoring the lungs and bronchial system during a detox program is traditional Thai herbal steam, as discussed in chapter 2. All of the herbal steam blends given in appendix 1, page 302 of the "Recipes and Formulas" guide help cleanse and clear the lungs, promote elimination of phlegm and pollutants from the bronchial tubes, and facilitate breathing and respiration.

If you don't have access to an herbal steam room, you may improvise a steamer at home by placing a large pot of water on the stove and bringing it to a boil, then reducing the heat to a medium simmer. Add some aromatic herbs or essential oils with decongestant, bronchiodilating properties to the boiling water, such as cinnamon, eucalyptus, peppermint, camphor, and clove, then stand by the steaming pot and hold a heavy bath towel like a tent over your head to trap the steam as you bend over the pot to inhale the aromatic vapors. Use caution that you don't burn the skin of your face by leaning too close to the steam. This method is an excellent way to clean the lungs and clear the bronchial passages on a daily basis during a detox program, and it also may be used any time in daily life to quickly decongest the lungs and open up the bronchia.

BRAIN AND NERVES: CLEANING AND BALANCING THE CIRCUITS

Brain and nerve tissues are particularly susceptible to heavy metal and mineral toxicity. Owing to their electrical potential, brain and nerve cells attract heavy metals and other toxic metals like magnets. People who live and work in densely populated urban areas and highly industrialized regions, where factory and automobile exhaust pumps tons of toxic metals and minerals into the air every day, are very vulnerable to serious toxic damage to brain and nerve tissues from these sources. While virtually any type of detox diet or therapeutic fasting program helps eliminate toxic metals and minerals from the brain and nerves, people who live in places that are heavily contaminated with these pollutants may wish to take extra measures to purge these poisons from their brain and nerve tissues.

One of the best herbs for removing heavy metals from brain and nerve cells is cilantro (coriander), but it must be taken as a highly concentrated extract to be fully effective for this purpose. Cilantro has strong affinity for brain and nerve tissue, where it binds with and dislodges heavy metals clinging to neurons and nerve cells, allowing them to be flushed away in the blood and lymph. Dragon River Herbal produces a pure high-potency extract of cilantro made specifically for this purpose. Alternatively, you may ask someone who has the necessary skills and equipment to produce a concentrated cilantro extract for you.

Ginkgo biloba has long been known for its powerful antioxidant activity in the brain and nervous system, for which it has specific natural affinity. Ginkgo may be taken as a tea, tablet, or tincture to help clear the brain of toxic residues during a detox program. It may also be used as a regular daily supplement to provide long-term antioxidant protection to the brain against damage from environmental toxins.

"Nervine" herbs, which calm the nervous system, promote sound sleep, and restore balance to brain and nerve functions, can also be very helpful as supplemental support in a detox program. During detox, the bloodstream must carry an overload of toxic substances from the tissues to the excretory organs, and as these toxins circulate through the system awaiting elimination, they can aggravate and overexcite the brain and nerves, causing nervous tension, irritability, insomnia, and other symptoms of the "detox blues." When that occurs, the best solution is to take nervine herbal formulas that calm the nerves and soothe the brain, relax the mind and promote sound sleep. The body cannot remain in the state of rest and relaxation required to conduct detox and healing functions if the nervous system is "jumpy" from excessive toxic exposure and the brain is buzzing with toxic tension. Nervine herbs can therefore play a pivotal role in a detox program by preventing you from getting so wound up and impatient that you break your detox fast or cheat on your detox diet before completing the program.

Many excellent nervines in the herbal pharmacopoeia are available, including chamomile, passion flower, catnip, hops, St. John's wort, linden flowers, valerian, and lavender. These may be taken singly or in various combinations as teas or tinctures, and some of them, such as lavender, may be used as essential oils for aromatherapy. A formula for Nervine Tea that may be taken daily to calm the nerves and keep body and mind relaxed during a therapeutic fast or in a detox diet program is provided in "Recipes and Formulas," appendix 1, page 311. Several excellent nervine formulas in convenient liquid extract form are available from Dragon River Herbals, including a sound sleep formula called "Lights Out" and a relaxing nervine blend called "Peace & Quiet."

WORMS AND PARASITES

Worms, intestinal flukes, and dozens of other common parasites that enter and colonize the digestive tract generally don't cause much problem as long as they remain in the bowels, and the internal "climate" within the body remains properly balanced to keep them there. Serious problems can arise, however, when immune defenses weaken and the tissues enter a state of chronic acidosis and hypoxia. When the body is highly toxic and resistance is low, worms and parasites flourish out of control and spread quickly to parts of the body where they are not supposed to go, such as the liver and brain.

All parasites feed and thrive on the body's own nutrients, robbing the human system of the essential nutrition it requires to sustain health, and excrete their toxic metabolic wastes into the body's tissues. Parasites are therefore a major source of blood and tissue toxicity. As they multiply and spread, they gobble up an ever greater portion of the body's nutrients, further weakening the body's defenses and polluting the internal terrain. Herbs that destroy worms and other parasites so that they may be eliminated from the system are known as "anthelmintic," and they are very effective for ridding the body of these tenacious pests.

The most effective blend of herbs for overall worm and parasite control is the "Triplex" formula of unripened black walnut hull, wormwood, and clove. These herbs may be ground to a fine powder and taken in capsules, or taken as concentrated liquid extracts, which are far more convenient. The Triplex formula must be taken continuously for two to three months, in precise daily dosages, to achieve a complete eradication of all parasites, including the larva and eggs. When used in conjunction with the electronic "Zapper" device introduced in the next chapter, the Triplex formula effectively eradicates over a hundred varieties of parasite from every nook and cranny in the body. The Triplex tinctures are available in many herb shops and health stores, and may also be ordered by mail from Dragon River Herbal in the USA or Inner Glow Health Products in Australia. Be sure to ask your supplier to provide you with a copy of the proper dosage schedule.

Other herbs that help eliminate worms and parasites include pumpkin-seed extract, gentian root, quassia bark, neem leaves, garlic, and ginger. The latter two may be added fresh to all vegetable dishes during a detox diet to provide extra anthelmintic action. They may also be incorporated into your daily diet for ongoing protection against infestation by parasites.

"THE PEOPLE'S MEDICINE"

Traditional herbal medicine permits people to treat most of their own common health problems—including the root problem of tissue toxicity —safely and effectively at home, at far less cost and hazard to health than modern pharmaceutical drugs. In a study published by the World Health Organization (WHO) in 1992, medicinal herbs are described as "the people's medicine." The report states that "medicinal plants offer . . . immediate access to safe and effective products for use in the treatment of illness by self-medication," and that "the proper use of medicinal plants in therapy is a necessity, not a luxury." As pathogens grow ever more resistant to the effects of chemical drugs, these drugs become less and less effective in controlling even the most superficial symptoms of disease, while also making the root problem of toxicity much worse—all at ever-growing expense and hazard to the consumer.

The reason that herbal medicine still remains "the people's medicine" is because herbs cannot be patented, and thereby monopolized, by private pharmaceutical companies. Consequently, herbs remain affordable to almost everyone, and people can grow many of them in their own gardens at home. Moreover, some of the most effective medicinal herbs on earth are also among the most common and inexpensive, and this is especially true of internal cleansing herbs. When body and mind remain relaxed and at rest and the nervous system switches over to the healing mode of the parasympathetic branch, the hormones, enzymes, and other natural biochemicals produced in the body work in therapeutic synergy with the organic phytochemicals released into the system by medicinal herbs. As long as correct dietary principles and other guidelines are followed and medicinal herbs are properly selected and prepared, they always enhance the cleansing and healing process during detox, without causing the unpleasant and hazardous side-effects that chemical drugs invariably do. Owing to their specific natural affinity for various organs and tissues in the body, medicinal herbs may be selected and blended with great precision to achieve particular therapeutic results in specifically targeted parts of the body. With a bit of common sense and the aid of a good practical guide to the use of medicinal herbs at home, such as *A Handbook of Chinese Healing Herbs* and *A Handbook of Native American Herbs,** almost anyone can formulate and prepare their own basic herbal teas and boiled decoctions for detox purposes at home or can select the right blends of herbal tablets and tinctures in any health shop, exactly according to their own personal requirements. While it is always best to also seek guidance from a qualified health professional who specializes in herbal therapy, such guidance is not yet widely available in many parts of the world. So those who wish to harness the healing power of herbs for detox and healing at home must take "the people's medicine" into their own hands and administer it to their own bodies, along with the other "healing angels" of food, water, air, and sunlight.

---

*Published by Shambhala Publications, Boston, Mass., USA.

9

HIGH-TECH
ELECTRO-DETOX

In addition to traditional methods of detoxifying and healing the human body, such as fasting, hydrotherapy, heliotherapy, and herbs, a variety of high-tech "electro-detox" devices are now available. They have been developed by independent medical researchers using the latest advances in modern electronics and computer technology. In fact, the alternative health-care market has become flooded with new gadgets and gizmos that promise to cure you of everything from arthritis to zygomycosis and correct whatever else might be wrong with you as well, with the simple push of a button. Buyer beware! While traditional healing methods such as herbs and acupuncture are tried-and-true therapies that have been proven safe and effective over time, many of these new electronic devices, with all their impressive bells and whistles and blinking lights, have no therapeutic value whatsoever, and some of them can even do you harm. Therefore, it is always best to exercise caution when selecting new high-tech tools for detox, and to consult with someone who has experience in their use. Properly applied, some of these electro-detox devices can greatly facilitate the cleansing and healing process, while also correcting basic imbalances in the human energy system that are the root cause of many physical disorders. It is therefore well worth familiarizing yourself with some of these new technologies, and learning how to use them to assist the detox and healing process.

THE HUMAN ENERGY SYSTEM

Since most electro-detox devices work through the human energy system, it is helpful to understand the basic principles of human energy. The entire human body and all its myriad parts operate on energy in much the same way that a complex mainframe computer runs on electricity. As long as all the circuits are open and sufficient power is running freely through the system, all the various functional subsystems and moving parts operate smoothly. But as soon as there's a short circuit somewhere in the energy network, or a blocked relay, blown fuse, or rusted switch, the whole system goes haywire, and all sorts of strange symptoms begin to develop in the physical apparatus. It won't help to add some oil here, or change a part there, or fiddle with the dials. To restore proper function, you must fix the root problem by finding and clearing the blockages in the energy system, rebalancing the circuits, and restoring the power supply to all the parts of the system.

The human energy system (HES) constitutes an invisible template of energy that powers and regulates the entire physical body. By using external sources of energy to recharge and rebalance the HES, each cell in every tissue of the body is revitalized and all vital functions are restored to normal. The HES has three basic dimensions. The one most directly related to organic functions of the body is the system of twelve organ-energy meridians, which activate and control the vital organs and their related glands and tissues. This system is the energy network used for acupuncture therapy in TCM. Another dimension of the HES is the chakra system, comprised of seven chakras, or "energy wheels" stacked one above the other from coccyx to crown along the spinal column, like a pagoda of energy. Known as "elixir fields" *(dan-tien)* in TCM, the chakras function as energy transformers to "step down" the ultra-high frequencies of cosmic energy that radiate from sky to earth and enter the human system through the crown chakra on top of the head. Each chakra receives specific frequencies of these higher energies and transforms them into patterns and vibrational rates compatible with the HES. They are then transmitted to energize specific functions of both body and mind. Whenever a blockage or imbalance develops in a particular chakra, the related physical and mental functions become impaired, and the body grows vulnerable to disease and degeneration.

The third aspect of human energy is known in TCM as *wei-chi,* or "Guardian Energy." It travels around the whole body just below and above the surface of the skin, forming a protective shield against invasive external energies. This surface shield of Guardian Energy is the inner-most core of the multilayered human energy field (HEF), which has numerous additional shells of auric energy of increasingly subtler quality surrounding and overlapping it. For the purposes of physical health and healing, it is mainly this inner core of the HEF that is treated in bio-electric energy medicine. With all the hazardous unnatural energies and artificial electromagnetic fields in the environment today, the protective role of Guardian Energy in fending off negative energies and resisting harmful force fields is more important than ever to human health and longevity.

Internally, each and every one of the body's 75 trillion cells functions like a microbattery and has its own individual polarity and energy field. Collectively, the sum total of all this cellular energy determines the overall strength and radiance of Guardian Energy field and represents the net potential energy available to the whole system. If a blockage or imbalance in the flow of energy occurs in a particular part of the body due to damaged or toxic tissues, trillions of cells are "unplugged" from the energy system and go "off-line," deflating the Guardian Energy field and drastically reducing the power supply to the whole system. This results in low immunity and weak resistance and opens the gate to disease and invasive external energies.

The overall electrical potential of the HEF can easily be measured with an ordinary volt meter. A robust individual with the "glow of good health" will register a significantly higher electrical potential than a weak and ailing individual, while a corpse doesn't even budge the meter's needle. Electromagnetic energy is one of the fundamental energies that activate the universe and everything in it. The HEF functions within the greater context of the earth's and the sun's electromagnetic fields and is strongly influenced by any fluctuations in planetary and solar energies. The specific frequencies of electromagnetic energy that activate organic life are known to modern energy healers as "bioelectric energy," or simply "bio-energy." In TCM, electromagnetic energy is called "True Energy." Electro-detox devices generate this spectrum of bio-electric energy and transmit it into the HES to recharge and rebalance it. The potential significance of these recent discoveries to the future of human health and healing is incalculable. As Dr. Robert Becker, one of the world's leading authorities on human energy and bio-electric therapy, states:

> The data obtained in the past few years indicate very clearly that we must now include the earth's normal geomagnetic field as an environmental variable of great consequence when we deal with the basic functions of living things. . . . It provides us with a key to the mechanisms by which all electromagnetic fields produce biological effects.

Dr. Becker's research provides scientific confirmation of the ancient Chinese view of the human energy system as a complex network consisting of hundreds of energy channels and overlapping energy fields that may be manipulated to transmit therapeutic energies into the human system to heal the body, balance the mind, and correct deviations in the HES. Dr. Becker has developed techniques to activate the body's innate self-cleansing and healing responses by applying electrical stimulation to the HEF. He has invented electronic devices that may be used to accelerate the mending of broken bones and the healing of traumatic wounds. These units produce precisely the correct wave patterns and energy frequencies required to signal the brain to activate and sustain internal cleansing and healing responses.

THE HAZARDS OF ELECTROMAGNETIC
ENERGY POLLUTION

In traditional medicine, the human energy system (HES) serves as a functional bridge between body and mind, and energy is the therapeutic medium that heals and balances both physical disease and mental malaise. Today, the HES has come under intensive attack from an entirely new phenomenon that the human system has never before had to face. This new threat to human health and longevity is the rapidly growing hazard of electromagnetic "energy pollution." Since the industrial revolution and the subsequent electronic age, the earth's electromagnetic energy environment has become intensely polluted with artificial electromagnetic fields (EMF), unnatural radio frequencies, microwave radiation, nuclear radiation, and many other forms of aberrant energy that cause severe deviations and imbalances in the HES. Today, there are 250 million times more artificially generated radio frequencies in the earth's atmosphere than there were in 1930. These invisible but highly reactive energy waves and artificial EMF from high-voltage power lines, transformers, and home appliances have become the big unknown factor in all the vital equations of human health, and they constitute the hidden cause in many common human ailments, from cancer to schizophrenia. This pollution of our energy environment is even more hazardous to the human system than chemical and ecological pollution, and it calls for an entirely new approach to healing, an approach that effectively protects the HES from distortion by artificial energies and EMF and cures the conditions they cause.

Let's take a quick look at some of the most widespread and hazardous forms of electromagnetic energy pollution on the earth today. High-voltage alternating current power lines and transformers, which operate at 60 hertz, create an artificial EMF of one hundred milligauss extending twenty-two yards around them. At a range of twelve inches from the human body, three milligauss has been determined to be the level of exposure to EMF above which cancer and brain damage can occur.

As Dr. Robert Becker, one of the world's leading authorities on energy medicine, writes in his book *Cross Currents:*

> At this time, the scientific evidence is absolutely conclusive: sixty hertz magnetic fields cause human cancer cells to permanently increase their rate of growth by as much as 1,600 percent and to develop more malignant characteristics.

The two types of human tissue most seriously damaged by artificially generated EMF are brain tissue and rapidly developing tissues, such as those in growing children, because these tissues display the most electrical activity and are therefore most strongly affected by external EMF.

Common household appliances produce artificial EMF that brings energy pollution straight into your own home and expose every member of the family to danger. Electric blankets create fields of 50–100 milligauss, far above safe levels, and pregnant women who use them are known to experience a far higher than normal rate of miscarriage. Electric razors operated from a plug-in power line generate highly hazardous fields ranging from 200–400 milligauss, a risk to the brain behind the beard that is hardly worth the "convenience" of not having to use shaving cream and a razor. A 10-watt fluorescent light tube produces an artificial EMF that is twenty times stronger than an ordinary 60-watt bulb, and in offices and school rooms lit by multiple banks of fluorescent tubes, everyone in the room is exposed to aberrant EMF far above the level of safety for human health. Electric hair dryers produce a harmful field of 50 milligauss at six inches, and this factor is suspected as the cause of the abnormally high rate of breast cancer among professional beauticians and hair dressers, who operate these devices all day only inches from their chests. At 12 inches, an electric stove will expose you to an EMF of 50 milligauss, far above the 3 milligauss safety limit, so if you do a lot of cooking at home, it is much safer to use gas. The list goes on and on, but by now you probably get the picture.

All of these artificial energy fields and unnatural energy frequencies to which humans are today routinely exposed also catalyze extremely harmful reactions between toxic chemical pollutants and natural biochemicals within the human body. These reactions create all sorts of noxious poisons in the tissues and have extremely strong acid-forming effects in the bloodstream and other bodily fluids, thereby upsetting the all-important natural pH balance in the blood and tissues and causing a state of chronic acidosis. Acidosis of blood and tissues is a primary precondition for the development of *all* cancers.

Despite the proven risk of exposure to artificial EMF over 3 mG, very few countries have legislated legal limits to the EMF produced by machines and appliances at home and in offices and factories. In Sweden, strict laws prohibit EMF exposure to humans above 2.5 mG, and in Russia, where this hazard has been extensively researched, the limit is an even safer 1.5 mG. Compare that with the legal limit of 1,000–5,000 mG exposure to EMF for people in homes, offices, and schools in Australia, and similar hazardous levels in America, Canada, and the UK, as well as most of Asia. Small wonder that one in four people today develop some form of cancer, and that brain disorders and mental malaise have become rampant throughout the world.

The net result of chronic exposure to these various forms of invisible EMF energy pollution is an ongoing onslaught against the balance and integrity of the HES and its surrounding bio-energy field. This exposure, in turn, poses a constant challenge to health that drains the entire system of vital energy. Abnormal EMF fields and unnatural frequencies disrupt all of the body's vital functions, weaken immune response, disturb the mind, and contribute much to the development of a chronic state of acidosis and tissue toxicity. Traditional energy medicine such as acupuncture, heliotherapy, aromatherapy, and breathing are usually insufficient to deal with the deep deviations in the human energy system caused by abnormal EMF and microwave pollution. The only way to counteract these new hazards to health and repair the damage they cause is to "fight with fire" by applying the latest advances in high-tech, electro-detox therapies.

THE GLOBAL MICROWAVE "OVEN"

Brain tumors have also been conclusively related with microwave pollution, and the worst offenders are wireless cell phones, which drive a powerful beam of microwave radiation straight into the brain. During the Cold War, the Soviet Union beamed microwaves at the American Embassy in Moscow from a rooftop across the street. As a result, one American ambassador and several staff members developed cancer. The level of microwave radiation they used for that purpose was *less* than that at which an ordinary household microwave oven operates. Here's what Dr. Robert Becker has to say about microwaves:

> The scientific data at this time indicate that microwaves have major biological effects at power levels *far below* those required to cause heating [such as microwave ovens]. The majority of these effects are productive of various disease states, primarily cancer and genetic defects, in those exposed and in their unexposed offspring. . . . The hazard comes from the fact that exposure to microwaves, like exposure to any abnormal electromagnetic field, produces stress, a decline in immune-system competency, and changes in the genetic apparatus. Thus the levels of exposure that governments say are "safe" are in fact not safe at all.

Think about that next time you receive a call on your cell phone or heat up a pizza in a microwave oven.

The human body, particularly the electrically active brain, is extremely sensitive to disruption from the high-frequency electromagnetic radiation produced by cell phones and cell-phone transmission towers. Our brains and bodies depend on hundreds of delicately balanced, internally generated, electrical impulses to conduct the vital functions of life, and these are thrown into disarray by the invasive ultrahigh frequencies generated externally by cell phones and phone towers. As Blake Levitt states in his book *Electromagnetic Fields,* "When it comes to mobile phones, a worse frequency could not have been chosen for the human anatomy." Researcher Carolanne Patton has found that "the brain reaches peak absorption in the UHF bands, right where cellular (mobile phone) telecommunications operate."

Since the advent of cell phones, there has been a 600 percent increase in automobile accidents among drivers who use these devices. This alarming rise in road fatalities and injuries is not due to the "distraction" of speaking on a cell phone. The increase in driving accidents is due to impairment of brain function and nerve response while such phones are being used. Tests conducted by the U.S. Department of Energy found that "using mobile phones impairs memory and reaction times. 'Hand-free' mobile speakerphones cause even more crashes because they typically emit 10-times more brainwave interference than handheld units." This elevation of intensity is due to the metal frame of the car, which amplifies the field frequencies produced by cell phones and speakers used in automobiles. A University of Toronto study concludes that "the heightened probability of crashing your car persists for up to 15 minutes after completing a call," and Dr. Chris Rumball of the B.C. Medical Association notes, "This is comparable to driving while dead drunk."

One of the leading experts on cell-phone hazards was the late biophysicist Dr. Neil Cherry of Lincoln University in New Zealand, where mobile-phone towers are prohibited on school grounds due to their hazardous influence on human health, particularly the rapidly developing nervous systems of children. His research showed accelerated aging, rapid cell death, and an increase in cancer rates caused by microwave radiation from cell phones and phone towers. He warned that frequent exposure to these frequencies disrupt the delicate balance of the brain's electro-chemical communications and can result in chronic headaches, fatigue, lethargy, nausea, dizziness, depression, arteriosclerosis, and possibly Alzheimer's disease. "There is also a higher incidence of cardiac problems," states Dr. Cherry. "It has now been shown in many studies that mobile-phone users get more heart attacks and more heart disease." He also discovered that the imbalances in the brain of essential minerals such as calcium, various trace elements, and neurotransmitters such as serotonin caused by mobile phones can easily alter moods and result in depression, suicide, rage, and violent behavior.

Another scientist who has issued public warnings about the hazards of mobile phones is Dr. George Carlo, who found that rare types of brain tumors have more than doubled among mobile-phone users, particularly on the side of the head where they use their phones. "Mobile phones cause genetic damage leading to cancer," states Dr. Carlo bluntly, and he recommends "prudent avoidance" of these devices after finding that every type of mobile phone tested exceeded U.S. Federal Communications Commission's own standards for EMF absorption rates. Dr. Carlo notes that "the more a person uses a mobile phone, the more cellular destruction and health risks they incur. Mobile-phone-confused cells can go crazy. Experiments on captive animals show that this cumulative DNA damage is passed on to succeeding generations." A study conducted at Adelaide Hospital in Australia confirmed Dr. Carlo's conclusions when it demonstrated a doubling in the rate of B-cell lymphoma cancer in mice after eighteen months of only one-hour exposure daily to the frequencies used in mobile-phone technology.

Studies conducted by Dr. Peter French in Sydney, Australia, show that "cells are permanently damaged by mobile-phone frequencies and inherited unchanged, from generation to generation." Dr. French also found that "the production of histamine, which triggers bronchial spasms, is nearly doubled after exposure to mobile-phone transmissions." Mobile phones also reduce the effectiveness of anti-asthmatic drugs and retard recovery from illness. Since the introduction of mobile phones, metropolitan Sydney has experienced a 25-percent increase in the incidence of asthma and a 5-percent increase in asthma-related deaths.

One of the most disturbing effects of exposure to mobile-phone transmissions is the disruption of the delicate, protective mechanism known as the "blood brain barrier," which is designed by nature to prevent toxins and other dangerous substances from entering the brain from the bloodstream. Swedish neurologist Professor Leif Salford stated to the Daily Mail his finding that after a two-minute conversation on a mobile phone, "It seems that molecules such as proteins and toxins can pass out of the blood, while the phone is switched on, and enter the brain. We need to bear in mind diseases such as MS and Alzheimer's, which are linked to proteins being found in the brain." The accumulation of toxic residues in the brain due to the malfunction of the blood brain barrier caused by exposure to radiation from mobile phones and phone towers can also lead to the formation of tumors in the brain, which then grow even faster than normal as a direct result of exposure to abnormal EMF, as noted above by Dr. Robert Becker.

You don't even have to be using your cell phone to receive or make a call to suffer serious damage. In one hospital in Australia, nurses noted a direct correspondence between which side of the body kidney cancer occurred in patients and which side of the body they habitually wore their cell phones on their belts. Men who carry cell phones in their front pockets run the risk of sterility, impotence, and even testicular cancer, and women who keep mobile phones in their pockets risk the same problems with their ovaries. As EMF researcher Dave Ashton states, "Because mobile phones constantly search for the nearest repeating tower, long-term damage comes from mobile phones in the stand-by mode." And if you think the analogy of a global microwave oven is an exaggeration, then consider this: if you place a mobile phone on stand-by mode in the cavity of a fresh raw chicken and leave it there for about three days, the microwave radiation from the phone will cook the chicken.

The telecommunications industry is trying very hard to prevent these facts from coming to light to protect what has become a $50-billion-dollar-a-year industry. But the scientific research is conclusive: artificial electromagnetic fields, microwave radiation from cell phones, and transmissions from phone towers pose a serious hazard to human health and cause particularly serious damage to the brain and immune system. Only two ways exist to avoid these serious threats to your health and longevity: either stop using these high-frequency electronic devices, or else start using high-tech devices that are designed to transform harmful EMF and microwave radiation into harmonious patterns that are compatible with the bio-electric energies of life.

It is quite obvious by now that the chemical/mechanical model upon which modern allopathic medicine is based does not accord with the real facts of human health, for it fails to account for the most important factors of all in health and healing—energy and energy fields. The human body is an integrated system of energy networks. Those networks collectively produce a human energy field that interacts with the earth's own energy field and other natural EMF from sky and earth. The recent rapid rise in the earth's own vibrational frequency is perhaps the most significant factor of all for human health today, because it means that to remain in a state of vibrant health and vitality, people must take measures to raise the vibrational rate of their own personal energy fields if they are to remain in a healthy state of resonant harmony with the planet. To do this, people today must progressively detoxify their systems—both physically and energetically—to rid their systems of dense, low-frequency energies. We must utilize devices that counteract dangerous EMF radiation from our daily living and working environment, thereby strengthening our immunity to disease and raising our resistance to the invasive influence of exposure to hazardous artificial energy fields.

Today, the human energy system is under severe frontal attack from a wide range of unnatural EMF and artificial energy radiation produced by broadcasting stations, power lines, cell phones, microwave transmission towers, military installations, and other conventional technology. The damage these sources have done, and continue to do, to human health throughout the world is incalculable. Here's what Dr. Becker has to say about the medical significance of these recent discoveries regarding the dangers of EMF, and the current developments to counteract these risks :

The data obtained in the past few years indicate very clearly that we must now include the Earth's normal geomagnetic field as an environmental variable of great consequence when we deal with the basic functions of living things. In my opinion, this knowledge is probably the single most important discovery of the century. It provides us with a key to the mechanisms by which all electromagnetic fields produce biological effects, and it may enable us to determine more accurately the risks involved in our technological uses of such fields.

"Forewarned is forearmed!"

PRESCRIPTION FOR "BIO-ELECTRIC ENERGY MEDICINE"

The primacy of energy over matter as the most decisive factor in human health and life in general has been proven beyond a doubt in scientific theory and clinical practice, but the mainstream medical industry still clings stubbornly to its vested interests in the chemical/mechanical approach of allopathic and surgical medicine and continues to turn a blind eye to these new discoveries. But that fact has not prevented the inventive wizards of high-tech alternative medical science from forging ahead on their own to develop new healing technologies based on the view of the human body as a dynamic, interactive bio-electric energy field, and to invent devices that allow prescriptions for bio-electric energy medicine to be delivered safely into the human energy system.

The tricky part of this new bio-electric medical technology is to accurately replicate the precise frequencies, currents, and wave patterns of human energy, to reproduce their intricate pulses and complex rhythms, and then to introduce these externally generated energies into the human bio-field. While many of the new gadgets on the market today are useless and sometimes even hazardous, several recently developed bio-electric energy devices have demonstrated remarkable results as therapeutic tools for detoxifying, repairing, and rebalancing the human body.

In previous chapters, we briefly discussed how two of these new inventions—the GEOMED Activated Air System, and the alkalized, ionized microclustered water system—which use electric energy to boost the potency of air and water as cleansing and healing elements in the body. In the following pages, we'll take a look at five more high-tech electro-detox devices that may be safely and effectively used in conjunction with traditional therapies to enhance and hasten cleansing and healing functions during a detox program. These methods have all been extensively tested and proven therapeutically effective in clinical practice, and they may all be safely used at home as well.

THE "JAI" ELECTRO-PRESSURE REGENERATION THERAPY

The "Jai" device is a small, pocket-sized unit operated by battery that produces a gentle wave of electrons that sweep through the body's tissues and recharge each and every cell with "electro-pressure." Driven by currents that are compatible with the natural bio-electric energies of the HES, the Jai delivers detoxifying antioxidant activity to the whole system and stimulates rapid healing of wounds and damaged organs. Clinical studies have shown that the Jai unit accelerates the rate of healing in elderly people and brings it up to par with that of youth by regenerating the body's ability to cleanse and repair itself.

As previously noted, water has a unique capacity to record and transmit any energy patterns and frequencies to which it is exposed. The Jai takes advantage of the natural conductivity of water by using it as a medium in which an externally generated electric charge interacts with the bio-electric charge of the human energy field to produce therapeutic effects in the human system. Acting as a sympathetic mediator between the body's energy field and the healing field produced by the Jai device, the water generates a bio-electric energy field that harmonizes the HEF with the incoming energy waves from the unit, thereby creating a therapeutically beneficial bio-electric field. This effect is achieved by soaking absorbent foam-padded bands in water, wrapping them snugly around the wrists or ankles, where the patterns and pulses of the HES broadcast most clearly, then attaching an electrode from the unit to each band. This process allows the incoming electric charge to interact and blend with the patterns of the HES imprinted in the water within the bands. Adapting the external charge to the precise conditions of human energy, the water then conducts the signals from the resulting balanced bio-field directly into the body, where it enters the energy channels, which in turn deliver the precisely programmed therapeutic energy pulses to the whole system.

Electro-pressure regeneration therapy provides manifold benefits to human health and longevity. The incoming bio-electric charge opens the energy meridians, increases energy flow, and balances energy distribution throughout the system. It relieves pain and reduces inflammation in the soft tissues of the body, promotes rapid healing of wounds, and elevates immune response. The Jai's potent antioxidant activity mops up free radicals and neutralizes toxins throughout the body, which makes it particularly effective as a supporting therapy for any type of detox program. Unlike nutritional and herbal antioxidants, which depend on the vagaries of the digestive and circulatory systems for delivery, electro-pressure regeneration therapy overrides the physical pathways and delivers its vigorous antioxidant activity directly to every tissue and cell of the body via the bio-electric template of the HES. The Jai may also be used in the course of daily life for a quick, convenient "minidetox," and to recharge and rebalance the whole system whenever energy runs low.

TESLA'S INNOVATIONAL TECHNOLOGIES

As modern quantum physics continues to verify the universal principles of energy dynamics that lie at the heart of traditional holistic-healing systems, modern technology is beginning to develop new techniques and devices that greatly amplify and expand the therapeutic applications of energy medicine, giving birth to the exciting new field of "Bio-Electro-Energy Medicine."

One of the most important new developments in energy medicine is the line of titanium products made by Tesla's Innovational Technologies in Australia. These products are based on the original scientific genius of Nikola Tesla, the man who invented modern electric power systems in the early twentieth century. After realizing the harm that EMF, from high-voltage AC electric power lines and other electromagnetic radiation, causes to human health, he developed a method to alter the atomic structure of titanium so that it becomes a transceiver of a very fine, bio-friendly energy known as "photon" or "tachyon" energy. A photon is energy from subatomic particles of light that radiate from the center of the universe and have the power to override harmful EMF and micro-wave radiation and transform them into patterns that are compatible with the energies of life.

Before his death, Tesla gave the plans for the device that alters tita-nium for this purpose to one of his most trusted students, who subse-quently brought it to Australia, where it was in turn passed on to the person who now utilizes this highly advanced technology to produce a variety of titanium products specifically designed to transform harmful electromagnetic fields and radiation from various sources in our daily living environment. Titanium was selected for this purpose because it has a similar molecular structure to human bone, thus allowing the bio-friendly frequencies emitted by the titanium plates to resonate through-out the human skeletal structure. The harmonious fields and frequencies that the titanium products create are therefore easily conducted by reso-nance throughout the entire human system.

Born in Europe in 1856, Nikola Tesla migrated to the United States in 1884 and worked for a while with Thomas Edison. Widely regarded as the greatest scientific genius of the early twentieth century, Tesla owned sixteen hundred patents on his many inventions and received twenty-seven honorary degrees for his work from universities around the world. In 1912, he demonstrated what he referred to as a "free energy" device, which would allow every building and household to provide its own electric energy, free of cost, and without hazard to human health. His invention was promptly suppressed by the banker J. P. Morgan, who had invested heavily in the conventional electric-energy generation system, whereby every home and building is linked to a meter and must pay for every minute of power. While most of Tesla's papers were confiscated after his death, his design for a device to alter certain metals so that they become transceivers of photon energy to counteract the harmful effects of EMF radiation was fortunately passed safely to the hands of a young physicist whom Tesla trusted. Today this technology is the basis of the entire line of Tesla's Innovational Technologies energy products.

Each titanium plate in Tesla's device is specifically designed and energized for specific functions, with variations in diameter, thickness, circumference, and time spent in Tesla's energizing chamber. A selection of the most useful products in daily life are briefly described below:

Phone Tag

This is a small octagonal disk about the size of a standard button. It adheres to the back of a cell or cordless phone, near the antenna, to alter the hazardous frequencies coming to and from cordless, handheld phones. This small plate may also be used to help heal eye injuries, by sticking it to an eye patch (concave side toward the eye), and wearing the patch over the injured eye.

Users of the phone tag report fewer headaches and less mental confusion when they use phones with the titanium button attached.

Personal Pendants

The personal pendant is designed to be worn around the neck, so that the pendant rests concave-side down over the thymus gland. This plate is about 1 inch in diameter and is designed to take on the unique vibrational signature of the person who wears it. Therefore, it should be worn constantly for at least the first twenty-four hours, after which your individual frequency patterns will be imprinted on it. This plate then becomes your personal pendant and should not be lent or given to anyone else.

This pendant comes in three levels of strength: children; teenager; and adult. Each is designed for the specific requirements of humans in different stages of growth, and all of them strengthen the human energy field, boost immunity, and transform harmful electromagnetic radiation to which the wearer may be exposed. One of its most important functions is to keep the personal field vibration of the wearer in tune with the swiftly rising vibrational rate of the planet (Schumann Resonance). The pendant does this by first adjusting its own vibration to the planet's rising pulse, then transferring that elevation to the human energy field. The plate's harmonizing effect between the fields of the wearer and the whole earth gives a big boost to overall health and vitality, increases immunity and resistance, and is particularly beneficial for practitioners of energy work and spiritual awareness. The pendants come in a variety of shapes, sizes, and colors. Your selection reflects your personal energy traits, so we encourage you to pick the pendant that somehow "turns you on."

Travel Plate

Travel plates are designed to be carried in the pocket, wallet, or purse, to counteract harmful EMF radiation, especially when traveling or walking around a crowded city. It may also be placed concave-side down over a wounded area of the body, to accelerate healing and relieve pain. In a restaurant or at home, you can energize your water and other beverages, as well as your food, by placing the travel plate concave-side up under the glass or plate for a few minutes.

Computer Plate

Specifically designed to counteract various forms of harmful EMF radiation from computers, this plate has a powerful pulse that is not suitable for keeping in a pocket or purse. It should be placed on top of the computer screen, concave-side down over the area just behind the screen.

House Plate

This is a large thick plate of energized titanium that is programmed to transform harmful EMF and microwave radiation for an entire house, extending for an area of one-acre around the house. It may be placed concave-side up or down depending whether the source of the EMF is below ground (Ley lines, underground streams, etc.) or above ground (power lines, phone towers, transformers, etc.).

Car Plate

The car plate covers an area extending 3.3 yards from the concave side and 1 yard from the convex dome. It was developed to alter the EMF inside a car, which can be harmful to drivers and passengers. In other uses it can be placed: under a massage table (concave-side up) to help put the client in a calm alpha state; in a small room (such as a hotel bedroom) to counteract EMF; in a person's energy aura to counteract damage from X rays, microwaves, and other EMF; and close to water and food, to energize them.

The Tesla's line also includes a variety of other energized titanium products designed to counteract harmful effects from artificial EMF and microwave sources in our environment. Products include a Farm Plate to cover an entire farm, a power stabilizer to harmonize the EMF from household appliances by transforming the electric-current patterns through the entire electric wiring system in a house, Practitioner's Plates for healers and energy therapists, and a device to restore vital energy to piped water that enters a house through taps. A complete listing of the products and prices may be found on the Tesla's website: www.teslas.us.

THE BEFE "BIO-ELECTRIC BATH"

Q-Tech of Australia has recently developed an electromagnetic device that programs ordinary water as a powerful tool for detoxification and healing. This system, known as the "Bio-Electric Field Enhancer" (BEFE), utilizes bath water as a medium to cleanse the lymphatic system and rebalance the entire human energy field. In TCM, the "True Energy" that activates the human body is regarded as the essential force of life, the fundamental foundation of health, and the primary key to healing. This is the energy that the BEFE unit manipulates to stimulate detox and healing responses in the human body.

Like the Jai device, BEFE technology utilizes water as a medium to transfer healing energy signals into the body and rebalance the human energy field. Since water reproduces and holds the precise patterns and vibratory rates of any energy field to which it has been exposed, when the adult human body—which itself is 70 percent water—is submerged in a tub of water, the body's bio-energy field imprints itself and produces an exact personal "energy profile" in the water, including all the imbalances and deviations that require correcting. At the same time, the

BEFE unit introduces a perfectly balanced, properly tuned bio-energy field into the water, where it interfaces and interacts with the body's energy field, correcting imbalances and adjusting abnormalities in the latter until the two fields harmonize and resonate as one in the water. When the body's bio-energy field has been recharged and rebalanced by the externally generated bio-electric field in the water, the physical body responds immediately to the properly balanced signals by detoxifying and repairing itself. Note that BEFE therapy may be applied in a foot bath as well, with equally effective results.

By correcting faulty circuits in the HES and restoring balance in the body's bio-field, BEFE therapy triggers a major cleansing response through the skin, drawing toxic residues and acid wastes out from the subcutaneous tissues and lymph channels, and excreting them through the skin into the bath water. Naturopathic healers in Australia who have used this device in their clinical practice report that some of their more toxic clients turn the bath water brown with toxic wastes excreted through the skin, after only twenty to thirty minutes of therapy. This therapy is powerful detox technology; it is best to seek some professional guidance when using it at home, or else try it at a naturopathic clinic or spa first.

THE "ZAPPER"

In the course of her research into the hazards posed to human health from infestation by common parasites, particularly the nasty "fluke" (*Fasciolopsis buskii*), which uses the human intestinal tract as a breeding and picnic ground, Dr. Hulda Clarke has developed a small, battery-operated device that generates an eight-volt current of 30Khz with a square wave pattern, precisely tuned to destroy, or "zap," these tenacious parasites, without harming the human body. Popularly known as the "Zapper," this device may be used in conjunction with the "Triplex" herbal parasite formula introduced in the previous chapter, for even better results.

According to Dr. Clarke and many other naturopathic healers, one of the primary causes of some of the world's most virulent and often fatal ailments is the extreme tissue toxicity produced by the poisonous secretions and metabolic wastes that flukes and other parasites release inside the body. Common debilitating conditions such as asthma, cancer, chronic fatigue syndrome, and candida fungal infections often develop as a direct result of parasite infestation, and whenever parasites are the primary cause of these ailments, the only effective cure is a complete eradication of all parasites in the body. The elimination of parasites is the specific purpose for which the Zapper was invented. Victims of chronic asthma and candida infection usually respond quickly to antiparasite therapy, and several lifelong asthmatics in Australia who used the Zapper for this purpose report that they no longer needed to use inhalers and could breathe freely again after only ten weeks of treatment.

When using the Zapper, carefully follow the treatment protocol. Treatments are usually done in three consecutive sessions of seven minutes each, with a fifteen-minute pause in between. The reason for this sequence is that some of the parasites inside the human body carry smaller parasites within themselves, and when they're "zapped" and killed by the incoming electric wave, they release these other parasites directly into the body, and some of the new parasites are even more toxic to human tissues than their hosts. Therefore, the second round of treatment knocks out these hidden fellow travelers, and the third round mops up any survivors of the first two. Dr. Clarke's recommended treatment schedule for a complete elimination of parasites is as follows:

Week 1:   One session per day of three consecutive seven-minute periods, with a fifteen-minute pause in between.

Week 2:   One session per day of only one seven-minute period.

Week 3:   One session every two days of only one seven-minute period, for a total of three times in the week.

Week 4:   One session per week of only one seven-minute period, in conjunction with commencement of the Triplex Herbal Formula.

For even better results, this program may be done while following a strict detox diet to accelerate elimination of the dead parasites and all the metabolic garbage they leave in the blood and tissues. Once a complete eradication of parasites has been achieved, a series of treatments of one-to-three weeks duration every six-to-twelve months usually suffices to keep the body free of parasites, especially if daily diet is reformed to eliminate the internal conditions of acidosis and toxemia in which parasites thrive. Other maintenance protocols with the Zapper include one session once a week, or three consecutive days of one session every month. While the Zapper is very effective used alone, when combined with the Triplex herbal formula, it eliminates a wider range of parasites and penetrates more deeply into the tissues.

The Zapper should not be used by people with pacemakers or other electronic implants, or by pregnant women. Other than that, it is safe to use any time by people who wish to rid their bodies of parasites and eliminate the diseases and degenerative conditions the organisms cause. Several models of this device are on the market as are a variety of treatment protocols, so be sure to get one that has been properly manufactured and tested for quality control, and always follow the directions provided with the unit.

THE NET: NO MORE "COLD TURKEY"

One of the most important new inventions in the field of electro-energy medicine, particularly in terms of its potential applications for dealing with a major worldwide health crisis, is "Neuro-Electric Therapy," or NET. It is a perfect example of how the "Best of East and West" may be successfully blended in medical therapy, and of how fusing the ancient healing principles of Asia with the modern technology of the West can achieve greater therapeutic results than either one could ever produce alone.

The NET technology was inspired by a fortunate stroke of serendipity when Scottish surgeon, Dr. Margaret "Meg" Patterson, was working in residence at a hospital in Hong Kong during the late 1970s. It was there that Dr. Patterson observed Western-trained Chinese surgeons using electrically enhanced acupuncture to help their patients recover more swiftly and less painfully in postsurgery. She also observed that some of these patients persistently pestered their doctors to keep them hooked onto the electro-acupuncture unit all the time, day and night, and that without it they became extremely restless and irritable. Later, a few of them finally admitted that they were in fact long-term heroin or opium addicts whose habits had been abruptly interrupted by their surgery, forcing them to endure acute drug withdrawal symptoms that were all the more agonizing after the trauma of surgery. They explained that whenever the electro-acupuncture therapy was applied, the "cold turkey" withdrawal symptoms vanished within minutes.

Subsequently, Dr. Patterson went to America and approached Dr. Robert Becker to research this phenomenon. Before long, they discovered that the key factor that produced the immediate relief from withdrawal symptoms was neither the acupuncture needles nor the points needled, but rather the pulsing electric current that the needles transmitted into the body. Soon thereafter, Dr. Patterson developed the NET device, which is about the same size as the "Jai" unit and attaches to the body with two small electrodes patched to the mastoid bone behind each ear. The NET device generates a gentle microcurrent of precisely the same frequencies and wave patterns produced by the brain when under the influence of a particular addictive drug. The genius of Dr. Patterson's work lies in the fact that she managed to precisely map the exact energy frequencies and brain wave patterns associated with each addictive drug—heroin, cocaine, amphetamines, barbiturates, and alcohol—and then produced a small computer chip for each one, which preprograms the NET device for the specific drug addiction to be treated.

After the addict takes his or her last dose of the drug and is ready for detox and withdrawal, the NET is patched to the body and remains attached day and night, except for showers, for the full ten days required to effect complete withdrawal. During this time, it delivers a continuous current of soothing neuro-electric therapy to the brain. While the frequencies and wave patterns produced by the NET prevent the patient from experiencing the worst symptoms of drug withdrawal, the body nevertheless remains completely drug-free throughout the course of treatment, allowing it to swiftly and effectively detoxify itself. By the time the treatment is terminated ten days later, the body has already passed painlessly beyond the most critical stage of drug withdrawal, without the intolerable trauma of withdrawal symptoms, and without the need to use substitute drugs such as methadone or sedatives, which not only reenforce addictive behavior but also stop the detox process.

Despite a consistent cure rate of over 90 percent in frequently repeated clinical trials, the FDA and medical establishments in the United States and most other Western nations still refuse to approve the NET for official drug-withdrawal programs. Because NET therapy requires no expensive drugs, no clinical treatment, and no dependence on doctors— i.e., because it works so well—it poses a major threat to many powerful vested interests in the medical industry, and so far only Ireland, Germany, and one or two other countries have officially certified its use.

The NET definitely works, as Rolling Stones guitarist Keith Richards, singer Boy George, and numerous other rock celebrities who were once stubbornly addicted to heroin can attest. "Dr. Meg," as she's affectionately known to those whom she has helped, has gifted the world with the most effective drug-detox method ever developed, one that manages the acute symptoms of addictive drug withdrawal without the intense agony of having to go cold turkey, or the need for anodyne drugs that block the detox process. Until government health agencies and medical establishments acknowledge the proven efficacy of NET therapy and sanction its clinical use for drug and alcohol withdrawal programs, however, those who wish to use this method must seek treatment through private channels.

RADIONICS: REBALANCING THE BODY'S BIO-ELECTRIC FIELD

Radionics is a new energy medicine technology that works with the specific spectrums of universal energy associated with the human system.

Radionics therapy is based on the scientifically proven principles that everything in the universe, from atoms to stars and microbes to humans, ultimately boils down to the same fundamental component—energy— and that each particular form of energy is governed by its own unique "Intrinsic Data Field" (IDF), which determines its characteristics and regulates its activity. Dr. Karl Jacobs, an energy healer who specializes in radionics therapies at his "Villa Deva" energy medicine clinic in Chiang Mai, Thailand, explains it as follows:

> The references to this spectrum have been given many names, such as radionics, psionics, dowsing, bioplasm, bio-electric energy, bio-fields, and Intrinsic Data Fields, as well as chi and prana in traditional Asian medicine. Regardless of the name, these subtle energy fields, or "bio-fields," are said to contain the essential intelligence, or information, that provides the distinctive pattern, or "energy matrix," that determines the organization of a particular form of matter. We call these informational patterns "Intrinsic Energy Fields," and in many instances they explain phenomena that cannot be explained by conventional medical science.

The device most commonly used to apply radionics therapy is called the SE-5. It is a compact, computer-based electronic instrument about the size of a laptop computer. This device, also known as a "bio-field analyzer," is programmed to detect and correct imbalances in the HEF and clear negative energies from the HES, thereby eliminating the root cause of many physical, mental, and emotional disorders and restoring optimum energy balance to the whole human system.

The SE-5 may also be used to increase the therapeutic potency of essential oils and herbal extracts to produce therapeutically energized elixirs, to program crystals with specific healing energy frequencies, and to clear negative energies from homes, offices, and other human habitats. Generally, the radionics therapist will ask the client to provide a lock of hair or a fingernail clipping, which is used to tune in the SE-5's sensors to the unique identifying frequencies of the client's personal energy system.

"Radionics is a powerful tool for healing," states Dr. Jacobs. "When you sign up for a consultation or a private cleansing retreat with me, I will ask for a sample of your hair, and from this I will determine which elixirs to create specifically for you, and prepare a comprehensive program of personal priorities designed to help you achieve your optimum state of health and well-being."

Since radionics therapy operates entirely in the dimension of energetics, consultations may be done long-distance, simply by mailing a hair sample to the therapist, who then analyzes the client's bio-energy field, prepares precisely the proper energized elixirs required to correct imbalances and clear blockages in the client's energy system, and mails them back to the client for use. Anyone interested in further information about radionics, or in arranging a consultation, may visit Dr. Jacobs's website: www.cleanse4life.com.

"NEW WAVE, SAME SEA"

High-tech energy medicine is certainly a "new wave" of the future in human healing and preventive health care and is particularly effective for repairing damage and correcting deviations in the HES caused by high-tech energy pollution, such as artificial EMF, microwaves, and unnatural radio frequencies. Nevertheless, regardless of how sophisticated and "advanced" this new wave of high-tech devices become, the therapeutic energies they generate still come from the same sea of basic universal energy of which the human body has always been composed and of which traditional holistic medicine has been aware for thousands of years.

Rarely does high-tech, electro-detox therapy by itself suffice to achieve effective and lasting results in healing the human system. For these new bio-electric energy technologies to achieve optimum results and effect permanent cures, they must always be applied in close conjunction with diet and nutrition, breathing and exercise, water and sunlight, and other traditional therapies that work directly with the fundamental energies and elements of the human system. High-tech electro-detox, and bio-electric energy medicine in general, are still in their infancy, and so far only a few of these new technologies have established a proven track record of therapeutic efficacy. The devices introduced above are among those that have demonstrated the most consistently positive results in clinical use as well as at home.

In fact, in some cases these new technologies can make the crucial difference between success and failure in a detox and healing program. Neuro-Electric Therapy (NET), for example, has repeatedly proven itself to be the key factor in curing the most stubborn cases of drug and alcohol addiction, because it permits detox to proceed without trauma and without resort to other drugs. The Zapper can be a decisive factor in curing conditions caused by long-term parasite infestation, and the GEOMED Activated Air System promises to become an indispensable tool for treating respiratory and other ailments that arise from chronic deficiency in the essential energy of negative ions in the air, especially in polluted cities. Still, when choosing detox and healing therapies, it's always best to begin with the most basic elements of life in the body, such as food, herbs, water, air, and sunlight, then amplify and accelerate those therapies with synergistic high-tech, electro-detox methods.

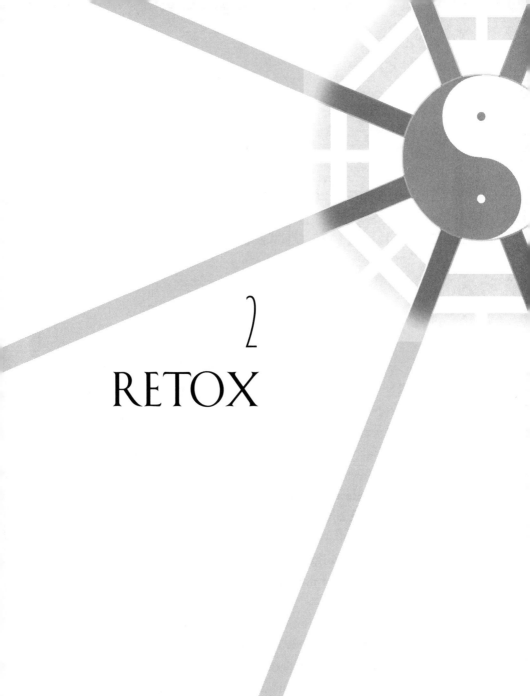

2

RETOX

10

THE ART OF
RATIONAL RETOX

Let's face it, life on earth is toxic. No sooner is detox done than "retox" resumes. The moment you start eating normally again, your digestive system starts producing toxic wastes, cellular metabolism repollutes the bloodstream with carbon dioxide and acid residues, exercise sours the muscles with lactic acid, and the whole process of progressive tissue toxicity begins once more.

The body's internal self-cleansing mechanisms are designed to deal with these natural sources of tissue toxicity on a daily basis through normal excretory functions, but the body is not equipped to handle the heavy overload of inorganic toxins and putrefactive wastes produced by unnatural sources of internal pollution such as chemically processed foods and medicines, toxic air and water, and indigestible combinations of denatured foods. For most people today, tissue toxicity is further aggravated by relentless enervation of the nervous system from chronic stress, insufficient rest and relaxation, overstimulation of the senses, and excessive dependence on stimulants and intoxicants. These stress factors keep the autonomous nervous system constantly racing in the "fight or flight" sympathetic mode, exhausting the adrenal glands, weakening immune response, and flooding the bloodstream with the highly acid-forming residues produced by stress hormones and the metabolic reactions they trigger. Unable to process and eliminate this growing overload of toxins through "normal channels," the body is forced to store them instead by tucking them away in joints, bones, liver, bowels, fat, lymph, and any other tissue where they cannot directly poison the bloodstream. If these toxic deposits are not periodically dislodged from the tissues in which they're stored and flushed out of the body, it will only be a matter of time before they do serious damage to those tissues and cause cellular malfunctions that can lead to cancer, heart disease, Alzheimer syndrome, and other fatal conditions.

The only viable solution to the vexing problem of toxicity in modern daily life is to cultivate the "Art of Rational Retox." In a nutshell, this means designing your daily lifestyle in ways that minimize internal pollution and maximize internal cleansing functions. It means reforming your daily diet, reordering your daily priorities, and refining your daily lifestyle. To do this, you must take the time to learn how your body works, and pay close attention to how it reacts to various things you feed it and do with it. You need to consider the "cost/benefit" factors involved in what you eat, drink, and do each day, and learn to avoid those things whose costs to health and longevity far outweigh their benefits. "Rational retox" in daily life can make the crucial difference between long-term health and longevity and their opposites, chronic disease and degeneration, especially when practiced in conjunction with periodic detox diets or therapeutic fasts.

The great advantage of doing a detox program first, prior to trying to eliminate harmful food addictions and reform bad eating habits, is that a preliminary detox makes it much easier to break unhealthy old food addictions and cultivate healthy new eating habits. People who suddenly stop eating sugar, meat, or dairy products without first purging their bowels, blood, and tissues of the toxic residues left by these foods in the body, usually find it difficult to resist the craving for these things. They find it almost impossible to stick strictly to their new diets because food addictions are very similar physiologically to drug addictions. The body grows accustomed to their metabolic effects and learns to tolerate the damage they do. In some cases, such as sugar addiction, the nervous system becomes dependent on the toxic by-products of sugar metabolism, which act as a nervous stimulant. When these substances are abruptly withdrawn from the body, their toxic residues remain in the blood and tissues, leaving a metabolic memory that causes the mind to crave those items. While the symptoms of withdrawal from food addictions are not as intense and dramatic as those produced by drugs, the basic symptoms are very similar, including hypertension, insomnia, headaches, indigestion, depression, and irritability. By doing a detox program to purify the blood and tissues and completely rid the body of all toxic "leftovers" from former food habits, all withdrawal symptoms are condensed into a single week of detox, during which time you have nothing else to do anyway but pamper yourself with hot saltwater baths, herbal steams, deep-tissue massages, and other soothing detox protocols. By the time you have completed these healing protocols, all cravings for former dietary trespasses will have totally disappeared, and healthy new eating habits may be cultivated to replace them.

If you find it difficult to give up all unhealthy eating habits and harmful food choices after your first round of detox, then just try eliminating one or two, and work on the others later, after your next detox program. As the novelist Nelson Algren observed, "Life is hard by the yard, but a cinch by the inch." This is especially true when it comes to making necessary changes in life, and replacing old ways with new. But if you take it step by step, replacing wrong choices with right ones, one by one, you will soon discover that good habits are as easy to develop as bad habits, and just as hard to break, and that healthy diets and wholesome lifestyles can be even more habit-forming than indiscriminate self-indulgence.

"DETOX/RETOX"

The first step in the art of rational retox is to redesign your diet and other daily lifestyle factors in ways that allow your body to unload most of its toxic wastes on a daily basis, rather than letting them accumulate inside and cause blood acidosis and tissue toxicity. The more efficiently the body detoxifies itself daily, the fewer toxins remain stored in the tissues, and the easier each periodic detox program becomes. To put it another way, the more you let your body cleanse and heal itself daily, the less severe is the "healing crisis" that manifests later, especially if you allow internal toxins to accumulate for too long. Efficient daily detox also makes daily life a lot more pleasant and productive by increasing available energy, boosting physical vitality, and enhancing mental clarity.

Although retox is a natural process of life that functions automatically, you can take rational measures to slow down the rate of retox and lessen the degree of internal pollution. The extent to which you practice such preventive measures can have a decisive influence on health and longevity. Detox is a natural, self-cleansing function of the body, but it is only designed to process toxic wastes from natural sources. To deal with the heavy overload of unnatural toxins that collect in the human body today from pollutants in food, water, air, medical drugs, and other environmental sources, you must take extra steps to help your body to eliminate these poisons on a daily basis, and thereby protect itself from the damage they produce if allowed to accumulate inside. These toxic chemical residues from industrial sources pollute the bloodstream and corrode the tissues far more swiftly and severely than natural metabolic wastes, and failure to flush them from the body paves a quick path to disease, degeneration, and premature death.

The key elements required to produce precisely the right climate within the body for detox and self-cleansing mechanisms to operate continuously day and night are alkali and oxygen. As long as the blood and tissues remain sufficiently alkalized and oxygenated, they will naturally cleanse and balance themselves, and the body will be able to neutralize and eliminate toxins as soon as they appear. Among the measures that may be taken to keep the blood and tissues alkalized and oxygenated on a daily basis, by far the most effective is proper utilization of life's two most basic elements—air and water—which enter and exit the body constantly throughout the day and night. Correctly used, air and water continuously alkalize and oxygenate the body as they enter and continuously eliminate toxins and acid wastes on the way out.

To facilitate daily detox in modern lifestyles today, nothing works faster and more efficiently than drinking the alkalized, ionized, micro-clustered water introduced in chapter 2 as microwater. Drinking this type of activated water throughout the day and using it to prepare all your foods and beverages provides continuous internal detox and cleansing activity that permeates all the tissues and fluids of the body and allows the cells to eliminate their metabolic wastes as soon as they're produced. The negative charge carried by ionized water neutralizes toxic residues in the blood and tissues owing to its potent antioxidant properties, and the microclustered minerals and water molecules easily penetrate cellular membranes to keep all of the tissues sufficiently hydrated and mineralized and to maintain proper pH balance in the cellular fluids.

Negative ions also constitute the essential element in air that helps keep the body alkaline and oxygenated and that facilitates continuous internal detox. When the oxygen molecules in the air we breathe are ionized, they become far more bio-active in the body, and their cleansing and healing properties become much stronger. The negative-ion count in air is an accurate measure of its capacity to support life, and without that energy, air is just a cocktail of inert gases. Breathing "dead air" with low or no negative-ion count is a major contributing factor in chronic fatigue, chronic toxemia, and chronic degeneration of the body, and it has become one of the biggest banes to human health throughout the world today. While living in a forest high in the mountains, or on an unspoiled beach by the open sea, is no doubt the best solution to this problem of bad air, it is simply not possible for most people to do that. The next best solution is to recharge dead air in homes and offices using negative-ion generators, or to spend twenty to thirty minutes each day breathing purified, super-charged air from the GEOMED Activated Air System.

In addition to breathing bio-active air, it is also very important to learn how to breathe correctly by using the diaphragm to draw the breath deep down into the abdomen, rather than breathing only in the narrow part of the upper chest. Correct diaphragmic breathing greatly increases oxygenation of the blood and tissues, as well as elimination of carbon dioxide, and it also has an immediate alkalizing effect on the bloodstream, thereby counteracting acidosis and assisting detox with each and every breath.

Besides air and water, other factors of daily life such as food and supplements may also be used to help keep the blood and tissues alkaline and assist the body's self-cleansing functions. Freshly extracted raw vegetable juices are particularly fast and effective alkalizers. Including a glass or two each day in your diet is a very good way to prevent acidosis and facilitate rapid elimination of toxic wastes. Various dietary supplements may also be used as sources of elements that alkalize and detoxify blood and tissues, including all green foods such as chlorella, spirulina, and cereal grass juices, Celtic sea salt and marine mineral extracts, and antioxidant nutrients such as vitamins C and E, beta carotene, zinc, and selenium. Sunlight, too, plays a vital role in this process by stimulating the body to produce enough vitamin D to assure maximum assimilation of calcium from food, water, and mineral supplements. Since calcium is the body's primary internal alkalizing agent and an essential element in all detox processes, sunlight can be an important supporting factor in maintaining the body's daily defense mechanisms against acidosis and toxemia.

In the final analysis, the primary factor in the complex "detox/retox" equations that determine human health is usually diet. "You are what you eat" is more than just a slick slogan; it's a basic fact of life. Rebalancing your daily diet according to the principles of "trophology"—the science of food combining—and reviewing your daily food choices in light of the effects they have on pH balance and other vital conditions in the body are the first and second steps on the path of rational retox. The reason that diet is the first priority is simple: wrong food combinations and wrong food choices have become the primary causes of blood acidosis and tissue toxemia, and these in turn are the primary conditions for the onset of disease and degeneration of the body. After giving up unhealthy food addictions and breaking acid-forming eating habits by doing a few detox diet or therapeutic fasting programs, it is both easy and enjoyable to cultivate healthy new eating habits and a taste for wholesome alkalizing foods that nourish and balance the body rather than derange and ruin it.

In the following chapter, we'll review the most important rules for combining food in ways that minimize internal toxicity and maximize digestive efficiency, then we'll examine the major categories of food in light of their effects and side effects within the body and decide what's really healthy and safe to eat today and what's not.

11

RETOX DIET AND SUPPLEMENTS

Diet and nutrition are the primary building blocks in the foundation of human health and longevity, and the essential elements of life provided by food cannot be replicated or replaced with any form of modern technology. Owing to mass production and corporate control of the world's food supplies over the past century, the human diet has become as polluted with toxic wastes as everything else produced by the modern-consumer industry. The industrially refined foods that most people consume today are contaminated with poisonous pesticides and preservatives, chemically altered with artificial flavors and coloring agents, and further denatured by irradiation and genetic modification. In the refinement process, most of the essential nutrients are stripped from the food, and the few that remain have little or no nutritional value. Prior to the advent of chemically processed foods, the famous American physician Dr. Charles Mayo, founder of the Mayo Clinic, described the central role of wholesome food in human health as follows:

> Normal resistance to disease is directly dependent upon adequate food; normal resistance to disease never comes out of pill boxes. Adequate food is the cradle of normal resistance, the playground of

normal immunity, the workshop of good health, and the laboratory of long life.

Modern Western eating habits, particularly the fast-food and snack-diet approach propagated by the American food industry, are far from adequate sources of nutrition for human health. These diets are composed almost entirely of the three most acid-forming types of food: animal products (meat, fat, eggs, and dairy products); refined white starch (white bread, pastries, potatoes, and starchy snack foods); and refined white sugar (candy, ice cream, sweet confections, and sugary soft drinks). In North America, Western Europe, and Australia, these three categories of food account for over 90 percent of the calories consumed by most people in those countries; they also contribute to at least 90 percent of the diseases and degenerative conditions people in those countries suffer. Overwhelmingly imbalanced in favor of highly acid-forming foods such as meat, milk, sugar, and starch, and virtually devoid of the alkalizing elements found in fresh fruit and vegetables, modern Western diets saturate the human body with toxic acid wastes, poison the blood and tissues, weaken resistance and immunity, and fling open the gates to chronic disease and degenerative conditions. The only way to deal with this daily dietary threat to health and longevity is to rationally redesign your diet and reform your eating habits in ways that reduce formation of acid wastes and ways that increase alkalinity. This means reordering your priorities in food choices and adopting the basic laws of food combining to govern your eating habits.

THE YIN AND THE YANG OF IT

The science of combining food in ways that prevent acid-forming reactions of fermentation and putrefaction in the digestive tract, while increasing alkalinity and reducing production of toxic wastes, is known in nutritional science as "trophology." Following these principles in your daily diet and personal eating habits is the first basic step in applying the "art of rational retox" to your daily life. Proper food combining is one of the most effective measures one can take to prevent the development of blood acidosis and tissue toxemia, and it provides a practical way to control the balance of acid and alkaline elements in the body.

In TCM, the "Great Principle of Yin and Yang," which lies at the heart of all functions of life, manifests its polar dynamics in diet and digestion in the form of alkaline (Yin) and acid (Yang) balance. As we can see from this terminology, traditional Chinese physicians regarded "alkaline" as a manifestation of the cooling, calming, nourishing "water" element of Yin, and "acid" as a reflection of the heating, agitating, depleting "fire" element of Yang. From this viewpoint, modern Western diets are extremely imbalanced with an excess of highly acid-forming Yang foods such as meat, milk, eggs, fat, sugar, and starch, and this imbalance is further aggravated by the acidifying effects of eating these foods in wrong combinations, which drives the internal organs ever deeper into the inferno of what TCM calls "fire-energy excess" *(huo-chi da)*. The obvious solution to this problem of excess acid-forming "Yang" is to rebalance the diet in the direction of more alkaline-forming "Yin" factors.

Strictly applied, trophology becomes a highly complex discipline that can interfere with the enjoyment of food. Since everything we eat reacts in a Yin or Yang way with anything else we eat together with it, as well as with whatever is already in the stomach, if we're too fastidious about food combining, we finally reach the point that we dare to eat only one single type of food at a time. Eating under such restrictions is impractical as well as boring, and it detracts from the natural pleasure food can provide. Fortunately, such a strict approach is also unnecessary. You may compose meals that are properly balanced trophologically as well as fully satisfying gastronomically by following the "75 Percent Rule," whereby the basic laws of food combining govern about 75 percent of your food choices whenever you compose a meal, with a 25 percent margin of error for indiscriminate self-indulgence. This is a rational approach to food combining that is both practical and effective, and it may be applied with equal ease at home or in a restaurant.

For example, if the rule states, "Don't combine meat and starch at the same meal," you don't need to be a fanatic about it and pluck out the few slivers of chicken or shrimp you find in a Chinese stir-fried noodle dish that is over 90 percent noodles and vegetables. Nor need you worry about having just one small whole-grain dinner roll with a meal of meat and lots of vegetables. On the other hand, eating a large baked potato slathered with sour cream together with a thick steak, or a greasy cheeseburger on a starchy white bun, is definitely a violation of the rules, punishable by acid indigestion and other gastric distress. By following the 75 Percent Rule in applying the laws of food combining to your daily diet, you'll avoid all of the worst acid-forming pitfalls in food, while still allowing yourself to enjoy a few dietary indiscretions.

To simplify the matter for those who wish to try trophology as a practical measure for preventing indigestion, controlling internal acidity, and reducing tissue toxicity, the most important rules for balancing alkaline-forming Yin and acid-forming Yang in a diet on the basis of proper food combining are presented below in terms of their practical applications to six major categories of food: complex animal proteins, starchy carbohydrates, fats, sugars, fruits, and vegetables.

Putrefactive Protein

What we're discussing here is the complex, concentrated protein found in foods from animal sources, such as meat, fish and fowl, eggs and dairy products, not the light, simple protein contained in nuts and seeds, beans and grains, and other vegetable sources. Vegetable proteins are far less complex than animal protein, and therefore they are much easier to digest. They also combine well with most other foods. Meat, eggs, and dairy products, however, cause digestive disaster when wrongly combined with other foods, or even when improperly combined with each other.

The first and foremost rule of food combining is, "Don't eat concentrated animal protein and starchy carbohydrates together." Yet this very combination forms the mainstay of modern Western meals—steak and potatoes, hamburgers and french fries, toast and eggs, spaghetti with meatballs. The earliest recorded prohibition against this digestively noxious food combination appears in the Hebrew scriptures in the Bible, when Jehovah instructs Moses to teach his people to eat their meat and bread at separate meals: "At evening ye shall eat flesh, and in the morning ye shall be filled with bread." This means that bread and other starchy carbohydrates are the foods that should be eaten for breakfast in the morning, without any meat, and that meat should only be eaten for dinner in the evening, without bread. This advice accords exactly with the first law of trophology.

Simply by following this single cardinal rule, a primary source of acid indigestion and toxic putrefaction in the stomach and bowels is eliminated from the diet. Whenever meat, eggs, or cheese are eaten together with bread, rice, or other starch, the starch starts to digest in the mouth with secretions of the alkaline enzyme "ptyalin," and this alkaline-forming digestive process continues when the starch reaches the stomach, blocking digestion of the protein by pepsin, hydrochloric acid, the other acid-forming enzymes required to digest animal proteins. Consequently, the alkaline requirements of starch digestion conflict in the stomach with the acid requirements of protein digestion, resulting in the digestion of neither and the fermentation and putrefaction of both. This internal struggle in turn produces more toxins and acid wastes that further inhibit digestion and allow bacteria to gobble up all the available nutrients in the food and dump their own acid wastes into your digestive tract.

The second basic rule regarding consumption of animal proteins is, "Don't combine meat and dairy products at the same meal," such as meat and milk, fish and cheese. This rule is so important that it, too, is mentioned in the Bible. It became known as the "second Mosaic law" of diet, whereby Moses forbade his people to consume meat and milk together at the same meal. Moses's advice in food combinations is wise and is based on sound science, for the strongest gastric enzyme activity on meat occurs during the first hour of digestion, whereas milk is digested mostly during the last hour of digestion, and eggs somewhere in between. Consequently, if animal flesh and dairy products are eaten together at the same meal, neither can be properly digested, and both putrefy instead. While it is fine to combine two types of meat, such as beef and chicken, lamb and fish, tuna and shrimp, no meat should be eaten together with milk, cheese, or eggs.

Starchy Carbohydrates

Starch is the culprit in carbohydrates that causes acid indigestion, and since most carbohydrates eaten today are highly refined, their starch content is unnaturally elevated. Whole grains, which contain far less starch, gram for gram, than refined varieties, are easier to digest and combine much better with other foods, but anything that consists mainly of refined starch, such as white bread, pastries, white rice, or noodles should be eaten separately from all concentrated animal proteins such as meat, eggs, and cheese.

Most people today eat starchy carbohydrates in the morning, in the form of toast, porridge, or cereal. Whole-grain versions of these foods are by far the better choice: they contain less starch and supply more vital nutrients than refined varieties, and they cause fewer severe acid-forming reactions when improperly combined with other foods. One of the worst breakfast combinations today is packaged dry cereal made from factory-processed grains, heavily sprinkled with refined white sugar and soaked in pasteurized cow's milk. Children suffer most from the ravages of this indigestible food combination for breakfast. A breakfast made of such sweetened carbohydrates is a major factor in the obesity, constipation, skin problems, and low resistance to disease that plague children today.

Since proper digestion of starch must begin in the mouth with thorough insalivation by the ptyalin enzyme, chew all carbohydrate foods very well before swallowing, and do not drink any liquids with them. Any beverage taken together with starch dilutes salivary secretions of ptyalin in the mouth, preventing proper predigestion of starch in the mouth and resulting in fermentation in the stomach.

Fat

Fats such as butter and oil may be combined with most carbohydrates and all vegetables, but they should be used sparingly with concentrated animal proteins such as meat and eggs. Fat impairs the digestion of meat in the stomach by inhibiting the gastric secretions required to digest meat. Consequently, for two to three hours after ingesting significant amounts of fat, levels of pepsin and hydrochloric acid in the stomach are sharply reduced, resulting in the putrefaction of any meat or eggs eaten along with the fat. You should therefore eat fats and proteins separately, or combine only very small amounts of one with normal portions of the other, and avoid eating "marbled" meats such as bacon and fatty steaks. The only exception is lamb: the fat in lamb is readily digested by the human body.

Sugar

Refined white sugar is the single most acid-forming food substance in modern diets, and its presence in the stomach interferes with the proper digestion of almost all other foods. When sugary desserts or soft drinks are consumed at the same meal with meat, for example, the sugar blocks secretion of the gastric juices required to digest meat, resulting in putrefaction, fermentation, and extreme acidity. When eaten with starchy carbohydrates, sugar shuts off salivary secretion of ptyalin in the mouth, and the starch lands in the stomach without the essential enzyme required to predigest it, resulting in fermentation production of acid wastes. To a lesser degree, sugar also causes fermentation and "acid indigestion" when eaten with fruits and vegetables. Therefore, the best policy toward foods and beverages that contain a lot of refined sugar is not to combine them with proteins, starchy carbohydrates, or any other category of food at the same meal. If you wish to occasionally indulge your "sweet tooth" by eating ice cream, cake, pastries, and other sweet confections made with refined sugar, it is best to eat them alone, preferably with some hot tea, and it also helps to flush the stomach with a glass or two of alkaline water an hour or two later.

Fruit

Fresh fruit requires virtually no digestion in the stomach. Instead, it moves quickly into the duodenum, where it dissolves and releases its nutrients for rapid assimilation. If its swift passage through the stomach is blocked by the presence of any other food, however, fruit gets delayed in the stomach, and its rich stores of natural sugars are immediately raided by the ever-present bacteria in the stomach. This causes everything in the stomach to quickly ferment, producing acids, generating gas, and disrupting the entire digestive process. Melons and citrus fruits ferment even faster than other fruits and cause even worse gastric distress when combined with other foods, including other types of fruit. They should never be eaten together with anything else. Wait at least one hour after eating any melon before eating any other type of food, and half an hour before eating another variety of fruit.

If eaten in sufficient quantity and variety, fresh fruit can provide all the essential nutrients required for life, including amino acids, which are the basic building blocks of protein, as well as vitamins, minerals, and active enzymes. Besides nourishing the body, fresh fruit also alkalizes the digestive tract, cleans the bloodstream, and detoxifies the tissues.

Vegetables

Vegetables are the great common denominator in most food-combination equations. They combine very well with all proteins, including meat and eggs, as well as with starchy carbohydrates like noodles, bread, and rice, as well as with fats. Vegetables assist digestion and assimilation of other foods by supplying essential minerals and enzymes that facilitate digestive functions. They also assist elimination by providing fibrous bulk to propel digestive wastes through the bowels. Most vegetables have strong alkaline-forming properties as well. Vegetables may therefore be eaten in unlimited amounts to complement meals based on either proteins or carbohydrates. The only food with which they don't combine well is fruit.

When raw vegetables are eaten whole, as in salads, they can take a long time to digest and release their nutrients owing to their high cellulose content. When extracted as pure juices, however, with the cellulose pulp removed, their nutritional value and alkalizing benefits increase significantly and are delivered more swiftly. The best way to eat fresh vegetables whole is to cook them very briefly by steaming, stir-frying, or poaching, which softens the cellulose content sufficiently to allow easy digestion without destroying their nutritional value with prolonged exposure to heat.

SHORT LIST OF ALKALINE- AND ACID-FORMING FOODS

To assist readers in learning how to compose harmoniously balanced meals based on the relative alkaline- and acid-forming properties of various foods, the chart on page 242 divides a wide selection of common food items into alkaline and acid categories, and lists them in order of their relative strength. The number next to each item indicates the degree of its alkaline- or acid-forming effects, compared with the base number 1 for the least alkalizing or acidifying item on the list. For example, tofu is the least alkaline-forming food in the alkaline category and therefore has a rating of 1. Strawberries, with a rating of 56, are 56 times more alkalizing than tofu, and ginger is 211 times stronger. Similarly, oysters are 80 times more acid-forming than asparagus, but only slightly more acidifying than salmon. This chart is based on information from Herman Aihara's excellent booklet, *Acid and Alkaline*.

LIVE FOOD FOR LIVING PEOPLE

It stands to reason that "dead food" hastens death, and "live food" prolongs life, which is indeed the case. The rational choice for the "retox diet" is to eat only live foods. The best definition of "live food" was formulated back in the 1930s by Dr. E. V. McCullum, the pioneering nutritional scientist at Johns Hopkins University in prejunk-food America. McCullum's advice was: "Eat nothing unless it will spoil or rot, but eat it before it does!" That eliminates all processed and packaged foods produced with chemical preservatives, artificial flavors, synthetic dyes, and other unnatural additives, as well as any food that has been highly refined, irradiated, or genetically modified. Such food products

ACID-FORMING FOODS		ALKALINE-FORMING FOODS	
rice bran	852	wakame seaweed	2608
bonita flakes	371	kombu seaweed	400
dried squid	296	ginger	211
dried fish	240	kidney beans	188
egg yolk	192	shitake mushrooms	175
oatmeal	178	spinach	156
brown rice	155	soybeans	102
tuna	153	bananas	88
octopus	128	chestnuts	83
chicken	104	azuki beans	73
pearl barley	99	carrots	64
oysters	80	mushrooms	64
salmon	79	strawberries	56
buckwheat	77	potatoes	54
scallops	66	cabbage	49
pork	62	radishes	46
peanuts	54	squash	44
beef	50	sweet potatoes	43
cheese	43	turnips	42
abalone	36	orange juice	36
whole barley	35	apples	34
shrimp	32	egg white	32
peas	25	pears	26
beer	11	grape juice	23
bread	6	cucumbers	22
butter	4	watermelon	21
asparagus	1	eggplant	19
		coffee	19
		onions	17
		tea	16
		string beans	11
		tofu	1

are designed with only one purpose in mind: to extend the "shelf life" of the product. They do nothing to extend the life of the consumer.

One way to trim dead food from your diet is to eat 40–50 percent of your daily fare in the form of raw or very lightly cooked foods. Raw and "rare" cooked foods are only edible when fresh and complete with the essential elements of life. This natural freshness and vitality cannot be duplicated with the artificial flavors, chemical preservatives, and other additives used to produce processed foods. Live raw foods help clear the stagnation and eliminate the toxic debris produced in the digestive tract by dead, processed foods by supplying the active enzymes and vital trace elements required to digest this inert toxic sludge, and by providing fresh fiber bulk to dredge these wastes quickly through of the bowels and out of the body.

Another way to insure the life in the food you eat—as well as your own—is to strictly eliminate all items from your diet that contain chemical preservatives, dyes, flavoring agents such as MSG, and any other non-nutritional additives. Thousands of toxic chemicals, including some that are known carcinogens, are commonly used to manufacture junk food, fast food, and other so-called convenience foods. All of these synthetic additives are extremely acid-forming and leave toxic residues that are very difficult to excrete lodged in the tissues. This policy applies equally to fresh produce grown with pesticides, herbicides, and chemical fertilizers, all of which contribute heavily to acidosis and toxemia. Although organically produced foods are more expensive and difficult to find than factory-farmed food, they are well worth the extra cost and effort. If the price of organic foods is a bit "rich" for your budget, the solution is to buy them anyway, but to buy less. Eating just a small serving of organically grown, nutritionally complete food does more to nourish the body and prolong life than eating a whole bushel of processed factory food.

Last but not least deadly on the list of dead foods that should be banished from your diet are the "impostors": artificial food substitutes that pose prettily on the supermarket shelves, brightly packed and labeled to catch your eye, pretending to be "healthy alternatives" to real foods.

Among the worst offenders here are margarine, "non-dairy creamer," and all other fake foods made from hydrogenated vegetable oils, as well as all synthetic sugar substitutes such as saccharin and aspartame. Not only are these fake foods dead, they were never alive to begin with, so they contain nothing whatsoever that supports life. All of them wreak havoc with human metabolism. These phony fat and sugar substitutes are all extremely acid-forming, extremely toxic to the tissues, and, if consumed to excess, can also become highly carcinogenic.

THE CRON DIET: CALORIE RESTRICTION/OPTIMUM NUTRITION

The "CRON" diet, which stands for "calorie restriction/optimum nutrition," was developed by Dr. Roy Walford as a means of extending the lifespan of any species. Dr. Walford, "Biosphere" veteran and author of *Beyond the 120 Year Diet,* based the CRON diet on extensive, long-term studies he conducted with rats, dogs, and other mammalian species. He designed the CRON diet to take advantage of the scientifically proven correlation between low calorie/high nutrient diets and longevity. The basic rationale for this direct link between the CRON diet and long lifespan is simple: maximum nutrition with minimum calories means maximum metabolic energy with minimum toxic waste. It also means that the body requires less energy to digest food and eliminate wastes, allowing more energy to be reserved for sustaining internal cleansing and immune functions. By reducing internal acidity and tissue toxicity to minimal levels while supplying optimum nutrition, the CRON diet counteracts the conditions that give rise to disease and degeneration, and provides the proper balance of essential elements and energy needed to support health and prolong life.

Traditional Chinese physicians have known about the life-prolonging benefits of calorie restriction for thousands of years. Their dietary prescription for health and longevity is succinctly summarized in the ancient dietary axiom to eat until only *chi-ba fen bao,* or "70–80 percent full." Traditional Chinese cuisine was exquisitely well balanced to provide optimum nutrition, so the only dietary factor that required attention in Chinese food was quantity. The "Chinese Rule," to eat only until you're 70–80 percent full, is still a convenient measure for determining how much to eat at any meal, and for knowing when to stop.

Another effective way to reduce the quantity of food eaten while also increasing its nutritional value is to chew, chew, chew your food until it is well enough masticated to dissolve in the mouth before swallowing. This technique is particularly helpful when eating carbohydrates, which require predigestion in the mouth to properly digest in the stomach. Chewing food well helps prevent the acid-forming reactions of putrefaction and fermentation in the stomach, increases assimilation of nutrients, and reduces transit time of digestive wastes through the bowels.

Remember, however, that to effectively extend the human lifespan, both aspects of the CRON diet must be equally implemented—not just "calorie restriction" but also "optimum nutrition." Following a low-calorie fad diet consisting mainly of denatured, "convenience" foods and eating them in indigestible combinations provides the body with nothing but "empty calories" and has the opposite effect: it ruins health and shortens life. In the following pages, we'll take a brief look at several major categories of food commonly consumed in modern diets, and establish a few rational guidelines for determining what foods to include and which ones to strictly eliminate when designing a new diet balanced for health and longevity.

GUIDE TO EATING MAMMALS, BIRDS, AND FISH

In prehistoric times, when the human species still depended on meat to survive, people got their meat not at the supermarket but by killing mammals, birds, and fish in the wilderness and eating them raw or slightly cooked the same day, fresh off the bone. Today, most humans still retain this primitive taste for the flesh of other species, even though meat products have become totally unnecessary and often very harmful factors in the human diet. Moreover, the meat that people get on their dinner plates today is a far cry from the fresh flesh of healthy, wild animals that their ancestors ate.

The meat sold in markets today is loaded with powerful synthetic hormones and chemical steroids that are fed to livestock to stimulate rapid growth, increase weight, and bring entire herds into heat simultaneously for breeding purposes. When humans eat this meat, the hormones are absorbed into their bodies and stimulate rapid growth in their tissues as well. Consumption of such chemically contaminated meat has become a major contributing factor in the widespread obesity today in the wealthy, meat-eating countries of the West. These chemical growth stimulants and synthetic sex hormones also severely disrupt the delicate hormonal balances within the human body, especially in ovulating women and growing children. The extraordinarily high incidence of breast and cervical cancer, ovarian cysts and other reproductive disorders among women in the Western world is due in large part to this contamination of the human food chain.

Owing to the appalling conditions in which commercial livestock is raised, these animals must also be heavily dosed with antibiotics to keep them alive long enough to reach the slaughterhouse. Over 40 percent of the antibiotics produced in the USA are fed directly to cattle, pigs, chickens, and even to commercially farmed salmon and trout, and whoever eats these products regularly receives a continuous infusion of powerful antibiotic drugs that weaken natural immune responses, kill all the friendly lactobacteria in the digestive tract, and produce a state of chronic acidosis. In addition to all these toxic drugs and hormones, commercial livestock also assimilates all the poisonous pesticides, herbicides, and chemical fertilizers used to grow the crops for their feed, and these toxins, too, pass into the body of the consumer. Anyone who wants to know more about the atrocious conditions livestock today suffer and how these hapless creatures are systematically drugged, poisoned, and fed on dead, denatured food that often includes such delectables as sawdust, paper pulp, and the processed cadavers of other animals that died of disease, should read John Robbins' latest book, *The Food Revolution,* and its prequel, *Diet for a New America.* The conditions Robbins describes prevail in the commercial meat industry throughout the world, not just in the United States, and anyone who still eats factory-farmed meat or fish after reading these books has no one to blame but themselves for the consequences.

Even without all the toxic contamination in modern meat products, beef and pork have always been difficult for the human body to digest and process. In addition, both are extremely acid-forming. The main digestive challenge of these products is in the fat content: the type of fat in beef and pork inhibits gastric secretions in the stomach, clogs digestion, and puts a huge strain on the liver, where all fat must be processed. After conducting extensive studies in sixteen countries, researchers in Canada established a close causal link between high consumption of pork products and cirrhosis of the liver. In countries where pork is commonly consumed together with alcohol, such as beer and wine, the incidence of cirrhosis soared to one thousand times higher than average. Daily consumption of beef and pork can also establish the conditions that lead to development of bowel cancer.

Other than wild game, which is almost impossible to get these days, the only red meat that is both beneficial to health and relatively safe to eat is lamb. Sheep generally graze in open pasture and get plenty of fresh air and natural sunlight, rather than being cooped up day and night in cages and pens and fed on dead industrial feed. Surprisingly, it is still possible to buy lamb that has not been poisoned with drugs and steroids. And unlike the fat from cattle and pigs, lamb fat digests quite easily in the human body. Lamb fat is a rich source of carnitine, an amino acid that transports fat into the cells for metabolism. Since the human heart is the biggest burner of fat in the body, carnitine carries fat from the liver to fuel the heart. This process, which can only be performed by carnitine, helps prevent cirrhosis and other liver damage caused by excess accumulation of fat in the liver. In the Himalayan, Middle Eastern, and Mediterranean regions, where lamb has always been the main meat food, arteriosclerosis, heart disease, bowel cancer, and other ailments associated with high consumption of beef and pork in Western countries, are relatively rare.

When eating red meat, cook it on the rare side to preserve some of its enzymes to assist digestion and prevent damaging the proteins with excessive exposure to high heat. Additionally, using some strong mustard, horseradish, or fresh ginger as a condiment for meat stimulates secretions of the gastric juices required to digest it.

Consumption of poultry is even worse for humans than eating beef and pork. The way chickens are produced for market today is far more of a horror story than the conditions under which pigs and cows are raised. In the standard, commercial chicken farm, up to forty thousand chickens are cooped up in steel cages in their multistoried poultry prison, with two or three birds jammed together in each cell. The chicks are fed on dry pellets of noxious industrial feed laced with hormones and antibiotics. Anyone who wants to learn the whole, ugly truth about this foul business is again referred to John Robbins's books.

Ninety percent of the broiler chickens produced in America today are so jacked up on growth hormones that they cannot even stand up under the bloated weight of their obesity, and those that try to stand often break their legs. Could this possibly be a factor in the rampant obesity seen today among chicken-chomping children in America and other wealthy societies that have adopted Americans' fast-food diets? The average tissue mass of a typical chicken breast in America today is seven times greater than it was only twenty-five years ago. Again, one wonders what effects the hormones that produce these big-breasted chickens have on the breast tissues of the women who eat those chickens.

"Free-range" chicken is certainly much safer to eat than "jail-bird" chicken, but the term has become so abused by the commercial chicken industry that it is difficult to find a chicken these days that has been allowed to range freely in nature, foraging for its own food. In many cases, the free-range label only means that caged chickens are occasionally let out of their cells and allowed to range freely around a fenced, concrete yard that is barren of vegetation, just like convicts in a prison yard. Then they are locked up again and fed the same denatured commercial feed that fully confined chickens eat. The only label designation that now assures you of getting a real chicken that has been naturally raised without drugs and other chemicals is the term "non-caged, free-range chicken." If you cannot find these genuine free rangers in your local markets, the only remaining options are to delete chickens from your diet, or else to raise them yourself.

If you wish to make flesh a regular part of your diet, the best choice is fresh seafood. Deep-water ocean fish such as tuna, swordfish, and salmon are rich sources of essential fatty acids that cleanse the blood vessels of excess cholesterol and other fatty plaque deposits, dissolve clots, and prevent sludging of red blood cells. These cleansing effects help prevent arteriosclerosis, heart attacks, and strokes. Fresh seafood also supplies the essential minerals and trace elements from the sea that are required for balanced brain and nerve functions, which is why fish has long been known as "brain food." Frozen seafood is an equally good source of nutrition, as long as the fish has been "fresh frozen" soon after the catch and not processed in factories. Commercially farmed seafood, however, is not a good food choice. Like other commercial livestock such as pigs and chickens, farmed fish are fed on industrially processed feed and heavily dosed with drugs and hormones that pass into your body when the fish is eaten. Similarly, unless you catch it yourself in a clean river or lake, freshwater fish is usually contaminated with the toxic pollutants that industry—particularly the commercial beef industry —dumps into public waterways.

FAT AND OIL

The first and foremost rule that governs healthy, rational choices in dietary fat and oil is this: strictly avoid *all* artificial substitutes for butter and cream, including margarine, "shortening," nondairy creamer, and nondairy whipped cream. All of these gummy, plasticine products are made with hydrogenated vegetable oils, which are forged at searing heats of over 500 °F, then bubbled through with hydrogen and hardened with nickel. When natural fats are replaced in the diet with these artificially synthesized fats, the body incorporates them into the construction of new cells, which become defective and malfunction as a result.

Because the cells of the brain and immune system require the most fat, these are the tissues that suffer the most damage from regular consumption of hydrogenated vegetable-oil products. Here's how Dr. Cass Igram, author of *Eat Right or Die Young,* describes the damage done to white blood cells and immune response when artificial fats made from hydrogenated oils are consumed:

> These cells incorporate the hydrogenated fats you eat into their membranes. When this happens, the white cells become sluggish in function, and their membranes actually become stiff. . . . This (response) leaves the body wide open to all sorts of derangements of the immune system. . . . In fact, one of the quickest ways to paralyze your immune system is to eat, on a daily basis, significant quantities of deep-fried foods, or fats such as margarine . . . [which] is associated with a greater incidence of a variety of cancers.

Real dairy butter, which is the only part of cow's milk that the human body can properly digest, is actually a rich source of metabolic energy. If butter comes from cows that are healthy and allowed to graze in green pastures, it is an excellent dietary source of fat nutrition. Ghee, also known as clarified butter, is made by skimming off all of the white protein particles from melted butter to produce a pure, clear "butter oil." This oil may be used for cooking at high heat without scorching the oil and producing free radicals. Fat rendered from beef (tallow) and pork (lard) should be eliminated entirely from the diet; both are highly acid-forming, extremely hard to digest, and damaging to the liver.

The best overall choice in oil for cooking food, mixing dressings, and other culinary purposes is high-grade olive oil. Olive oil can be used to cook food at high temperatures without producing an excess of free radicals, and it contains only the "good fats," such as the monounsaturated variety. Other healthy choices in edible oils include sesame, sunflower, peanut, and various other nut oils, preferably cold-pressed from organic sources. Many of the mass-produced, processed cooking oils on supermarket shelves today, including corn, soy bean, canola, and the dubious "blended vegetable oils," are not beneficial to human health, and some of them are downright hazardous to health, especially any oil that has been "hydrogenated." To be sure, always read the label.

DAIRY PRODUCTS

If health is the first priority in choosing foods for the human diet, then there's so much good reason not to consume pasteurized cow milk products from commercial dairies that it is difficult to understand why people who wish to stay healthy still do. Cow milk contains 400 percent more protein than human milk, including large amounts of casein, a tough protein substance so strong and sticky that it is often used to make book-binding glue and postal paste. Imagine what this stuff does to your bowels.

Pasteurization kills the active enzyme in milk that is required to digest it. Since most people don't produce this enzyme in their bodies, the milk stagnates in the stomach and the indigestible protein putrefies into a slimy sludge that oozes through the digestive tract and plasters gummy layers of mucus to the intestinal walls, forming a tough, rubbery lining that increasingly binds up the bowels. The reason that babies froth at the mouth and regurgitate foamy white phlegm after being fed pasteurized cow's milk is because their newly functioning stomachs, which are genetically designed to digest human milk, cannot digest the bovine casein protein in cow milk.

Today, commercial dairy milk is rendered even more hazardous to human health by the high doses of synthetic hormones that are fed to dairy cows to make them produce more milk. Residues of these powerful hormones, which can force a cow's mammary glands to produce five to six times more milk than untreated cows are able to, enter the human system when this milk is consumed. The residue can cause severe imbalances in the human endocrine system, especially in women and children. Women are particularly sensitive to these bovine hormones because they interfere with the delicate balance of female hormone cycles in the body, and in growing children these bovine growth factors can cause abnormal development, causing excessively rapid growth of tissues. Synthetic bovine hormones in commercial dairy milk, for example, has been indicated as a major factor in premature puberty in young girls.

In recent years, family physicians throughout the United States have reported an alarming rise in premature puberty among girls as young as eight and nine, including full breast development, sexual fertility, and pregnancy. Dairy hormones in the daily diet have become the major suspect in this abnormal development. These dairy hormones cause glandular deviations in adult women, as well. In *Food and Healing*, nutritional therapist Annemarie Colbin writes, "The consumption of dairy products, including milk, cheese, yogurt, and ice cream, appears to be strongly linked to various disorders of the female reproductive system, including ovarian tumors and cysts, vaginal discharges, and infections." In many cases, these problems quickly disappear soon after all dairy products are strictly eliminated from the diet.

Women in the Western world are advised by their doctors to drink pasteurized cow milk as a source of calcium to prevent osteoporosis, and yet the incidence of osteoporosis among dairy-consuming Western women continues to grow unabated because the human body cannot assimilate the calcium in cow milk. Owing to its high phosphorus content, which blocks absorption of calcium in the bowels, cow milk is definitely not a viable source of calcium for the human body. In fact, the acidity produced in the body by the putrefaction of milk products forces the body to leach calcium *out* of the body's own bones to restore alkaline balance in the bloodstream, and this process contributes further to osteoporosis. Doctors properly trained in basic nutritional science would never recommend cow milk as a dietary source of calcium for human nutrition, especially when so many richer, more bio-available sources of dietary calcium than milk are available, none of which causes the digestive distress produced by processed dairy products and all of which deliver far more calcium.

For example, while 100 grams of cow milk contains 118 mg of calcium, the same amount of almonds supplies 254 grams of calcium. Many other foods also deliver significantly more calcium than cow's milk. For example, 3½ ounces of broccoli delivers 130 grams of calcium, while the same 3½ ounce weight for each of the following foods delivers the following weights in calcium: kale 187 grams, sardines 400 grams, kelp has a whopping 1,093 grams; and 100 grams of the humble, organic sesame seeds supply a megadose of 1,160 mg of organic calcium to the body. So who needs cow's milk?

People who wish to include dairy items such as milk, cheese, and yogurt in their diets should choose products made from goat's milk, which has slightly alkalizing properties and contains the same basic proportions of protein, calcium, phosphorus, and other nutrients as human milk. And since it contains very little fat, goat's milk is relatively easy to digest and is low in calories.

GRAINS

Most grains are warming, acid-forming "Yang" foods and are best eaten with cooling, alkaline-forming vegetables to insure digestive and metabolic balance. The only major food grain that is alkalizing is millet, which was the first grain to be cultivated as food in ancient China. Wheat, on the other hand, which has for centuries been the most popular grain food in the Western world, is one of the most highly acid-forming grains, and it can cause allergic reactions in people who consume it daily. Rye is a much better choice than wheat, especially for making bread, because it is less acid-forming, supplies more well-balanced nutrition, and rarely causes allergic reactions.

Grains are easier to digest and more nutritionally complete when consumed in whole form rather than refined. Whole grains are truly "whole foods": they contain carbohydrates, proteins, fats, vitamins, minerals, and fiber. Newcomers to the science of food-combining often ask why a protein food such as meat and a carbohydrate food such as bread must be eaten separately to avoid indigestion and acidosis, whereas foods that contain both protein and carbohydrate, such as whole grains, may be eaten without causing trouble in the stomach.

Dr. Herbert Shelton, author of the booklet *Food Combining Made Easy*, answers this question as follows:

> There is a great difference between the digestion of a *food*, however complex its composition, and the digestion of a *mixture of different foods*. To a single article of food that is a starch-protein combination [e.g., whole grains], the body can easily adjust its juices, both as to strength and timing, to the digestive requirements of the food. But when two foods are eaten with different, even opposite, digestive needs [e.g., meat and bread], this precise adjustment of juices to requirements becomes impossible.

When boiling grains in whole form as a staple food for meals, they should first be washed well, drained, then soaked in pure water for two to three hours or overnight before cooking. Alternatively, you may first toast the grain till golden brown in an oven or a dry pan over a medium-hot flame, prior to boiling. This toasting process, known as "dextrinization," converts much of the starch content into simple sugars, making the cooked grain easier to digest and less acid-forming in the stomach. The chart below gives the cooking times, proportions of dry grain to water, and cooked yield for boiling brown rice, wild rice, buckwheat, and bulgur:

GRAIN	COOKING TIME	AMOUNT DRY	WATER	COOKED YIELD
Brown rice	35–40 min.	1 cup	2 cups	2 ½ cups
Wild rice	60 min.	1 cup	4 cups	3 ½ cups
Buckwheat	20 min.	1 cup	5 cups	3 cups
Bulgur	15 min.	1 cup	2 cups	2 ½ cups

The other way to prepare whole grains as food is to grind them into flour and bake bread. Bread is one of the most ancient and widely consumed foods in the Western world, but virtually all of it today is made with baker's yeast, which ruins much of the bread's nutritional value and causes allergic reactions in people who are sensitive to yeast. The problem with yeast as a leavening agent for bread is that it renders the calcium and magnesium in the flour insoluble and therefore unavailable to the body. Calcium and magnesium are the two most important macrominerals required for human health, and they play especially important roles in detox and alkaline balance. Whole grains are one of the best dietary sources of these essential nutrients. Even when high quality organically grown grains are used to make bread, if the dough is leavened with yeast, it robs the body of an important source of dietary calcium and magnesium and makes bread more acid-forming in the digestive tract.

The solution here is to "go back to the basics" and eat only whole-grain breads that are prepared with natural "sourdough" leavening. Sourdough produces precisely the right balance of pH and other vital factors that allow calcium, magnesium, and other minerals in whole-grain flours to become soluble during digestion and makes them easy to assimilate into the bloodstream. When Celtic sea salt is used in making sourdough bread, it further increases the bread's bio-available magnesium content and improves the fermentation of the dough, making the bread even more digestible. Using sourdough cultures to ferment flour for bread, pancakes, and other leavened-grain products is similar to using lactobacteria to ferment milk and make yogurt: the bacteria predigests the protein and starch in the flour, rendering it far easier to digest in the stomach.

Whenever eating grains, don't forget to chew well before swallowing. Chewing grains thoroughly saturates the starch with ptyalin enzyme from the salivary glands in the mouth, without which the grains cannot be properly digested in the stomach. When grains are wolfed down without sufficient mastication in the mouth, they ferment rather than digest in the stomach, producing acid indigestion and gas.

FERMENTED FOODS

Fermentation has been used as a way to prepare food for at least as long as fire has, and fermented foods play an important role in healthy human diets. Fermentation by "friendly" bacteria breaks down complex carbohydrates and proteins in food, predigesting them so that they are easier to digest and assimilate. Fermentation also increases the vitamin content in food, especially B vitamins, and provides abundant supplies of bio-active enzymes that assist digestion and help regulate pH balance in the digestive tract. The bacteria cultures used in fermented foods support the colonies of "friendly" flora in the lower bowels, which facilitates regular bowel movements.

In Western diets, yogurt and sauerkraut are good examples of fermented foods that provide both nutritional and digestive benefits. Traditional Asian cuisines feature a wide range of tasty, nourishing foods made by fermentation. Koreans eat a fiery fermented side dish called *kimchee*, made with cabbage, carrot, garlic, and chili, at almost every meal. Thai dishes are liberally laced with a pungent, fermented fish sauce called *namphla*. Chinese cooks use lots of fermented soy sauce, chili pastes, and bean curd products and prepare a variety of fermented vegetable side dishes known as *pao-tsai*. Indonesians eat a delicious, nutrient-rich ferment of soy beans called *tempeh*, and Japanese cuisine features richly fermented miso paste for soups and sauces, fermented fish and vegetable side dishes, and the remarkably nutritious, strongly flavored ferment of whole soy beans called *naddo*, which is one of the few nonanimal dietary sources of vitamin B12. All of these traditional Asian, fermented beans and vegetables are easier to digest and richer in nutritional value than commercial yogurt made from pasteurized cow milk, and they are therefore the best choices in fermented foods.

"SUGAR BLUES"

Sugar Blues is the title of a book by William Duffy, in which he states, "The difference between sugar addiction and narcotic addiction is largely one of degree." The average daily consumption per person of refined white sugar in the United States has reached an astounding fifty-three teaspoons, which amounts to about half a pound of sugar per person per day. This certainly qualifies as substance abuse. Such a high rate of sugar consumption definitely becomes addictive, causing symptoms similar to drug addiction.

Whenever such massive quantities of industrially refined sugar enter the body, the immune system treats it as a toxic substance, which it certainly is at those dosages, and this triggers a continuous autoimmune response that throws the whole system off balance. One of those emergency responses is the constant secretion of insulin from the pancreas, which is needed to break down the massive overdose of sugar in the bloodstream. Over time, this causes the pancreas to swell up from overstimulation, and to finally collapse from depletion, at which point diabetes develops. Meanwhile, the excess insulin activity in the bloodstream suppresses release of growth hormone in the pituitary gland, which weakens immune response and lowers resistance.

Refined sugar is one of the primary causes of obesity and arteriosclerosis in the Western world. When sugar is consumed to excess, the liver converts most of it into triglycerides and stores it as fat, transforming the rest of it into the "bad" cholesterol that gets deposited as a sticky sludge in the walls of the arteries. Sugar is also a primary cause of osteoporosis and tooth decay because the extreme acidosis it produces forces the body to re-alkalize itself by leaching calcium from bones and teeth.

In addition, excessive consumption of refined white sugar has extremely deleterious effects on human behavior, particularly in children. The hyperactivity, learning disabilities, and other behavioral disorders experienced by so many children today is largely due to excessive intake of sugar. Studies conducted by Dr. C. Keith Connors at the Children's Hospital in Washington DC have established what he calls a "deadly link" between excessive daily consumption of sugar—especially when combined with starch—and the development of hypertension, violent behavior, and learning impediments in children. In 1991, to reduce the exposure of children to this health hazard, Singapore banned the sale of all sugary, carbonated soft-drinks at schools and youth centers, setting off a howl of protest from peddlers of the most popular and profitable brands of these addictive drinks. By contrast, many public schools in the

United States sign exclusive contracts with the major producers of these acidifying, enervating, habit-forming drinks, in exchange for a cut of the profits, allowing children to freely nurse their sugar habits throughout the day from vending machines. Trial studies have shown that chronic violence among inmates in prisons drops dramatically when all foods made with refined sugar are withdrawn from prison diets. There's no reason to think that the same would not hold true for chronic violence in schools.

Artificial sweeteners such as saccharin and aspartame are even more hazardous to health than refined white sugar. These synthetic sweeteners should be strictly avoided, particularly in light of evidence linking them with a wide range of disorders, including cancer, nerve damage, immune dysfunction, and metabolic problems that lead to obesity. The best alternatives to refined white sugar are whole, natural sweeteners such as unrefined, raw cane sugar, honey, and maple syrup. The latter is an especially good choice because it is a complete whole food in itself, brimming with many essential vitamins, minerals, trace elements, and other nutritional factors drawn from deep within the earth by maple trees.

For weight-watchers and diabetics, nature provides the perfect herbal sweetener in the form of a plant called "Stevia." Stevia is extracted from the leaves of a shrub native to South America, and gram-for-gram it is one hundred times sweeter than sugar. A serving the size of a match head suffices to sweeten any hot or cold beverage, and Stevia may also be used for cooking, sweetening porridge, and other culinary purposes. It also tastes good. Not only is Stevia harmless to diabetics, it actually helps them by improving the efficiency of insulin activity in the bloodstream. Stevia is by far the most rational and healthy choice as an alternative sweetener for people who have a "sweet tooth" but who don't want to gain weight from all the extra calories in sugar, or who worry about developing diabetes from excess consumption of refined white sugar. The product is not expensive and may found at most well-stocked health shops or may be obtained from mail-order suppliers.

"THE SALT OF LIFE"

Salt has always been one of the most basic pillars of life in the human diet. Like so many other fundamental foods, modern food processing methods have denatured commercial salt supplies and stripped them of their most essential nutrients. The salt sold today in supermarkets for kitchen and table use is over 99 percent sodium chloride, and like refined white sugar, it is this industrially processed salt that is harmful to human health, not natural, whole salt.

The most important element missing from refined salt is magnesium, a deficiency of which contributes to heart disease, nervous system disorders, and immune deficiency. Clinical studies in Canada and the United States have shown a dramatic decline in the mortality rate among heart-attack patients who were given intravenous injections of magnesium. Magnesium is also an essential supporting factor in phagocytosis, an important immune response whereby white blood cells destroy infectious bacteria and scavenge other pathogens in the body. Perhaps most important of all, magnesium regulates the balance of acid and alkaline elements in the cellular fluids, thereby keeping the biochemistry of the entire body properly balanced by automatically adjusting cellular pH levels. Dr. Jacques de Langre, author of *Sea Salt's Hidden Powers,* cites magnesium as the single most vital element required to maintain proper pH balance in the body:

> The human organism functions at its peak only when the balance between acid and alkaline is maintained. All substances that nourish the body are either acid or alkaline. Magnesium possesses the remarkable ability to maintain the acid/alkaline balance within the organism.

The best sources of magnesium and other essential minerals and trace elements are whole Celtic sea salt and Himalayan Glacial Salt, as discussed in previous chapters. Celtic sea salt is only 87 percent sodium chloride, plus the full spectrum of eighty-one other macro- and microminerals from the sea, all in precisely the proportions required by the human body. Himalayan Glacial Salt contains 30 percent less sodium than other forms of sea salt, and it may therefore be consumed in larger amounts for extra mineral supplementation. Those who wish to increase their intake of magnesium to correct blood acidosis and alkalize the cellular fluids may use the fluid bittern of Celtic sea salt, the liquid blend of magnesium chloride and Celtic sea salt, or pure magnesium chloride oil, mentioned in chapter 2.

SUPER SUPPLEMENTS

Debate continues to rage regarding the efficacy of vitamins and other concentrated nutritional supplements, and like most health issues, both sides have their valid points. For one thing, there's a big difference between the benefits of synthetically manufactured supplements and those extracted from natural sources without the use of heat or industrial solvents. The efficacy of any given supplement also depends to a great extent on other supporting factors, such as diet, consistent dosage, use of medical and recreational drugs, exercise, and overall lifestyle. One thing can be said for certain: even the very best supplements cannot compensate for the ill effects of poor diet, malnutrition, excessive smoking and drinking, frequent use of pharmaceutical drugs, and a high-stress lifestyle. Unless you're willing to systematically adjust all the basic factors of life, there's no point in going to the expense and trouble of using costly supplements.

The supplements recommended below are all derived from natural sources, and each provides specific forms of protection against various factors that contribute to acidosis and toxemia. While some of these supplements also have excellent nutritional benefits, the primary reason for their inclusion here is their facilitating role in daily detox functions. All of them have potent alkalizing, detoxifying, and digestive properties that assist in the elimination of toxins and acid wastes from the tissues and that continuously purify the bloodstream, thereby helping to keep the whole system properly balanced.

Antioxidants

Antioxidants scavenge and neutralize free radicals, which are highly reactive molecular fragments produced internally by natural metabolic processes as well as by pollutants assimilated from external sources, such as contaminants in food, water, and air. Free radicals are the cellular terrorists of the body, roaming randomly through the tissues, blasting holes in cell walls, damaging DNA codes, disrupting vital functions, and laying waste to the internal terrain of the body. Antioxidants are the special "commandos" introduced into the body with food, water, and air to hunt down free radicals and terminate their destructive activity. With the steep rise in free-radical activity today caused by toxic contamination within the body, antioxidants have become one of our strongest allies in the ongoing war against the cellular terrorism of free radicals.

Certain nutrients such as vitamins C, E, and beta carotene and the minerals zinc and selenium, play key roles in the body's antioxidant defenses. Vitamin E breaks the self-generating chain reactions whereby free radicals operate, and it boosts the body's overall immunity and resistance. Vitamin E also helps protect the tissues against damage from toxic chemicals such as mercury, lead, benzene, and other poisons and has inhibiting effects against the development of cancer and heart disease. Vitamin C effectively scavenges a wide range of free radicals and works within the cells as well to protect DNA from free-radical damage. Vitamin C also provides specific protection against cardiovascular disease and enhances overall immune response. Beta carotene is the strongest antioxidant for scavenging an extremely reactive type of free radical known as "singlet oxygen," and it also inhibits the formation of cancerous tumors.

Selenium is a trace element that has been almost totally leached out of the food chain by modern farming and food-processing methods. Selenium is essential for the synthesis of peroxidase, one of the body's most important antioxidant enzymes, which neutralizes hydrogen peroxide and other peroxide radicals that are produced in the body by fats. Selenium itself bonds with mercury, lead, cadmium, and arsenic, neutralizing these heavy toxins and carrying them away for excretion. Selenium has become so scarce in food that supplementary supplies are the only viable source for most people today. Zinc is the key element in the body's other major antioxidant enzyme, superoxide dismutase (SOD), which scavenges free radicals in all of the body's tissues and vital fluids.

Whatever other vitamin and mineral supplements you may wish to take as part of your daily diet, include therapeutic doses of vitamins E, C, and beta carotene, plus the minerals selenium and zinc, to insure sufficient antioxidant activity, especially if you live in polluted urban environments.

Recent studies in Japan, China, and the United States have shown that unfermented green tea from Japan and semifermented High Mountain Oolung Tea from Taiwan have very potent antioxidant properties and provide significant protection against cancer. While both green tea and High Mountain Oolung Tea have strong antioxidant activity, green tea can irritate the stomach when drunk in sufficient quantities to have therapeutic effects, and it is not nearly as fragrant and flavorful as the top grades of High Mountain Oolung Tea, which may be consumed freely throughout the day without upsetting the stomach.

The anticancer effect in those teas is produced by compounds known as polyphenols. Research in Japan has demonstrated that High Mountain Oolung Tea provides particularly strong protection against toxic damage and cancer formation in the lungs. In East Asia, where people smoke heavily, High Mountain Oolung Tea has long been the tea of choice among smokers, and those who drink it daily have a consistently lower incidence of lung cancer than smokers who don't. One of the ways in which this tea suppresses growth of cancerous tumors is by inhibiting angiogenesis, a process whereby tumors generate growth of their own blood vessels to allow them to expand and multiply. Green and High Mountain Oolung teas also contain half a dozen types of catechins, which are potent phytochemicals that strengthen antioxidant defenses by stimulating production of peroxidase, SOD, and other important antioxidant enzymes in the body. On top of all that, these teas aid digestion, alkalize bodily fluids, purify the bloodstream, and gently stimulate the nervous system without racing the heart, as coffee does.

Another primary source of an antioxidant defense in the body comes from the negative ions that are derived from ionized air and water. The best way to enlist this ally into your army of antioxidants is to drink ionized water and breath ionized air, as discussed in foregoing chapters.

Green Food

Green food has already been mentioned in chapter 5 as a potent cleansing supplement for detox diets, but it is also very useful in daily diets as a source of essential nutrients and blood purifiers. Green food's strong alkalizing and internal cleansing properties make it an excellent supplement for counteracting the internal pollution and acidity produced in the body by modern diets and eating habits. Its full-spectrum profile of essential nutrients compensates for common nutritional deficiencies in modern diets, insuring the body a daily supply of all the vital elements it needs to function properly.

Enzymes

Enzymes are the "spark plugs" of human metabolism, providing the ignition that catalyzes every metabolic reaction in the body. Over five thousand different enzymes have so far been identified in the human body, and without them the whole system would grind to a halt. Here's how Dr. Edward Howell, one of the world's foremost authorities on enzymes, describes their importance in his book *Enzyme Nutrition:*

> No mineral, vitamin, or hormone can do any work without enzymes. Our bodies, all of our organs, tissues, and cells, are run by metabolic enzymes. They are the manual workers that build our bodies from proteins, carbohydrates, and fats.

Among the thousands of enzymes in the body, the three most important types for detox and cleansing purposes are antioxidant enzymes, such as peroxidase and SOD, digestive enzymes such as those secreted by the pancreas to handle the advanced stages of digestion, and food enzymes, which are not produced in the body and can only be obtained from fresh raw foods. Food enzymes, which are destroyed by heat in cooking and by chemical additives in processed foods, are required for the first stages of digestion in the stomach, and if they are missing, complex foods such as proteins and carbohydrates cannot be completely digested. Unless your daily diet consists of at least 30–50 percent fresh, enzyme-rich raw foods, you should take capsules of food enzymes with all meals that consist mainly of cooked foods. The four primary food enzymes required for digestion are the following:

Protease

This enzyme digests protein as well as pathogenic bacteria, damaged cells, the membranes around viruses, inflammatory fluids such as pus and phlegm, and any other harmful substance that contains protein.

Amylase

Amylase digests carbohydrates in food and helps dissolve pus and phlegm in damaged tissues. Combined with lipase, amylase digests a wide range of viruses and helps eliminate impacted mucus from inflamed lungs and bronchial passages.

Lipase

This is the enzyme responsible for digesting fats. It also dissolves the fatty part of the membrane that envelops many types of viruses, and the fatty deposits in the arteries.

Cellulase

Cellulase digests the cellulose content in food, so that it may pass easily through the digestive tract as fibrous bulk to assist the elimination of wastes.

Food enzymes have strong alkaline-forming properties, which help reduce acid-forming reactions throughout the digestive tract and prevent blood acidosis. Because they improve digestive efficiency, food enzymes also reduce production of toxic wastes in the digestive tract, thereby preventing the development of toxemia. In addition to taking them for digestive purposes with cooked meals, food enzymes may also be taken on an empty stomach when ill, in which case they enter general circulation in the bloodstream, assisting other immune factors such as white blood cells on search-and-destroy missions against pathogens and pollutants and breaking down mucus, phlegm, and pus in ailing organs and damaged tissues.

Supplements containing both digestive enzymes and food enzymes are available in tablet or capsule form for convenient daily use.

"ALKA-AID"

In case of sudden gastrointestinal distress caused by excess acidity from wrong food combinations, highly acid-forming foods such as sugar and meat, excessive use of pharmaceutical or recreational drugs, or intake of poisonous substances, the following supplements may be taken for fast, effective alkalization in the stomach and digestive tract. All of them are natural products and perfectly safe to use. You may take more than one at a time for even stronger alkalizing effects.

Fresh Lemon Juice

Mix the juice of one large or two small fresh lemons (not limes) with four ounces of water, and take one teaspoon every fifteen to twenty minutes until the acid crisis passes. This is particularly effective therapy for kidney stones.

Apple Cider Vinegar

A great stomach alkalizer and digestive aid, apple cider vinegar contains malic acid, not the acidifying acetic acid found in other vinegars. It increases the flow of gastric juices in the stomach and counteracts acidity throughout the digestive tract. As a digestive aid, take 2 tablespoons with 1 teaspoon of honey in warm water, twenty to thirty minutes before meals; or take it any time of day or night on an empty stomach for swift alkaline relief.

Cream of Tartar

A highly alkalizing source of natural potassium, ½ teaspoon of cream of tartar may be stirred into a few ounces of water and taken for immediate relief of acid-forming reactions in the body, including the acidity produced by stress and anxiety.

Charcoal powder

Pure powdered charcoal in capsule or tablet form may be used in cases of extreme stomach acidity due to food poisoning, fermentation and putrefaction, or poor digestion. Take four to five capsules, or stir one teaspoon of the powder into a glass of water, for quick symptomatic relief of strong acid reactions in the stomach.

Baking Soda

Sodium bicarbonate swiftly neutralizes almost any sort of excess acidity in the stomach, and it may be used as often as required for such relief. Take 1 level teaspoon stirred into a glass of water, and repeat again later if necessary.

SHORT LIST OF SUGGESTIONS FOR CULTIVATING RATIONAL EATING HABITS

Many people these days prefer to have important new information on healthy lifestyle habits succinctly summarized in list format, so that they can tack it to the kitchen cupboard or family bulletin board for quick and easy daily reference. The dozen dietary precepts listed below may serve this purpose:

1. Don't eat unless you're hungry, and when you do eat, follow the "Chinese Rule" of eating only until chi-ba fen bao, 70–80 percent full.
2. Whether cooking food at home or ordering it in a restaurant, keep your meals as simple as possible by not combining more than three or four different categories of food at the same meal,

and by combining those properly in accordance with the laws of trophology.

3. Strictly avoid eating all products made with hydrogenated vegetable oils.

4. In addition to balancing your individual meals by the rules of food combining, balance your whole diet according to season and climate. In the heat of summer, eat more cooling fresh vegetables and fruit; in the cold of winter, eat more warming proteins and carbohydrates. And always try to eat food that's in season.

5. Try to eat at least 30–50 percent of your daily diet in the form of fresh raw foods—more in summer, less in winter.

6. Strictly avoid consuming any form of artificial sweeteners, and strictly limit intake of refined white sugar. If you like sweet things and are worried about calories or diabetes, use natural Stevia as your sweetener.

7. Try to chew your food thirty to forty times before swallowing, especially when eating starchy carbohydrates. Brown rice, which is acid-forming, actually becomes alkaline-forming if chewed at least one hundred times, due to abundant salivation with the alkaline enzyme ptyalin in the mouth. You may not wish to chew all bread, rice, and noodles that many times, but at least be aware that the more you chew them, the further they move toward the alkaline side of the scale, and the less acidity they produce in the stomach.

8. Don't drink juice or water together with your meals because it dilutes salivary and gastric secretions, which delays digestion and permits fermentation. A glass of beer or wine sipped slowly with meals is fine, because beer and wine are fermented beverages, which means that they are "predigested" and contain enzymes that assist digestion in the stomach—hence the old saying, "Take a little wine for the stomach's sake."

9. Try to drink at least six, eight-ounce glasses (1½ quarts) of pure, alkaline water every day, but drink the water only between meals. A good regimen is to drink two glasses immediately upon

arising in the morning; one glass late-morning, before lunch; two glasses in the afternoon between lunch and dinner; and one glass between dinner and bedtime.

10. Eat the sort of food that fits your lifestyle and work habits. Unless you do hard manual labor every day, or engage in strenuous physical exercise, don't eat too much animal protein and fat, because most of it will rot in your bowels and poison your body with toxic by-products of putrefaction, rather than being used to build new muscle and connective tissue. If you do a lot of mental work, eat plenty of complex whole carbohydrates to provide sustained cerebral energy, but take it easy on refined sugar and starch. "You are what you eat," and therefore you should eat to suit the way you are.

11. Eat your meals only when you can take the time to sit down, relax, and eat properly; don't eat in a hurry or "on the run." The faster you eat food, the more slowly it digests.

12. Do not eat solid food when you're sick, especially when you have a fever or chills, or when you feel acute pain. And don't eat when you're feeling emotionally upset or mentally unbalanced, such as when you're angry, anxious, worried, or confused. The digestive system shuts down under these conditions, so whatever enters the stomach just sits there and decays, forming acids and toxins, which only makes your condition worse. Fasting is the best cure for most ills.

Last but not least, always try to follow the "golden mean" of moderation in food. An ancient Chinese adage states, "Disease enters the body through the mouth," and this dietary wisdom is echoed in a similar Western maxim, "We dig our graves with our teeth."

Toward the end of the nineteenth century, a group of scientists spent the better part of a decade traveling through Europe, Scandinavia, and the British Isles, searching out and investigating as many cases as they could find of individuals who had already lived past the age of one hundred and were still alive. Altogether they located nearly two thousand living centenarians, some of whom were already well past 150 and on their way to becoming "bicentenarians." After carefully questioning these venerable elders and their families regarding their personal lifestyles and daily eating habits, the common factor discovered in all cases was moderation in food. Here's an excerpt from their report, as quoted in Baroody's book *Alkalize or Die*:

> On reviewing nearly 2,000 reported cases of persons who lived more than a century, we generally find some peculiarity of diet or habits to account for their alleged longevity; we find some were living amongst all the luxurie . . . others in the most abject poverty . . . some drank large quantities of water, others little; some were total abstainers from alcoholic drinks, others drunkards; some smoked tobacco, others did not; some lived entirely on vegetables, others to a great extent on animal foods . . . some worked with their brains, others with their hands; some ate one meal a day, others four or five . . . in fact, we notice a great divergence both in habits and diet, but in those cases where we have been able to obtain a reliable account of the diet, we find *one great cause* which accounts for the majority of cases of longevity: *moderation in the quantity of food.*

Let's leave the final word on this topic to the ancient Greek philosopher Diogenes, who left us so much other sage advice regarding the foibles and follies of human behavior. "As houses well stored with provisions are likely to be full of mice," he wryly noted, "so the bodies of those who eat much are full of diseases."

12

ADVICE ON SMOKING AND DRINKING

Smoking and drinking are the most common and widespread forms of so-called recreational drugs that are used throughout the world today. If we're going to discuss these issues rationally within the context of human health and longevity, then we must be perfectly clear about two basic points. The first is the fact that tobacco and alcohol are potent, habit-forming drugs, and smoking and drinking are essentially methods of delivering these drugs into the human system. Most people who use tobacco and alcohol daily wince when reminded that these substances are "drugs," and many of them deny it on the assumption that because tobacco and alcohol are legal and don't require a prescription, they are neither drugs nor dangerous. This is wishful thinking, and anyone who smokes or drinks on that basis tends not to exercise the caution and self-discipline that should govern the use of any potent drug.

The second point we must bear in mind here is this: the distinction people make between recreational and therapeutic use of drugs, including tobacco and alcohol, is tenuous at best, and the difference between the recreational and therapeutic effects of a particular drug is usually more a matter of semantics than substance. Who's to say whether a woman sitting in a cafe and lighting up her third cigarette over her second cup of coffee is smoking "like a chimney" because smoking is so much fun and tastes so good (recreational), or because it instantly relieves her tension, calms her nerves, and helps her think more clearly (therapeutic)? And who can tell whether a man drinking his third martini during "Happy Hour" at his favorite bar after work is doing so as a friendly social gesture and an epicurean experience (recreational), or as a quick-fix remedy for stress, anxiety, or depression (therapeutic)?

From the viewpoint of health, it doesn't matter whether the reason people smoke or drink is recreational or therapeutic, because the basic effects they have on the body and mind are the same either way. Both tobacco and alcohol belong to a class of drugs known as intoxicants, and as the name clearly indicates, they are not only intoxicating but also toxic. The reason that people take such drugs, despite the fact that they are toxic to the body, is because a side effect of these substances is to intoxicate the mind by altering brain chemistry. All intoxicants have a strong natural affinity for brain and nerve tissues, and the "high" (or "low") that they produce in the mind is a direct result of their toxic effects on brain and nerve cells; that's why this psychoactive effect is known as intoxication. By altering the body's brain chemistry and interfering with nerve transmissions, intoxicants change the way the mind experiences the world through the body's physical senses, thereby producing an altered state of mind. People who use intoxicants do so because the way they normally experience the world causes them to feel pain, anger, sadness, fear, anxiety, or sheer boredom, and they know that they can alter these unhappy feelings instantly with a quick nip of whatever turns them on.

Among the many intoxicants found in nature, modern societies have chosen, for reasons that we shall not speculate upon here, to make tobacco and alcohol the primary and only legal forms of recreational drugs. The point remains, however, that like all toxic substances that have intoxicating side effects on the mind—including some of the most potent medicinal plants and minerals in traditional herbal medicine—tobacco and alcohol also have very specific physiological effects in the body, and these effects can be used beneficially as therapy for relieving the symptoms of various ailments and correcting internal imbalances, particularly in the nervous system. Therefore, like all toxic substances that have both therapeutic and recreational applications, tobacco and alcohol should always be used with caution and moderation to insure that the user may enjoy the benefits of the desired effects, regardless of why the substances are used, without causing permanent damage to the body.

"SMOKE SIGNALS"

From the point of view of health, the best advice on smoking is this:

"Don't!"

While not every substance that's smoked is addictive, smoking itself is highly habit-forming, and while some forms of smoking may be marginally more or less harmful than others, the real damage to health is caused by smoking itself, not by the particular substance smoked. Smoking involves the inhalation of highly toxic by-products of combustion, many of which are carcinogenic. "Where there's smoke there's fire," and when the fire is burning dried plant material such as tobacco, not only does it produces searing hot smoke, it also produces extremely poisonous chemicals that damage the delicate lining of the bronchia and lungs, cause highly acid-forming reactions in the blood, and leave harmful toxic residues in the tissues. So unless you have valid medical reasons for smoking, it is simply not worth the risk.

Nevertheless, all kinds of people throughout the world choose to smoke, and like everything else in life, there are relatively good ways and bad ways to conduct a smoking habit, especially for those who smoke primarily as a means of balancing the nervous system and stimulating cerebral functions. During the 1950s, the renowned clairvoyant healer Edgar Cayce sometimes advised clients to smoke three-to-eight cigarettes of tobacco per day to control the symptoms of nervous disorders and to compensate for inherent imbalances in neurochemistry. It didn't matter whether the client already smoked or not, but Cayce stipulated that to gain the desired therapeutic effects without harming health, it was essential not to exceed his recommended daily dosage of three-to-eight cigarettes. Tobacco is a potent medicinal herb with strong natural affinity for brain and nerve tissues. Even in very moderate doses such as those recommended by Cayce, tobacco stimulates abundant secretions of a wide range of vital neurotransmitters that are essential for balanced brain functions. In Cayce's time, cigarettes were not yet contaminated with dioxin and the hundreds of other carcinogenic chemical additives that are used to manufacture cigarettes today. Cigarettes then were still a relatively safe product, especially when used according to Cayce's guidelines. For people who cannot think clearly or function properly in society due to nervous disorders caused by inherent or acquired imbalances in their neurochemistry, the moderate risks to health posed by smoking three-to-eight cigarettes made with pure tobacco and rolled in chemical-free paper are certainly acceptable, if that's what it takes to control their symptoms. As long as smokers don't exceed such a moderate daily dosage, they can gain significant therapeutic benefits from smoking tobacco, at minimum cost to health, and the smoking habit can become more helpful than harmful.

Similarly, many people today who are suffering from the advanced stages of cancer and AIDS report that smoking a bit of cannabis hemp stimulates their appetites and restores their capacity to digest food and assimilate nutrition, while also relieving the intense physical pain caused by their conditions, and allowing them to sleep soundly at night. Prior to its prohibition, opium was also smoked as much for its therapeutic medicinal benefits as for recreational pleasure. In fact, during the eighteenth and nineteenth centuries in China, traditional doctors often recommended that elderly people suffering from chronic pain and incurable degenerative conditions associated with the aging process start smoking opium in moderate daily dosages to control their discomfort and permit them to continue enjoying life. While certainly addictive, opium is no more addictive than tobacco, and smoking opium the Chinese way, which involves distillation rather than combustion, is considerably less harmful to health than smoking either tobacco or hemp, as evidenced by the remarkable longevity of many old Chinese opium smokers who properly conducted their habits and never exceeded their daily measure.

Today, however, both opium and hemp are prohibited, and tobacco is the only neuro-active medicinal herb that may be smoked legally for recreational or therapeutic purposes. Smokers should be aware, however, that tobacco is at least as addictive as opium, and that smoking is an even more difficult addiction to break than using opiates. Smoking tobacco is also more hazardous to health than smoking either hemp or opium. Nevertheless, since tobacco remains the only legal and socially condoned form of smoking throughout most of the world today, we shall limit our discussion here to tobacco.

Cigarettes

If you smoke cigarettes, the best advice is not to exceed Edgar Cayce's recommended daily allowance of three-to-eight cigarettes, and to strictly follow the cardinal rule of, "Roll your own, or leave them alone!" Factory-made cigarettes today truly live up to their designation as "coffin nails," but what causes lung cancer and eventually kills the smoker is not the tobacco—it is the carcinogenic chemicals added to both the tobacco and the paper in the factory production process. Among the approximately two thousand toxic chemicals commonly found in commercially produced cigarettes today, dioxin poses the greatest threat to human health. Dioxin is a proven carcinogen that not only causes cancer but also produces genetic mutations, reproductive defects, and brain damage. According to the Environmental Protection Agency in America, "Dioxin is by far the most toxic chemical known to mankind." A report issued by a group of distinguished German scientists in 1998 concludes that dioxin alone is responsible for at least 12 percent of all human cancers in industrialized societies. Dioxin is definitely not something you want to inhale into your lungs from the burning tip of a cigarette—not unless you're trying to kill yourself.

Many popular brands of cigarette today also contain radioactive residues from the uranium dust that commercial growers add to the chemical fertilizers they use on their tobacco crops. Why on earth they add radioactive material to the soil in which tobacco is grown has not been explained, but traces of radioactive isotopes of uranium are present in their tobacco products as well as in the lungs of people who smoke them. No wonder the Marlboro Man succumbed to lung cancer at the height of his fame.

The paper used to manufacture ready-made cigarettes is even more contaminated with poisonous chemicals than the tobacco itself. Cigarette smokers who are still reluctant to take the time to roll their own cigarettes should try this experiment: cut open a typical popular brand of cigarette, remove the tobacco, flatten out the paper, and lay it in an ashtray. With the glowing tip of a lit cigarette, touch one corner of the paper and observe what happens. The edge of the paper ignites and the entire sheet gradually incinerates to ash, without bursting into flame, as the glowing edge fizzles and sparkles like the fuse of a firecracker, searing its way through the paper until it's gone. The chemicals added to cigarette paper to produce this effect are similar to those used in making fuses for firecrackers and other explosives, and the reason they're added is to make sure that the cigarette continues burning even when the smoker isn't puffing on it, to increase consumption and sales of cigarettes. Smokers accustomed to the convenience of ready-made factory cigarettes may find rolling their own inconvenient at first, but the task is not nearly as inconvenient as getting lung cancer. Here again, if health and longevity are important considerations, the "cost/benefit" ratio of smoking "coffin nails" compared with that of rolling your own cigarettes clearly dictates that you roll your own.

Good quality, organically grown tobaccos that are free of chemical additives and radioactive residues are now available on the market. They include such brands as "American Spirit" rolling tobacco, and while they may be somewhat more expensive than commercial factory brands, if you roll your own cigarettes and smoke moderately, your consumption will decline so much that it offsets the extra cost of buying pure tobacco. It is equally important to use pure cigarette papers that have not been chemically treated to make them burn faster, and these too are readily available in tobacco shops. One of the purest cigarette papers is "Club" brand, made by S. D. Modiano. These papers have no gum or glue, are thin as a butterfly's wing, and yield a minimum of toxic wastes when burned.

Cigars

"A woman is just a woman," wrote Kipling, "but a cigar is a smoke!" While this doesn't say much for Kipling's feelings toward women, it says a lot about the way dedicated cigar smokers feel about their preferred manner of smoking tobacco. Cigars rolled in natural whole tobacco leaves were the first form of smoking brought to England and Europe from its native habitat in the New World, and purists still feel that only a cigar is a real "smoke." Paper-rolled cigarettes were a later British and European development, which then replaced cigars as the world's most widespread form of tobacco smoking.

Assuming that they are made from pure tobacco that is uncontaminated by chemical additives and that they are rolled in natural leaves, cigars are significantly less hazardous to human health than cigarettes. Former President Clinton's claim not to have inhaled marijuana may be fatuous, but he probably didn't inhale the smoke from his cigars. Cigars are designed to allow nicotine to be gradually absorbed through the mucus membranes in the mouth and nasal cavities, as smoke wafts continuously through the lips and nostrils, without inhaling it into the lungs. Since it takes much longer to smoke a cigar than a cigarette, by the time the smoker has finished the cigar, he or she will have slowly but surely assimilated enough nicotine into the bloodstream to suffice the body's requirements for quite some time. To obtain therapeutic dosages of nicotine from cigarettes, the smoke must be inhaled all the way through the bronchia and into the lungs, a much more invasive way of smoking that damages the delicate lining of these organs with heat and carcinogenic chemicals. While good cigars made by hand with pure tobacco, such as the better brands produced in Cuba, are far more expensive than cheap dime store "stogies," the latter are every bit as hazardous to health as factory-made cigarettes owing to the toxic chemical additives and synthetic wrappers used to mass-produce them. The extra cost of a pure cigar may therefore be offset in exactly the same way as the extra cost of pure cigarette tobacco and pure food—consume less, enjoy more, and live longer!

Pipes

The third way to smoke tobacco is in a pipe. Here too, only pure tobacco that's free of chemical additives and artificial-flavoring agents should be smoked in pipes. Owing to growing awareness among smokers regarding the deadly dangers of chemical contaminants in tobacco, many tobacco shops these days stock a variety of organically grown pipe tobaccos flavored only with natural plant essences. Besides ordinary tobacco pipes, water pipes may also be used to provide an additional measure of protection against the harsh by-products of combustion by running the smoke through water first.

"FIRE WATER"

"Fire Water" is the term that Native American tribes used to describe rum and other liquors brought to North America by British and European colonists. Alcohol intoxication contributed heavily to the downfall of traditional tribal cultures in North America, just as it did in Australia when British settlers introduced "devil rum" to indigenous aboriginal tribes there. The blood, liver, and brain chemistry of these genetic groups are unable to properly metabolize alcohol, resulting in devastating destructive effects on their bodies and brains whenever alcohol is consumed. For this reason, alcohol still remains a "forbidden fruit" in many traditional tribal cultures, as well as in most Islamic countries and many parts of India, where its consumption is strictly prohibited and severely punished.

In the Western world, however, from early Greek and Roman times right down to modern European and American societies, alcohol has always been the main intoxicant of choice, and liquor is consumed in more variety and volume than anywhere else on earth. When Westerners began to colonize Asia and Africa during the seventeenth and eighteenth centuries, they brought their liquor and drinking habits with them, prompting native observers to remark, "Liquor is to the white man as mother's milk is to babies."

From the viewpoint of traditional Eastern medicine, "Fire Water" is actually a very apt term for alcohol. When alcohol is metabolized, it produces a lot of heat in the body, and if consumed daily in large amounts, this constant metabolic "fire" tends to "burn out" the internal organs, particularly the liver and brain. Alcohol is also a potent solvent of organic matter, which means it can dissolve organic tissue such as brain and liver cells, and its metabolism in the body is extremely acid-forming. As previously noted, high acidity is also regarded as a condition of "Yang" excess, so drinking "fire water" produces extremely "Yang" conditions of "fire-energy excess," both as excess metabolic heat and excess tissue acidity.

The first drink or two of any liquor has a swift stimulating effect on human metabolism, producing a fast flush of body heat and a big surge of extra physical and cerebral energy. However, if the drinker continues to drink, the excess acidity and toxic waste produced in the blood and tissues by the continuous metabolism of alcohol accumulate rapidly, overloading the system with toxic metabolites and rapidly depleting reserves of vital nutrients and energy. As the body struggles to process and excrete the toxic wastes and quell the metabolic "fire," more alcohol enters the bloodstream with each sip, adding more fuel to the fire and progressively weakening the body's vital functions. At the same time, the intoxication produced in the mind as a side effect of the toxic influence of alcohol on brain and nerve tissues continues to grow more intense with each drink, disorienting the drinker's mind and producing a drunken stupor that ends in loss of consciousness. The toxic metabolite of alcohol that causes the most damage to brain and nerve cells, and that destroys liver tissue, is acetaldehyde. This highly reactive, extremely toxic waste poisons the bloodstream and corrodes the cells and tissues. Crude cheap liquor, which produces far more of this toxic acid waste in the body than more refined forms of alcohol, is known among derelict drinkers as "rot-gut" precisely because of the highly corrosive effects of this compound on the internal organs.

Contrary to popular notions, the forms of alcohol that are most hazardous to human health are not hard liquors such as whisky and rum but rather the fermented varieties such as beer and wine. Although beer and wine have a lower percentage of alcohol than distilled spirits, fermented liquors retain all of the metabolic wastes produced by the yeast during the fermentation process—in effect "yeast poop"—and these fermentive wastes are highly acid-forming and toxic to the tissues. The liver bears the major burden of processing all the acids and toxic wastes that enter the body and pollute the bloodstream whenever beer and wine are drunk. If fermented liquors are consumed daily, the liver gradually succumbs to toxic overload, swelling up and hardening with residual toxic waste until cirrhosis develops. To make matters worse, most commercial beers and wines today contain chemical contaminants such as formaldehyde, preservatives, artificial dyes, flavoring agents, and other toxic additives, all of which contribute to blood acidosis, tissue toxicity, and the gradual erosion of the liver. In terms of their effects on health and longevity, except for an occasional glass of an exceptionally good vintage wine or naturally brewed beer with dinner, beer and wine are not good choices as intoxicants for daily use, especially for "social drinking," when one tends to drink to excess, because the cost/benefit ratio is far too high.

Distilled spirits, which are refined from fermented liquors, are a much cleaner form of alcohol for human consumption because the distillation process completely eliminates all the other toxic by-products of fermentation, leaving only pure distilled alcohol. While distilled spirits such as vodka and brandy have a higher alcohol content than beer or wine, they may be consumed in much smaller amounts per drink than fermented beverages and still deliver the same basic dose of alcohol into the bloodstream.

Known for centuries in Western Europe as *eau de vie,* the "water of life," and in ancient China as *jiou-jing,* the "essence of wine," distilled spirits were originally used more for therapeutic medicinal purposes than for recreational intoxication. Used properly and in moderation, spirits have potent medicinal properties that may be used to treat a variety of conditions, including sluggish circulation, insufficient body heat, low metabolic rate, and nervous tension. The slightly intoxicating effect on the mind produced by small doses of spirits adds an extra dimension to its therapeutic applications, and this psychoactive influence is well reflected in the term chosen to denote distilled alcohol: spirits.

All distilled spirits, including brandy and whisky, are crystal clear and completely pure after the distillation process. The distinctive amber color and characteristic flavor in various types of whisky, brandy, and other tinted spirits come from the resins leached from the wooden casks in which these liquors are aged. This aging process leaves tannins and other toxic resins suspended in the spirits, and these must all be processed by the liver along with the toxic metabolites of alcohol itself. Therefore, the healthiest choice in spirits are the clear varieties that have not been aged in wooden casks, such as vodka, gin, tequila, and white rum.

Throughout East Asia, people drink a type of medicinal spirit that is prepared by steeping potent tonic herbs in distilled spirits for three to six months. They then strain the infused liquor into bottles and take it in measured dosages, on a daily basis, particularly in the winter. Known in China as *yao jiou* ("medicine liquor") or *chun-jiou* ("spring wine"), this ancient herbal tonic has been used for thousands of years throughout the Far East as a means of preserving health, boosting vitality, and prolonging life, as well as for its relaxing effects. The alcohol serves to extract and preserve all the essential active ingredients from the various tonic herbs, delivering them swiftly into the bloodstream directly through the stomach and providing a strong metabolic boost to the therapeutic potency of the herbal essences. Medicinal spirits are an excellent delivery system for the life-prolonging therapeutic benefits of herbal tonics such as ginseng, astragalus, and wolfberry, while also serving the recreational function of liquor. This is a good example of how the art of rational retox may be applied to transform a toxic intoxicant into a tonic intoxicant, thereby reducing the costs to health and increasing the benefits to longevity of drinking alcohol. Readers who wish to add a therapeutic dimension to their recreational drinking will find the formula for preparing excellent traditional Chinese tonic spirits in the "Recipes and Formulas" section, appendix 1, page 314.

TIPS FOR TIPPLERS AND SMOKERS

If you drink and/or smoke daily, take a few basic precautions to counteract the additional acidity, toxicity, and dehydration that alcohol and tobacco produce in the body. Alcohol in particular dehydrates the blood and tissues, and it is therefore necessary to drink a few extra glasses of alkaline water each day, both to flush out the toxic acid wastes and to rehydrate the blood and cellular fluids. If the water you drink is charged with negative ions, it has even greater detoxifying and rehydrating activity in the tissues and helps protect the liver from damage by the toxic metabolites of alcohol and tobacco in the bloodstream.

People who smoke and drink regularly should also take extra rations of antioxidant nutrients, particularly vitamins E, C, and beta carotene, plus a full-spectrum mineral supplement to replace the essential minerals and trace elements depleted from the tissues by alcohol and tobacco. If you partake of these habits, make sure that you take some form of green-food supplement as a source of organic chlorophyll and other cleansing elements to purify the blood and cellular fluids.

One of the most effective antidotes of all against the toxic damage caused by daily use of alcohol, tobacco, and other intoxicants is to drink High Mountain Oolung Tea *(gao-shan oolung cha)* as a regular daily beverage, especially first thing in the morning and again in the late afternoon. This tea consumption is how many smokers and drinkers in China, Taiwan, and Japan protect their bodies from the hazards of their habits. Recent scientific research has confirmed the efficacy of High Mountain Oolung Tea as a potent blood purifier, tissue detoxicant, alkalizer, and preventive against cancer. The purifying effects and protective properties of High Mountain Oolung Tea are particularly effective in preventing toxic damage to the tissues of the lungs and the liver, which are precisely the organs that smokers and drinkers must take special measures to purify and protect. Here again we see how the art of rational retox transforms an ordinary daily beverage such as tea into an extraordinary therapeutic drink that protects health and prolongs life.

13

ADVICE ON MEDICAL AND RECREATIONAL DRUGS

In the previous chapter, we discussed the dubious distinction between therapeutic and recreational use of the legal leisure drugs, tobacco and alcohol, and we saw how so-called recreational drugs can also have useful therapeutic applications. In this chapter, we'll expand the scope of this discussion to include all drugs—medical and recreational, chemical and herbal, synthetic and natural—and try to establish a few basic guidelines for a rational approach to using these substances.

To begin with, we must admit the fact that, just as lots of people smoke tobacco and drink alcohol for therapeutic reasons rather than recreational ones, so do many people take medical drugs more for recreational than therapeutic purposes. It is hard to tell whether people who've been taking the same pharmaceutical drug every day for over ten years continue to use it because they still have the same therapeutic need for it as when the drug was first prescribed, or because they've grown fond of its effects and continue to take it simply because they like it, not because they need it.

The reason this point is so important is that many people today assume that just because their doctors prescribe a particular drug for a particular condition at a particular time, that drug must therefore be safe to take any time, or even all the time for an indefinite amount of time, with or without the original condition. This assumption is a false and often dangerous one. In the United States alone, more than two hundred thousand people die each year as a direct result of using pharmaceutical drugs, and several hundred thousand more are hospitalized each and every year due to severe adverse reactions to these drugs. The same point applies to people who rationalize their heavy use of alcohol and tobacco by telling themselves these activities must be safe and sound because they are legal. In both cases, the consumer suffers serious, sometimes fatal harm as a result of ignorance regarding the basic facts about the drugs they use, facts that their doctors and commercial advertisers usually fail to mention.

People who wish to preserve their health and prolong their lives should exercise the same basic precautions when selecting medical and recreational drugs as they do when selecting food. Would you start eating a new food product and include it in your daily diet without first finding out what's in it, simply because the person who sells it assures you that it is good for you? The same rule that governs choices in foods applies to drugs: if the drug has been derived from natural plant, animal, or mineral sources, then it's acceptable; if it has been synthesized from artificial chemical sources, it should be rejected. This rule applies both to medical and to recreational drugs, for as noted in the previous chapter, it doesn't matter to the body whether a substance is taken for therapy or for pleasure. Either way, it produces the same physiological effects and psychological side effects in the body and mind of the user.

The next time your doctor prescribes a new pharmaceutical drug for you to take, ask him or her to tell you what the basic ingredients are. Most doctors today don't have a clue how to answer that question, because they have nothing to do with the production of the drugs they prescribe. As a consumer, however, it is your right to know what's in the drugs the doctor prescribes, and it is the doctor's obligation to know and to inform you. In TCM, doctors always tell their patients precisely what ingredients are used to prepare their herbal prescriptions, and how the herbs react with various foods and other medications, and patients can request that particular ingredients be deleted, added, or substituted, based on their own personal requirements. If people today really knew what most modern pharmaceutical drugs are made of, many patients would be so revolted that they'd refuse to take them and switch to traditional medicine instead. Swallowing a pill on faith in the word of a doctor who doesn't know what's in it, how it has been made, and how it will reacts with other things is definitely not a rational way to take medicine.

The primary consideration when deciding what sorts of drugs to use for medical or recreational purposes is whether the drug comes from natural organic sources and is free of toxic chemical additives. In traditional medicine such as TCM and ayurveda, medicinal drugs are always made from plants, minerals, and animal parts, and those with intoxicating side effects, such as opium, cannabis, and datura, are not separated into a special class known as recreational drugs. While it is certainly true that medical drugs with intoxicating properties are sometimes taken for recreational purposes, they still remain legitimate medicines with therapeutic properties, and their occasional recreational use is of no concern to anyone but the user. Since all herbal intoxicants are organic compounds from natural sources, their moderate use does not do serious harm to health, whether taken for medical or recreational reasons, and their metabolites are easily excreted from the body.

In the past, when a patient had a therapeutic need for a particular medicinal herb that happened to have intoxicating side effects, such as opium or hemp, the recreational side effect became either a bonus or a nuisance to the patient, depending on his or her individual proclivities, but it never became a legal issue, as it has today. A good example of this point is smoking cannabis hemp to control pain, restore appetite, and assist digestion and assimilation in cancer and AIDS patients, all of whom testify that this herb is only effective for this purpose when the whole natural herb is smoked, and that the orally administered synthetic substitutes prescribed by doctors are totally useless. For these patients, the high produced by smoking this herb for therapeutic purposes is a mere side effect, enjoyed by some as a pleasant sensation and simply tolerated by others as an annoying distraction, but the high is not their primary reason for using it. Indeed, doctors today routinely give AIDS and cancer patients extremely toxic chemotherapy and other dangerous pharmaceutical drugs that have devastating side effects on their bodies and that often kill them. That consequence, however, still doesn't prevent doctors from continuing to prescribe these drugs, nor has it prompted the prohibition of the drugs. And when these same patients request a medicinal herb with proven efficacy and harmless intoxicating side effects, doctors site the herb as dangerous and deny its use to them. It's no wonder that many people today are confused on this issue.

While traditional medicine still relies entirely on herbs and other natural products, modern allopathic medicine employs thousands of chemically synthesized drugs produced by the pharmaceutical industry and prescribed by doctors for virtually all ailments. Many of these drugs are made from highly toxic, often carcinogenic, chemicals, such as coal tar. Coal tar is a poisonous by-product of the petroleum industry and was originally disposed of as a "hazardous waste," until chemists discovered that it could be used to synthesize a wide range of chemical drugs, including some with intoxicating properties, such as painkillers and sleeping pills. Many pharmaceutical drugs are made from inorganic substances that are extremely difficult to excrete from the body, and their toxic residues do untold damage to the liver and other tissues in which they accumulate. All chemical drugs cause highly acid-forming reactions in the bloodstream and depress the body's internal self-cleansing and excretory functions, resulting in a state of severe toxemia throughout the body. Unless absolutely necessary for short-term therapy, synthetic pharmaceutical drugs should be strictly avoided, and natural herbal medicines used instead.

Precisely the same advice applies to the use of recreational drugs: if they come from natural sources and have not been contaminated with toxic chemicals, they are relatively user-friendly; if they are made of synthetic substances, they are truly dangerous drugs. Examples of the latter category are all amphetamines such as speed (methamphetamine), ecstasy, and other "uppers"; all sleeping pills, sedatives, tranquilizers, and other "downers"; and all chemical narcotics, including heroin and cocaine. Even though heroin and cocaine are extracted from natural plant sources—opium and coca leaf respectively—there are so many industrial solvents and other toxic chemicals used in the refinement process that these two drugs are just as hazardous as synthetic narcotics. If you're in serious pain and need a natural narcotic painkiller, ask the doctor for morphine or codeine, both of which are organic alkaloids extracted from whole herbal opium and are therefore compatible with human metabolism and easily excreted from the body.

Pharmaceutical drugs that are used for recreational purposes are the most dangerous of all because they are designed to directly stimulate or sedate the brain and central nervous system by overriding or bypassing natural neurological functions, their toxic metabolites can do permanent damage to highly sensitive brain and nerve cells, while also causing serious behavioral and emotional disorders. These neuro-active chemical drugs are very addictive, and because they're mostly inorganic, it is much more difficult to flush their toxic residues from the body than it is to eliminate the metabolites of natural organic compounds, This tenacity makes addiction to these drugs extremely difficult to break. Using such drugs is simply not worth the damage it does to the body, nor does it conform with the principles of rational retox.

The best tip regarding the use of medicinal and recreational drugs is to abstain from taking anything that's synthesized from chemical components, and to use only organic products extracted from natural sources such as plants, minerals, and animal parts. If you have a condition that requires the use of a synthetic pharmaceutical drug, however, you should take similar protective measures as those suggested for daily use of tobacco and alcohol. Drink a few extra glasses each day of alkaline, preferably ionized, water to help flush out the toxic metabolites that these drugs leave in the blood and liver. Take some extra antioxidant supplements, such as vitamins C, E, and beta carotene, as well as green food to keep the bloodstream clean. When using chemically produced drugs, especially for prolonged periods, take liquid bentonite ("clay water") for a few days each week, or for a full week each month, to thoroughly purify the bloodstream and cleanse the cellular fluids of the residual acids and inorganic toxins that these drugs leave in the body. The negatively charged bentonite molecules saturate the bodily fluids and absorb the positively charged toxic particles, like a vacuum cleaner sucking dust from a carpet. This action helps prevent the cellular damage that invariably occurs if such toxins are permitted to accumulate for too long in the tissues.

Another factor that sometimes requires counterbalance when using chemical drugs is the drastic drop in blood sugar that these drugs often cause, especially those drugs that directly influence the central nervous system and have intoxicant properties. Such drugs significantly increase metabolic activity in the brain and nerve cells, greatly increasing their demand for glucose, which is the only fuel that brain and nerve cells can utilize. Consequently, these drugs cause the brain and nerves to drain the bloodstream of all available supplies of glucose, depleting reserves and causing a sharp, swift drop in blood-sugar levels. This reaction, in turn, causes dizziness and lethargy, weakness and confusion, chills and palpitations, and other unpleasant symptoms of hypoglycemia; it often triggers anxiety attacks as well.

The best way to offset this effect is to quickly replenish the bloodstream's supply of glucose by eating something that contains a concentrated natural sweetener, such as honey, maple syrup, or raw cane sugar, or else some sweet ripe fruit, such as banana, papaya, or peach. Best of all is to eat fresh black grapes, or drink freshly extracted grape juice, which contains abundant supplies of natural glucose, or blood sugar. Unlike fructose and other complex sugars in most fruits and natural sweeteners, glucose does not require conversion in the body to become bio-available as fuel for the brain and nerves. The glucose in grapes is assimilated directly into the bloodstream from the stomach, providing swift relief from the symptoms of low blood sugar, and refueling the brain and nerves with fresh supplies of glucose. Black grapes also contain elements that detoxify the blood and liver, protecting the body against damage from the toxic metabolites produced by chemical drugs in the body. Eating fresh black grapes is therefore a quick remedy for the "sugar blues" of hypoglycemia, and a good way to take the raw edge off harsh pharmaceutical drugs.

One of the best antidotes for the toxic degradation of the blood-stream caused by chemical drugs is chlorophyll, which eliminates toxic residues from blood and restores its capacity to carry oxygen. With the exception of a single atomic element (magnesium in chlorophyll and iron in hemoglobin), chlorophyll has precisely the same molecular structure as hemoglobin, the substance in blood that transports oxygen to all the cells of the body. All green-food supplements such as wheat-grass juice, barley-grass powder, spirulina, and blue-green algae contain abundant supplies of chlorophyll, which is also available as a concentrated liquid extracted from alfalfa and other green vegetable sources. When using antibiotic drugs, take a lactobacteria supplement, such as acidophilus or bifidus, to replenish the essential intestinal flora that antibiotics destroy. Since green foods function as a sort of "fertilizer" for lactobacteria, both supplements may be taken together for best results in counteracting the damage caused by antibiotics and other chemical drugs.

14

SETTING YOUR
DETOX/RETOX CLOCKS

A key strategy for protecting health, preventing disease, and prolonging life is to align your personal lifestyle with the natural patterns of your body's basic biorhythms, and to regulate your daily habits in ways that set your body's internal detox/retox clocks to activate periodic cycles of internal cleansing and healing responses. Detox/retox is a cyclical process: blood and tissue toxicity gradually increases until it reaches the critical stage, at which point the body's built-in detox mechanisms are activated and quickly remove the offending toxins, thereby restoring the original state of purity and functional balance, after which another retox cycle begins, and so forth. This cycle is a physiological manifestation of the primordial interplay of Yin and Yang within the body, the same polar principle that runs throughout all dimensions of nature and operates within the body in overlapping cycles of time—daily, weekly, monthly, and yearly (figure 12).

When allowed to function naturally, without human artifice or external interference, the body's self-toxifying (retox) and self-detoxifying (detox) cycles operate smoothly and efficiently, maintaining a homeostatic state of balance that supports health and prolongs life. For every artificial factor that we add to nature's carefully balanced equations of life, however, such as denatured diets, chemical drugs, electromagnetic

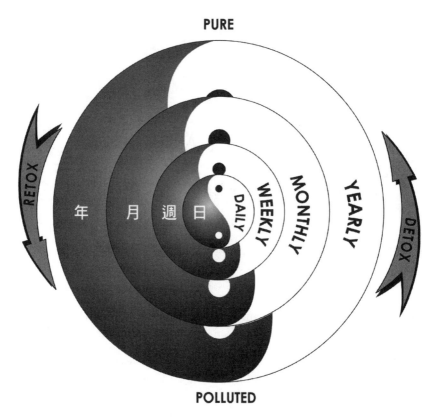

Fig. 12. Natural "detox/retox" cycles and the "wheels of time."

and microwave pollution, contaminated air and water, we must take specific counteractive measures to compensate for the imbalances and to correct the deviations that these factors produce in our internal detox/retox cycles. The most effective way to restore your body's natural detox/retox rhythms is to adapt your personal lifestyle to allow the body's internal self-cleansing mechanisms to catch up with the toxic overload on a daily, weekly, monthly, and yearly basis.

Let's briefly recall the analogy of maintaining a car, with which we launched this discussion in the preface. Just as a car needs to have its motor tuned, its internal parts cleaned, and its oil and other fluids replenished on a regular basis to perform properly, avoid break-downs, and prolong its mileage life, so the human body requires regular maintenance and internal cleansing work to stay healthy, prevent disease, and prolong its metabolic life. And like a car, in addition to major annual maintenance and repair programs, the human body must also be fed the right fuels and properly cared for on a day-to-day basis to prevent excessive wear and tear and to reduce production of toxic wastes. And in addition to annual and daily maintenance, some things may also be done on a weekly and monthly basis to improve the body's performance and reduce its rate of deterioration.

Yearly Maintenance

The seven-day detox and internal cleansing fast with colonic irrigation, as discussed in chapter 6, is the best way to periodically detoxify the blood and tissues, rebalance the body, and regenerate vital functions on a yearly basis. This length detox is also one of the most effective ways to prolong life. This program removes the hard, deeply impacted mucus and putrefactive waste that accumulate in the wall of the bowels, thereby eliminating the main source of blood and tissue toxicity in the body. Since these toxic wastes are a major cause of tissue degeneration, organ failure, fatigue, and other symptoms of aging, totally eliminating them from the body once a year with a seven-day fast and colonic irrigations is the best way to slow down the aging process and extend the human lifespan. Exactly seven days of fasting are required for this detox cycle to completely purify the bloodstream and detoxify the tissues and cellular fluids, and if you do this fast regularly once a year, all sorts of diseases and degenerative conditions are nipped in the bud and never have a chance to develop.

A yearly one-week cleansing fast may also serve as an annual withdrawal program to gradually give up old food addictions and break bad eating habits. Each time you do this program, it becomes progressively easier to adopt wholesome new food choices and cultivate better eating habits after the fast is done. This annual "house cleaning" program allows you to indulge in a bit of overeating, drinking, and other binging during the course of the year, then clears your body of all the residual toxic debris in one clean sweep, before it can do any serious damage.

Another yearly maintenance program that promotes health and

longevity is to take all or part of your annual vacation time in the form of a health holiday at your favorite resort, beach, or mountain retreat. This new style of vacation is becoming quite popular. Many spas and health resorts now provide packaged health-holiday programs that include various detox and healing therapies. Rather than exhaust your energy and pollute your body with all the hectic activity and overindulgence that characterizes conventional holiday plans, try giving your body and mind a real vacation from the stress and strain of daily life by resting quietly at a cozy spa, a deluxe beach resort, or a simple mountain cabin, eating only fresh, lightly cooked vegetarian food, drinking only pure alkaline water, and pampering your tired, toxic body with heliotherapy, herbal steam, hot mineral baths, massage, or just snoozes in a hammock. The money you save by not eating at expensive restaurants, not dancing in fancy nightclubs, not shopping, and not spending money on the other extravagances of conventional vacations may be used instead to pay for pure, simple foods and basic therapeutic services that cleanse and repair the body rather than pollute and damage it. Instead of returning to work tired and hungover from nonstop partying, you'll resume your daily routines with renewed vitality and fully replenished energy resources. If you like to party, do it on weekends, one party at a time, and give yourself a full day to recover afterward. Long vacations, however, are more wisely used for real rest and relaxation.

Monthly Maintenance

A traditional Asian regimen for monthly maintenance of the body is to ingest only water and fresh fruit juice for three days each month, starting on the day of the new moon to time the internal cleansing and regeneration process with the beginning of a new lunar cycle. To further increase the detox benefits of this regimen, you may also take a dose or two of ground psyllium powder shaken in water on each of these three days. This clears the bowels of putrid digestive debris and makes you feel less hungry owing to the bulking properties of psyllium. This is also a good time to do daily sessions with the "Zapper" to eliminate parasites from the body along with all the other toxic wastes.

Some people, especially heavy meat-eaters, cannot go for three days each month on nothing but fruit and water, without triggering a major detox reaction that interferes with work and other daily activities. In that case, a less rigorous monthly maintenance program is to take one full week each month in which they eat only a purely vegetarian diet, without any meat, eggs, or dairy products. While this plan is not as detoxifying as a three-day fruit and water program, it does effectively counteract acidosis in the blood and tissues, which is the biggest health problem caused by eating animal products. For someone accustomed to eating meat, eggs, and dairy products every day, eating only fresh vegetables, fruit, and whole grains for seven days each month serves as a sort of semifast, but without the intensive detox reactions and "healing crisis" triggered by a real fast. This approach is also a very good way for meat-eaters to discover how much better they feel when they cut down on animal products in their diets, and to gradually work their way toward trying a genuine therapeutic cleansing fast—first for only one day, then for three days, and finally for seven days.

Weekly Maintenance

An alternative way to allow your body to detoxify and rebalance itself on a regular basis is to spend one day each week consuming nothing but water and fresh fruit. This one-day program gives the bowels a chance to catch up with the backlog of waste elimination, it rests and rebalances the digestive organs, and it restores proper pH in the blood and tissues. Since no cooked food is consumed on that day, the enzymes normally used for digestive purposes are diverted to assist tissue cleansing and immune functions instead.

The cleansing and healing benefits of this weekly day of digestive rest may be further enhanced by soaking in a hot bath with Epsom or Celtic sea salts and a dash of detoxifying essential oils, such as grapefruit, rosemary, or sage. Even more effective for detox is the "Magnum Bath," with magnesium chloride crystals, magnesium oxide powder, and mica powder added to the water. Deep-tissue massage, herbal steam, and infrared sauna are other good ways to amplify the cleansing and rebalancing benefits of a weekly day of rest and relaxation. In fact, simply by remaining at rest for twenty-four hours and abstaining from cooked food, you permit your body to shift into the healing mode of the parasympathetic branch of the nervous system. This brief respite from the stress and strain of daily life suffices to recharge and rebalance the body and repair minor damage to tissues caused by weekly wear and tear. If you do this every week, that approach amounts to fifty-two days a year of rest rather than stress, waste elimination rather than waste accumulation, regeneration instead of degeneration. The cumulative benefits to health and longevity of such a weekly program are almost as great as a monthly three-day fast on fruit and water and make a good alternative for those who'd rather not spend three days in a row each month without eating solid food.

Daily Maintenance

The best way to support health and longevity on a day-to-day basis is to enlist the elements of air and water to assist daily detox and to help keep the bloodstream properly balanced. First thing each morning, before eating any food, drink two glasses of ionized, alkaline, microclustered water to flush mucus and acids from the stomach, give the bloodstream an alkaline boost, and rehydrate the cells and tissues. This infusion of energized alkaline water establishes proper pH balance in all the blood and other vital fluids of the body and boosts cellular metabolism with the ionized alkaline minerals required for optimum energy production. By starting each day this way, you flush out residual acids and toxins from the previous day and replenish your blood and tissues with pure, properly balanced water, establishing the conditions for optimum metabolic efficiency throughout the day.

The air element may be harnessed by practicing fifteen to twenty minutes of tu-na or other chi gung breathing exercises immediately after drinking those two glasses of water and before eating breakfast. Deep-breathing exercises practiced early in the morning expel residual carbon dioxide and other gaseous wastes from the bloodstream and replenish the blood and cellular fluids with abundant supplies of fresh oxygen and negative-ion energy. Deep diaphragmic breathing also alkalizes the bloodstream and helps establish proper pH balance throughout the body. Two glasses of pure alkaline water followed by twenty minutes of deep breathing is the true "breakfast of champions." This simple morning regimen will not only add more years to your life but also add more life to your years.

In addition to starting each day with an alkaline and oxygen boost from air and water, proper daily health care requires that the diet be regulated according to the basic rules of food combining, and complemented with a few special supplements to facilitate internal cleansing and provide complete nutritional balance. Herbal detox teas, green foods, digestive enzymes, and various full-spectrum vitamin and mineral supplements may all be judiciously used to help keep the body balanced and properly nourished on a daily basis. By eating food in a way that delivers optimum nutrition with minimum production of toxic waste, the body's daily elimination and self-cleansing cycles don't get overloaded and tissue toxicity never builds up to damaging levels. The lower you keep the level of toxicity in your body, the longer you extend the duration of your life.

15

"DON'T WORRY, BE HAPPY, FEEL GOOD"

These six words are printed across the top of the calling card of actor Larry Hagman, who portrayed the nefarious, pugnacious character "JR" in the popular television series *Dallas*. After spending fifty years of his life drinking champagne and orange juice for breakfast and lunch, then continuing throughout the afternoon and evening with vodka and orange juice, Hagman finally burned out his liver, which collapsed and ceased functioning as a result of chronic alcohol toxicity. His only hope of survival was to have a complete liver transplant, an operation with statistically slim chances of success, especially for a life-long alcoholic in his late-sixties.

Nevertheless, Hagman survived the ordeal, and today he still flashes that winning roguish grin that made "JR" famous. Having restored his vitality and reformed his lifestyle, Hagman continues to enjoy his new way of life as much as he did his old ways. By applying his "Don't Worry, Be Happy, Feel Good" philosophy as much to his present thera-peutic recovery stage as he did to his former recreational drinking days, Hagman has managed to survive the hazards of both and enjoy one as much as the other. As Norman Cousins, another man who laughed his way to a complete recovery from a supposedly "incurable" disease, wrote in his memoirs, "The will to live is not a theoretical abstraction, but a physiologic reality with therapeutic characteristics." So potent is the "power of positive thinking" that it can stimulate the body to cure itself of conditions that modern medicine regards as irreparable and fatal.

The "JR Attitude" of carefree, happy-go-lucky hedonism reflected in Hagman's motto is a lot more than just a cheerful slogan. When you "don't worry," your adrenal glands don't secrete stress hormones, such as cortisone, which suppress immune response and enervate the nervous system with hypertension. When you "be happy," your brain secretes neuropeptides, the "happy hormones" that communicate directly with the glands of the endocrine system and signal them to "turn on the juice" of healing responses and other immune factors. The invariable result of this biofeedback between the neuropeptides produced by a happy mind and the healing hormones required for a healthy body is that you "feel good" both in body and in mind. This balanced state of health and happiness is sustained by specific neuropathways and endocrine channels through which these secretions communicate in every part of the body.

While the right attitude is without a doubt the most fundamental factor in health, as it is in all aspects of living, some things in life require technique and discipline as well, and detox is one of the most important of these practical matters. Detox is no tea party. The process is a tiresome, sometimes grueling experience, especially if you're highly toxic when you start. As the internal cleansing process moves progressively into deeper layers of tissue and releases more and more toxic residues into the bloodstream for excretion, all sorts of unpleasant detox symptoms can manifest, including headache and body pain, insomnia and fatigue, fever and chills, irritability and anger. It is reassuring to know that the worse you feel during detox, the better the program is working for you and the more toxins you're draining out of your body, but you still have to endure the process. It is also rewarding to realize that the cumulative toxicity from years of indiscriminate eating, drinking, chemical medicines, and other careless habits can be completely flushed out of the body, and much of the damage may be repaired with just a week or two on an intensive, disciplined detox program. Of course, following a detox program requires more than just the right techniques—it also requires the right attitude. And it calls for time, patience, and a period of real rest and relaxation.

Activating the complementary relationship between a happy mind and a healthy body is one of the great achievements made possible by the power of positive thinking. Today, the neuroimmunological link between a positive state of mind and a positive state of health has become known in modern medicine as psychoneuroimmunology, or PNI. In traditional, holistic medicine it has been recognized as a basic fact of life for thousands of years. The two thousand-year-old Chinese medical text known as the *Internal Medicine Classic* states, "If one maintains an undisturbed spirit within, no disease will occur." In *Maximum Immunity*, Dr. Michael Weiner echoes the same premise in more technical terms when he writes, "By learning how to control our mind, subtle hormonal changes emerge that control our biochemical reality."

Among the subtle hormonal changes stimulated in the body by the mind is the so-called placebo effect, whereby a patient who's given a sugar pill, but is told that he's taking a marvelous new medicine that will cure his disease, becomes so hopeful and happy that his mind triggers his own internal healing responses, and he completely recovers. The placebo effect is produced entirely by the healing biofeedback between "happy neuropeptides" from the brain and "healthy hormones" in the endocrine system. In many double-blind clinical trials to test new drugs, the placebo cures the patient just as often as the drug itself. Pharmaceutical companies regard this all-too-human healing response as an unfortunate nuisance and are quick to discount it as an insignificant quirk, but in fact a positive outlook is the first and most important step in curing any ailment, and the main "active ingredient" comes from the mind, not from a pill.

The corollary principle to the power of positive thinking is the power of pessimism and negative emotion, which is every bit as destructive to health and longevity as a positive attitude is constructive. Stress and all the negativity it engenders in the mind have become primary causes of disease and degenerative conditions throughout the Western world, as well as in many newly developed Asian societies. Cortisone and other stress hormones set the stage for heart disease, cancer, stroke, hypertension, chronic infections, ulcers, immune deficiency, and many other crippling conditions. Stress factors like cortisone have also been linked to high rates of suicide in modern industrialized countries. As Dr. Weiner points out in *Maximum Immunity,* "Psychological stress releases powerful hormones that suppress our immune defenses." In *Eat Right or Die Young,* Dr. Cass Igram cites stress and negative emotions as the main causes of cancer and immune deficiency:

> The role played by stress in the causation of cancer is so great that it would not be an exaggeration to say that 80 percent or more of cancer cases have their immediate origin in some form of mental pressure or strain. Grief, distress, fear, worry, and anger are emotions that have horrible effects on the body's functions. Researchers have discovered that these emotions cause the release of chemicals from the brain . . . [that] have a profound immune-suppressive action. Scientists have traced a pathway from the brain to the immune cells proving that negative emotions can stop the immune cells dead in their tracks.

Just as the powers of positive and negative thinking have decisive effects on human health and longevity, so the "power" of proper pH has a strong influence on balance in body and mind. Alkaline blood and cellular fluids support a healthy body and promote a happy mind, while acidosis of the blood and tissues paves the way for disease and decay and gives rise to depression, tension, anger, fear, and other negative mental and emotional states. A good example of this response is the extreme state of acidosis suffered by many children today due to excessive consumption of refined sugar, starch, and dairy products. Not only does this sort of diet cause diabetes, obesity, tooth decay, and other physical defects but also the high acidity it produces in the blood and tissues is also a major factor in hyperactivity, attention deficit disorder, violence, depression, suicide, and other debilitating behavioral disorders experienced by so many Western children today. Doctors in the United States have responded to this growing blight of childhood malaise by giving these children powerful amphetamines and anti-depressants to suppress their symptoms, but this chemical drug therapy only further aggravates the root cause of the problem and does nothing to cure it. Usually in such cases, a thorough detox and a complete re-alkalization of the blood and tissues, followed by strict dietary reform, are all that's needed to correct both the physical and the mental and emotional disorders caused by chronic acidosis in children as well as in adults. For any real healing to occur, the state of the body and the state of the mind must be considered as two sides of the same coin and treated as inseparably linked aspects of the same conditions.

Almost everyone likes to "eat, drink, and be merry," but few of us wish to "die tomorrow." The human body is a complex engine that serves us both as a work horse and as a vehicle for enjoying life's plea-sures. It is therefore important to learn how to operate and maintain the body properly, so that it doesn't break down in the middle of life's journey and leave you stranded in a wheelchair or sickbed. The human body is genetically designed to last for about 120 years, and barring accidents and other unforeseen events, the body can remain fully func-tional for the full term of its natural 120-year lifespan—as long as it has been properly cared for along the way. There's no point in living long unless you are able to remain active and continue enjoying life until the end, and that requires careful attention to the basic facts and functions of life.

One of the most important factors, and the one upon which every-thing else depends, is the right attitude, without which health cannot be maintained for very long and healing can never be achieved. Patients who have an "attitude problem," whether it be cynical, resentful, angry, paranoid, pessimistic, or any other form of psychoemotional "dis-ease," must first purify their thoughts and detoxify their emotions before they can benefit much from any sort of physical cleansing therapies. Negative emotional and mental states, not only block the body's detox and self-healing responses, they also produce a constant stream of toxic metabolites and acid-forming reactions, thereby negating the positive benefits of any healing therapy.

The human experience suggests that positive mental factors such as joy, love, and hope are even more decisive than therapeutic physical factors such as diet, herbs, and exercise in determining the state of human health and the length of human life. People who know how to relax and enjoy life, and who take "Don't Worry, Be Happy, Feel Good" as their guiding motto, often live longer, healthier lives—even while eating, drinking, and living precisely as they please—than people who constantly worry about their health and dread death. With the right attitude, you can push your body to amazing limits in the pursuit of fortune and pleasure, then pull back from the brink of disaster and repair the damage just in the nick of time to enjoy your sunset years as well. Celebrating her ninetieth birthday in California in 2005, Cynthia Williams, still full of pep and the joy of living, offered her well-wishers this piece of sage advice: "It's a great life if you don't weaken."

If you still have any doubts about the importance of "attitude" and the power of mind over matter in renewing one's lease on a life nearly lost, write a letter to "JR" and ask him to explain the real meaning of "Don't Worry, Be Happy, Feel Good!"

Appendix 1
RECIPES AND FORMULAS

THAI HERBAL STEAM FORMULAS

Any steam bath may be turned into an herbal steam simply by adding the appropriate herbs directly to the water in the boiler. The active herbal essences vaporize along with the steam from the water and enter the steam chamber along with the steam. When using fresh herbs, a total of about 14 ounces of the chopped herbs is sufficient for a small steam room; when the herbs are in dried form, use about half that amount. Fresh and dried herbs may also be used together. Precise proportions are not important, but generally you may use equal quantities of each herb, adding fewer or more of the ones that you personally prefer. Three popular formulas are given below, but feel free to experiment with other combinations and different aromatic herbs.

Basic Formula

Lemongrass (preferably fresh)   Galanga Root ("Thai Ginger")
Wild Lime   Black Peppercorn
Ginger   Morning Glory (preferably fresh)
Sage

Formula for Arthritis and Inflammation

Lemongrass (preferably fresh)	Galanga Root ("Thai Ginger")
Wild Lime	Greenbriar
Ginger	Rosemary
Sage	Cinnamon

Formula to Assist Sleep and Relaxation

Lemongrass (preferably fresh)	Lavender
Ginger	Mandarin Orange
Sage	Thyme
Jasmine	

MAGNUM BATH

Taking a Magnum Bath is an excellent way to supplement any detox program and may also serve as a maintenance program for overall health in daily life. The two forms of magnesium chloride penetrate the skin and are distributed quickly to all the cells of the body, thereby providing optimum cellular levels of magnesium, which is involved in over three hundred enzymatic reactions in the cells. Magnesium oxide draws toxins out of the cells and carries them in solution to the pores of the skin for excretion into the bath water. If you are particularly toxic, you may notice a sour, vinegary odor rising from the water after soaking in a Magnum Bath; this is the smell of acid wastes that have been drawn out of your tissues into the water.

The mica powder energizes the bath water by virtue of its crystalline structure, which resonates with ambient energies in the atmosphere and draws those energies into the water. The product Dew Beads (also known as "prill beads") microstructures the bath water so that it penetrates the skin as well as the cellular membranes more easily.

This therapy may be taken as a full-body bath, or as a footbath, if a bathtub is not available. For the footbath, use about half the amount of products given below for the full body bath.

Place a Dew Bead pouch into a bathtub (or a bucket) and add hot water.

To the water, add the following ingredients:

⅓ cup magnesium chloride Bath Crystals
1–2 tablespoons magnesium chloride oil
1 teaspoon "Ocean Frost" magnesium oxide powder
1 teaspoon "Mountain Crystal" mica powder
Optional: a few drops of your favorite essential oil

Relax in the hot bath with your body full immersed in the water for 20–30 minutes, then rinse off in a cool shower. For a footbath, add enough water to the bucket to immerse the feet to a few inches above the ankles, and soak for 20–30 minutes. Rinse feet in cool water after soaking.

CLEAR VEGETABLE BROTH FOR DETOX DIET

Place the following ingredients into a large nonaluminum cooking pot:

1¾ quarts pure water
1 tsp Celtic Sea Salt
5 slices ginger root
2 finely chopped carrots
3 stalks finely chopped celery
1 cup finely chopped cabbage
1 cup finely chopped spinach
1 cup finely diced pumpkin
1 finely chopped squash
5 finely sliced shitake mushrooms (fresh or dried)
1 cup chopped parsley

Bring to a full boil, then reduce heat to a simmer, cover partially with a lid, and let it cook until the liquid is reduced to about half. Line a colander with a piece of cloth, and strain the broth into a bowl. Discard the vegetable pulp, and drink the broth with meals or as a snack between meals.

JOB'S TEARS AND BROWN RICE PORRIDGE

Herbal porridges have been part of the Chinese diet since ancient times, serving the dual functions of food and medicine. They are very easy to prepare and lend themselves to infinite variations in flavor and therapeutic effects. The recipe below is one of the oldest on record and combines the balanced nutrition of brown rice with the decongestant, anti-inflammatory, and cooling therapeutic effects of Job's Tears *(Coix lacryma-jobi)*. A few additional variations are given at the end of the recipe.

Wash and rinse 1 cup of brown rice together with 1 cup of Job's Tears, then place the two grains in a large, nonaluminum cooking pot with 2.2 quarts of pure water and set aside to soak for 3–4 hours, or overnight. When ready to cook, add 1 teaspoon Celtic Sea Salt, bring to a full boil, cover with a lid, and lower heat to a simmer. Let it cook for about 1¼ hours, until the mixture is soft and the liquid begins to thicken.

For savory porridge, add ½ teaspoon Celtic Sea Salt, 1 teaspoon Chinese sesame oil, and 1 tablespoon chopped scallion to individual serving bowls, then fill bowls with hot porridge and stir to blend.

For sweet porridge, add your choice of sweeteners such as maple syrup, raw sugar, honey, chopped dates, raisins, or banana to individual serving bowls, then fill with hot porridge and stir to blend.

Variations

1. Add ½ cup of dried lotus seeds to the rice and Job's Tears, plus an extra 1 cup of water to the cooking fluid. Lotus seeds add cardiotonic and nervine properties to the porridge and also function as a sexual tonic.
2. Add 8–10 Chinese Jujubes ("red dates") to the pot when cooking. These add both nutritional and tonic value to the porridge and are known in China for their long-term benefits to health and longevity.
3. For richer flavor, better texture, and extra nutritional value, try using ½ cup wild rice and ½ cup brown rice, rather than 1 cup brown rice.
4. If you're not vegetarian, you may substitute a rich chicken broth for the water when cooking the porridge, but be very sure to only use broth prepared from organically raised chickens. This increases the tonic properties of the porridge and provides extra warming effects in cold weather.

SAGE TEA

According to Dr. Rudolf Breuss, Sage Tea is the single most effective herbal tea for detoxifying the body and strengthening immunity and resistance on a daily basis. He recommends preparing a batch of Sage Tea first thing each morning, and drinking it throughout the day, every day, for life. His recipe for one day's dosage for one person is given below:

Bring two generous cups of pure water to a boil in a nonaluminum pot. Lower the heat, and add 1 teaspoon of dried sage to the boiling water. Allow to simmer for precisely 3 minutes, then remove from heat. Add ½ teaspoon St. John's Wort and ½ teaspoon peppermint, cover with lid, and let steep for exactly 10 minutes. Strain the tea into a thermos or bottle, and discard the dregs. Drink about ½ cup, 3–4 times daily, on an empty stomach.

LIVER DETOX TEA

This tea may be used to decongest and detoxify the liver and improve the circulation of blood and energy through liver tissues.

Ingredients

10 g Dandelion Root

2 g Mugwort

5 g Fennel

10 g Burdock Root

5 g Ginger

5 g Milk Thistle

Preparation and Dosage

Mix the dried herbs with 1 ⅓ quarts of pure water and bring to a boil in a nonaluminum cooking pot. Simmer slowly for about 20 minutes, then remove from heat and let stand for 10 minutes. Strain into a bottle and take ¼ cup to ½ cup of warm tea, 3 times per day. Start at the lower dosage and gradually work up to higher doses. Extra tea may be kept fresh in the refrigerator, but each dose should be warmed up before drinking.

BREUSS KIDNEY TEA

This is an excellent way to cleanse the kidneys and bladder, especially during a detox program, when those excretory organs must work overtime to remove toxic wastes from the bloodstream. One-half cup of the tea should be taken three times daily, continuously for up to 3 weeks, but no longer than that. For a complete kidney cleanse, do the full 3 weeks, and to follow a detox diet during this time. The amounts given below are sufficient for one person for 3 full weeks, but each day's dosage should be prepared fresh each morning.

Ingredients

Horsetail	3¾ teaspoons
Stinging Nettle	2½ teaspoons
Knotgrass	2 teaspoons
St. John's Wort	1½ teaspoons

Mix the chopped dried herbs together until they are well blended, and keep in a clean, well-sealed jar.

Preparation and Dosage

To prepare one day's dosage, steep one pinch (the amount held between the thumb and first two fingers) in one cup of boiling hot water for 10 minutes, then strain off the tea and set aside. Put the dregs into a nonaluminum pot, add 1½ cups pure water, bring to a boil, then lower heat and let simmer for 10 minutes. Strain off the tea, discard the dregs, and mix with the first cup. Drink ½ cup first thing in the morning, another ½ cup before lunch, and a third ½ cup at bedtime. Discard any leftover tea, and prepare a fresh batch the following day.

LIVER DETOX FORMULA FOR ALCOHOL AND DRUG POISONING

This is a classical Chinese liver cleansing formula that has been specially adapted to deal with severe toxicity of the liver due to poisoning from excessive long-term use of alcohol and/or drugs. Known as Major Bupleurum with Artemisia Decoction, this formula is a very strong liver detox liquid that must be used with considerable care. It has strong purgative properties for both the liver and the bowels, and it often prompts voluminous fluid bowel movements containing yellow-orange bile drained from the liver and gall bladder. It is very important to remain completely at rest while taking this formula, to avoid all excitement and stress, and to eat properly. During the course of treatment (7–14 days), do not eat any refined sugars and starches, avoid chili and other stimulating spices, and eliminate chicken, eggs, red meat, dairy products, and deep-fried foods from your diet. Eat only fresh vegetables, whole grains, and fruit, or select one of the detox diets given in chapter 5.

The proportions given below are for one day's dosage for one person. When ordering the formula in a Chinese herb shop, ask the clerk to mix individual one-day dosages and wrap each one in separate packets. A ten-day course of treatment would therefore require ten one-day packets of the mixed herbs, each containing the amounts given below.

Ingredients

Bupleurum falcatum (Hare's Ear)	1½ teaspoons
Artemisia cappilaris	1 teaspoon
Pinellia ternata	1 teaspoon
Zingiber officinale (Ginger, fresh)	1 teaspoon
Scutellaria macrantha	¾ teaspoon
Paeonia lactiflora (White Peony)	¾ teaspoon
Ziziphus vulgaris (Chinese Jujube)	¾ teaspoon
Gardenia florida	¾ teaspoon
Poncirus trifoliata (Trifoliate Orange)	½ teaspoon
Rheum officinale (Rhubarb)	½ teaspoon

Preparation and Dosage

Place all ingredients into a clay Chinese herb cooking pot, or use a heatproof glass vessel, but do not use a metal pot. Add 4 cups of pure water. Bring to a full boil, then lower heat, cover with lid, and let simmer slowly until the fluid is reduced by about half. Strain into a bottle or bowl, and discard the dregs. Divide into 3 equal doses and take one dose three times a day, on an empty stomach. Continue for 7–14 days.

BLADDER AND URINARY TRACT CLEANSING TEA

This blend promotes the elimination of wastes through the kidneys, urinary tract, and bladder and cleanses the tissues of these organs. It is particularly useful for flushing residual toxins and acids out of the bladder and urinary tract during an internal cleansing program, or after a period of excessive eating and drinking. It may be used in conjunction with therapeutic fasts and detox diets, or as a quick urinary system cleanser in the course of daily life.

Ingredients

Yarrow	1½ teaspoons
Elder Flowers	1½ teaspoons
Cleavers	1½ teaspoons
Dandelion Leaf	1½ teaspoons
Sarsaparilla	1½ teaspoons
Peppermint	1½ teaspoons

Preparation and Dosage

Place all the ingredients except peppermint into a nonaluminum pot, add 1⅓ quarts of pure water, bring to full boil, then lower heat and simmer for 10 minutes. Remove from heat, add the peppermint, and let steep for 10 more minutes. Strain into jars and keep refrigerated. Drink ½ cup, warm or cold, three times a day, on an empty stomach. After one week, dosage may be increased to 1 cup, three times daily.

LYMPHATIC DETOX TEA

This herbal tea may be used during a short fast, or in conjunction with a detox diet, to specifically detoxify the lymphatic system. The proportions given below are sufficient to make enough tea for about three days. Keep the tea stored in the refrigerator, but be sure to warm up each dose before drinking.

Ingredients

Red Root	½ teaspoon
Red Clover	1¼ teaspoons
Echinacea Root	¾ teaspoon
Lemon Peel	1¼ teaspoons
Ginger	½ teaspoon

Preparation and Dosage

Place all ingredients into a nonaluminum pot, add 4¼ cups pure water, bring to a full boil, then lower heat, cover, and simmer for 20 minutes. Strain tea into a bottle, and drink ½ cup twice daily, on an empty stomach. A bit of honey may be added for taste, if desired.

CHINESE HERBAL CONSTIPATION FORMULA

Known as "Moisten Bowel Decoction," this formula was first recorded in a Chinese medical text in AD 1249. It is designed to remedy chronic constipation caused by dry bowels, insufficient secretion of bodily fluids, and blood deficiency, all of which are common conditions today, especially among the elderly and postpartum women. This formula lubricates the bowels and helps clear blockages in the intestinal tract, thereby facilitating regular bowel movements.

Ingredients

Hemp seeds, roasted *(Cannabis)*	1¼ teaspoons
Peach kernels	1¼ teaspoons
Rhubarb *(Rheum officinale)*	¾ teaspoon

| *Angelica sinensis* | ¾ teaspoon |
| *Angelica pubescens* (purple) | ¾ teaspoon |

Preparation and Dosage

In a clay Chinese herb cooker or heatproof glass pot (but not metal), place the above ingredients and add 3 cups pure water. Bring to a full boil, lower heat, cover with lid, and simmer until fluid volume is reduced by about half. Strain out the fluid, add one more cup of water to the dregs, boil and simmer again until reduced by half, and strain again. Combine the two strained fluids, and divide into 3 equal doses. Take one dose, three times daily, on empty stomach, for one week, or until normal bowel movements are restored.

NERVINE TEA

This relaxing herbal tea may be used to counteract insomnia and irritability during an intensive detox program, or in the course of daily life to relieve anxiety or nervous tension, and to promote sound sleep at night. It may be used daily for long periods without any negative side effects.

Ingredients

Chamomile	1½ teaspoons
Lavender	1½ teaspoons
Passion Flower	1½ teaspoons
Hops	1 teaspoon
Catnip	1 teaspoon
St. John's Wort	1 teaspoon

Preparation and Dosage

Place all ingredients into a nonaluminum pot, add 1⅓ quarts of pure water, bring to a full boil, reduce heat, cover with lid, and let simmer for 10 minutes. Remove from heat and let steep for another 10 minutes. Strain the tea and discard the dregs. Drink ½ cup of the warm tea, 2–3 times daily, or as often as required. Store extra tea in refrigerator, and warm up each dose before drinking.

CARMINATIVE HERBAL TEA FOR GAS AND FLATULENCE

This tea may be taken daily as often as needed to help control gas and flatulence. To increase its carminative (gas-expelling) properties, you may add two or three drops of pure peppermint oil to each cup of the herbal tea.

Ingredients

Peppermint	2 teaspoons
Ginger	1¼ teaspoons
Fennel	1¼ teaspoons
Lemon Peel	¾ teaspoon
Cardamom	¾ teaspoon
Licorice	¾ teaspoon

Preparation and Dosage

Place all ingredients in a non-aluminum pot, add 1⅓ quarts of pure water, bring to full boil, then reduce heat, cover with lid, and simmer for 20 minutes. Remove from heat and let steep for 10 more minutes, then strain. Drink as required throughout the day, and store any extra tea in the refrigerator.

LEMON FLAX SHAKE

Grind 2 heaping tablespoons (about 1 ounce) of whole flax seed in a coffee grinder or food processor, then place into a blender with 3–4 ice cubes and 1 cup of water. Add the juice of 1 whole lemon, and blend until smooth. Pour into a glass and drink slowly on an empty stomach. For extra liver detoxifying properties, add 1 tablespoon of ground milk thistle seed to the blend.

REJUVELAC

Drinking cabbage Rejuvelac is an excellent way to replenish the friendly flora of beneficial lactobacteria in the digestive tract. It may be used to restore healthy lactobacteria colonies in the bowels after therapeutic fasts, colonic irrigations, antibiotic therapy, or long periods of poor dietary habits. It may also be used to stimulate sluggish digestion and improve lower bowel functions, and as a remedy for chronic constipation. For best results, use continuously for 30–45 days, and repeat at least once a year.

The first batch of Rejuvelac should be prepared in the morning by placing 1¾ cups (14 ounces) of pure water and 3 cups (24 ounces) of coarsely chopped fresh cabbage in a blender, and blending them together for just 30 seconds. If you don't have a blender, simply chop the cabbage finely with a knife and mix with the water.

Pour the mixture of cabbage and water into a large jar, cover loosely, and let it stand at room temperature for exactly three days. Then strain off the liquid, and discard the cabbage dregs.

Immediately prepare your next batch by blending another 3 cups of chopped cabbage with 1½ cups of pure water, then add ¼ cup (2 ounces) of the freshly made Rejuvelac as a "starter." Pour this mixture into a clean jar, cover loosely, and let stand for just 24 hours to ferment. Repeat this process each morning to prepare the following day's batch of Rejuvelac, using ¼ cup of each day's batch as a fermentive starter for the next batch.

Store the remaining fermented Rejuvelac in the refrigerator and take ½ cup (4 ounces), three times per day, with meals. If you don't finish the batch by the end of the day, discard what remains, and use the fresh batch of Rejuvelac the following day.

Good Rejuvelac should have a slightly sour taste, like yogurt, and is sometimes slightly fizzy, like mineral water. If the first batch smells putrid and has a slimy texture, discard it and start over. Once you get a good batch going, it replicates itself easily and may be continued indefinitely, as long as you prepare it daily. And remember: the first batch takes three full days to ferment, while all subsequent batches take only 24 hours.

TONIC HERBAL SPIRITS, OR "SPRING WINE"

This formula for tonic herbal spirits is one of the most ancient on record in Chinese medical texts. Known as "The Duke of Chou's Centenarian Liquor," it is said to have been the personal elixir of the great Duke of Chou, who founded China's ancient Chou Dynasty in the year 1123 BC. Its potent tonic properties increase semen production in men and stimulate hormone production in women. It also enhances immune response, stimulates circulation of blood and energy, and strengthens the kidneys and adrenal glands. Its benefits to health are cumulative over time, and long-term use builds strong immunity, raises resistance to disease, and paves the path to longevity.

Ingredients

Polygonatum cirrhifolium	¼ cup
Astragalus hoantchy (Astragalus)	¼ cup
Rhemannia glutinosa	2½ tablespoons
Porio cocus (Tuchahoe)	¼ cup
Cinnamomum cassia (Cinnamon)	4 teaspoons
Angelica sinensis	2½ tablespoons
Codonopsis dangshen	2 tablespoons
Liriope spicata (Creeping Lilyturf)	2 tablespoons
Atractylodes macrocephala	2 tablespoons
Lycium chinense (Chinese Wolfberry)	2 tablespoons
Citrus reticulata	2 tablespoons
Cornus officinalis (Dogwood Tree)	2 tablespoons
Ligusticum wallichii	2 tablespoons
Ledebouriella seseloides	2 tablespoons
Chinemys reevesii	2 tablespoons
Schisandra chinensis (Schisandra)	5 teaspoons
Angelica pubescens (purple)	5 teaspoons

Preparation and Dosage

Place all the ingredients into a large glass or ceramic vessel of at least 2¼ gallon capacity. Add 6 quarts of vodka, rum, or brandy, and seal the vessel so that it is airtight. Set aside to steep for 36 days, giving the vessel a good shake once in a while to mix the ingredients. After 36 days, strain off half the liquor into clean glass bottles, then add 3 fresh bottles of spirits to the remaining brew. Seal again, set aside to steep for another 15 days, then strain off the entire batch into clean bottles and discard the used herbs. Add a few lumps of rock crystal sugar, or a few tablespoons of honey, to each bottle to balance the flavor and smooth the texture, then seal with cork or cap. The herbal spirits may be stored indefinitely without losing therapeutic potency.

Take 1½ ounces (3 tablespoons) once a day in summer, or twice a day in winter, on an empty stomach. To reduce alcohol content, place herbal spirits in a cup, add a few ounces of boiling water, and let sit for a few minutes to evaporate some of the alcohol. The best times to drink herbal spirits are just before dinner and shortly before bedtime, but in cold winter weather, the first dose may be taken at midday to help warm the body.

Tonic spirits should only be taken when you're feeling healthy and well balanced. When ill or disordered, discontinue all tonics and switch to curative therapies until health and balance are restored.

Appendix 2
SUPPLIERS

Most of the products mentioned in this book can be found in one form or another at health supply shops in major cities throughout the world, or by mail-order through various Web sites on the Internet. The suppliers listed below are those from whom the author has been ordering these products for many years. They supply top quality products at reasonable prices, and all of them offer worldwide mail-order service.

V. E. Irons Inc. & Colema Boards Inc.
P.O. Box 34710
North Kansas City, MO 64116 USA
Telephone: (800) 544-8147, (816) 221-3719
Fax: (816) 221-1272
Web site: www.veirons.com and www.colema.com
E-mail: info@veirons.com and info@colema.com

The Irons family supplies the entire line of V. E. Irons's "Vit-ra-tox" brand of internal cleansing products, which the author highly recommends as supplements for any sort of therapeutic fasting program. The company also supplies several models of the famous "Colema Board" for doing colonic irrigations at home and provides detailed printed material regarding the seven-day, internal cleansing-fast and colonic-irrigation program developed by V. E. Irons. The Irons program is the fastest and most effective way to conduct complete detox and internal organ cleansing programs at home.

Products: "Intestinal Cleanser" (psyllium powder); "Detoxificant" (liquid bentonite); "Greenlife" (cereal grass juice tablets); "Enzymatic Supplement" (digestive enzymes); "Herb Tablets" (herbal laxative); "Colema Board" (colonic-irrigation kit); and additional related items.

Dragon River Herbals

P.O. Box 28

El Rito, NM 87530 USA

Telephone: (505) 583-2348

Fax: (505) 583-2339

Web site: www.dragonriverherbals.com

E-mail: info@dragonriverherbals.com

Dragon River Herbals produces a wide range of high-potency liquid extracts and herbal tinctures from top-grade medicinal herbs, including traditional Western as well as Chinese varieties. In addition to dozens of single-herb tinctures, Dragon River also blends a line of its own herbal formulas specially designed for specific conditions by master herbalist Charlie Jordon. As pure concentrated extracts, these formulas produce swift therapeutic results and are very convenient to use at home, at work, or while traveling. For information and instructions regarding the use of these herbal remedies, you may order a copy of Charlie Jordon's *Restorative Herbal Guidebook* from Dragon River.

Products: Single herb extracts, including those required for parasite program (black walnut hull, wormwood, clove); "Rejuvenate" (liver detox formula); "Life Support" (immune enhancer); "Lights Out" (nervine relaxant for sleep); "Breath of Life" (lung and respiratory remedy); "Peace & Quiet" (antihypertensive relaxant); and many others.

Fruitful Yield

P.O. Box 6247

Bloomingdale, IL 60108-6247 USA

Telephone: (800) 469-5552, (630) 351-9156

Fax: (630) 351-9430

Web site: www.FruitfulYieldDirect.com

E-mail: sales@FruitfulYieldDirect.com

This company supplies the complete line of "NOW" brand vitamins, minerals, and other nutritional supplements, as well as herbal extracts, green foods, essential oils, and other health products. NOW supplements are among the purest on the market today, produced only with natural ingredients without the use of chemical additives, and new products based on the latest discoveries in naturopathic health research are added to their line regularly.

Products: alkaline vitamin C; vitamin E with selenium; beta carotene; multivitamin and mineral formulas; spirulina; chlorella; calcium citrate with magnesium; stevia powder or extract (natural herbal sweetener); lactobacteria supplements; digestive enzymes; antioxidant formulas; sage, lavender, rosemary, peppermint, and other essential oils; and related health products.

Sandent Company

514 Greenland Drive

Murfreesboro, TN 37130 USA

Telephone: (615) 890-9832

Web site: www.sandent.com

Sandent is the USA supplier for the "ESF" energized water supplement, which releases free oxygen and hydrogen into the bloodstream. This product is also known as "Liquid Life" and "Cell Food," depending on where it is being sold. For more details on this product, and the names of suppliers in other parts of the world, check the manufacturer's Web site: www.nuscience.com.

Product: "ESF" / "Cell Food" / "Liquid Life"

Unique Health Products

Lot 3, Jackson Road

West Woombye, QLD 4559 Australia

Telephone: 011 61 7 5442-3555

Fax: 011 61 7 5442-3555

Web site: www.uhp.com.au

E-mail: sales@uhp.com.au

UHP supplies a wide selection of high-quality health products, both for internal and external use, including skin and body care products. UHP has one of the most complete health catalogs in the business and supplies products by mail-order within Australia and overseas.

Products: Himalayan Glacial Salt, stevia, herbal teas, aloe vera, skin care products, cell food (ESF), Chinese herbal extracts, and a variety of green-food supplements.

Acuneeds

622 Camberwell Road

Camberwell, VIC 3124 Australia

Telephone: (800) 678-789, 011 61 3 9889-4100

Fax: 011 61 3 9889-1200

Web site: www.acuneeds.com

E-mail: info@acuneeds.com

Acuneeds supplies traditional Chinese herbal formulas, as well as single herbs, produced by the most reputable herbal-medicine makers in China and Taiwan. Available as tablets, powders, freeze-dried granules, teas, ointments, and creams, these remedies are convenient and economical to use for prolonged periods of herbal therapy at home. Acuneeds also supplies acupuncture needles, moxibustion, and other TCM supplies and offers a variety of books for sale on various aspects of Chinese herbal medicine.

Products: Traditional Chinese herbal formulas and single herbs.

Ion Life

Box 520
Byron Bay, NSW 2481 Australia
Telephone: 011 61 2 6685-6471
Fax: 011 61 2 6680-7308
U.S. office: (800) 677-6117
Web site: www.ionlife.info
E-mail: info@ionlife.info

Ion Life specializes in supplying various types of home ionizers for both air and water, including water ionizers for making microclustered alkaline water and the GEOMED negative-ion generator for concentrated negative-ion breathing therapy.

Products: Drinking Water Purifiers and Ionizers; GEOMED negative-ion air generator.

Siamese Traders

85, Sukaseam Rd, Soi 12
T-Patan, A. Muang
Chiang Mai 50300 Thailand
Telephone: 011 66 53 409705, 011 66 53 409703
Fax: 011 66 53 409113
E-mail: nikolaus@siamesetraders.com

Siamese Traders supplies a variety of high-quality health products organically produced in northern Thailand, including natural health foods and herbal teas, herbal body care products, Celtic-style sea salts, and High Mountain Oolung Tea grown in Thailand, from plants from the highlands of Taiwan. All products are attractively packaged and reasonably priced, and many of them may be used to support the various detox programs and daily dietary guidelines introduced in this book.

Products: whole sea salt (plain or blended with chili and other Thai herbs); Himalayan glacial salt; herbal teas; cooling herbal body powder; healing herbal skin balm; traditional Thai herbal steam formulas; High Mountain Oolung Tea and other Chinese teas; "Bliss Bio-Circuit" (silk energy balancer); Tea Leaf Pillows; and many other fine products.

Global Light Network

23505 Bat Cave Road

San Antonio TX 78266

Telephone: (888) 236-2108, (210) 651-0505

E-mail: GLN@GLNUS.com

Web site: www.globallight.net or www.GLNUS.com

Web site for additional information on magnesium therapy:

www.magnesiumforlife.com

Global Light supplies a variety of high-quality magnesium-chloride products extracted from sea water for internal use, therapeutic bathing, and massage, as well as products to restructure water into "microwater" form.

Products: Magne-Oil (magnesium chloride oil), Magnum Bath (magnesium-chloride bath crystals), Ocean Frost (magnesium oxide powder), Mountain Crystal (mica flakes), Dew Bead (prill) sachets and pouches, and Cosmic Ball (for making microwater).

Teslas Innovational Technologies

E-mail: info@teslas.us

Web site: teslas.us

Teslas produces a variety of specially energized, molecularly restructured titanium plate products to transform harmful electromagnetic fields and microwave radiation from power lines, phone towers, cell phones, radio and television broadcast towers, and home appliances.

Products: mobile phone tag, personal pendants, travel plate, car plate, computer plate, house plate, power stabilizer for home electrical system, and water energizer.

Taiwan High Mountain Oolong Tea

www.taiwanoolongtea.com

A variety of top-grade High Mountain Oolong Tea from Taiwan may be ordered on-line from this Web site.

Colonic Cleanse Web site

www.detox-cleanse.com

E-mail: info@detox-cleanse.com

Information, technical support, and communication with other people who are doing colonic cleansing are available from this site.

Author's Web site

www.danreid.org

INDEX

Page numbers in *italic type* refer to illustrations

abdominal lock during breathing
exercises, 85
acid in food, 114–17, 126
acidosis, 6, 17–18, 116–17
in children, caused by refined sugar,
effects of, 299
acupressure, 65–67, *66*
acupuncture, 198
adrenal glands, 39
and cortisone, 297
air, 76–112
activated, 107–8
negative ions (yin particles) in,
102–7, 263
oxygen levels in, 42
See also breathing
air travel and air quality, 106–7
alcohol, 29, 270–72, 277–81
and acetaldehyde, 278
and High Mountain Oolung tea,
281
Algren, Nelson, 228

alkaline, 6, 33, 117
alkaline- and acid-forming foods, list
of, 242
alkalization, 20–21, 35
See also alkaline; oxygenation;
water
Alkalize or Die (Baroody), 3–4, 34,
176, 269
allergies, 9
aloe vera, 144, 190, 320
Alzheimer's disease, 205, 207, 227
anal lock during breathing exercises,
83–84
animal sources of food, 115, 234,
236–38, 245–49
See also food
antioxidants, 35, 261, 105
as supplement, 36, 101, 286
aromatherapy, 50, 108, 109–10, 194
arthritis, 9, 20, 26, 64, 99, 128,
303
artificial sweeteners, 258, 267

asparagus, 121–22
asthma, 206, 217
astronauts, 106
autonomic nervous system, 4–5,
    26–29
avocado, 143–45
ayurveda, 284

Barley Green (green food), 136
    See also Appendix 2 for products
    and suppliers
Baroody, Dr Theodore, 3, 34,
    176–77, 269
    on sunlight, 176–77
basil, 51
Becker, Dr Robert, 200–2, 219
    on microwaves, 204
beetroot, 20
    See also food
BEFE bio electric bath, 215–16
    See also Appendix 2 for products
    and suppliers
bentonite, 138–39, 144, 148, 156,
    160, 168
beta carotene, 136, 231, 261–62,
    281, 286, 319
beverages for detox, 131–33
    See also alcohol, food
Beyond the 120 Year Diet (Walford),
    150, 244
bile, 17, 81, 140
bio-energy, 200, 215–16
    See also electro-detox; human
    energy system
bladder, 22, 187–88, 310
    herbs for, 188

blood system, herbs for, 186–87
body odor, 9, 23, 156, 157
bowels, see colon
Boy George, 220
Bragg, Paul, 150–51
brain, 98, 192–93
    intoxicants' effects upon, 271
    neuropeptide secretion by, 297
Breath of Life, 191
    See also Appendix 2 for products
    and suppliers
breathing, 19, 21, 23, 27, 73, 76–112
    abdominal lock during, 85
    anal lock during, 83–84
    anxiety and, 77–78
    bodily movement and, 95–96
    control of, 78–82
    diaphragmatic, stages of, 82
    and exhalation, types of, 92–93
    four-stage, 82
    neck lock during, 85–86
    negative ions (yin particles) and,
        102–7
    still, 86–94
    tu na, 92–94, 94, 294
    two-stage, 86
    See also air; exercise
Breuss kidney tea, 188, 310
Breuss, Rudolf, 124, 306
butter, 238, 242, 250
    See also food

calcium, 20–21, 116–17, 121–22,
    134, 143, 176–77, 231, 252–55
calorie-nutrient ratio, 244–45
    See also food

cancer, 7–9, 17
Breuss cure for, 158–59
diet and, 8–9, 115
fasting and, 8, 158
oxygen deficiency and, 42
water intake and, 32
candida, 217
cannabis, 273, 284, 313
See also smoking
carbon dioxide, 19, 23, 26–27, 73, 117
Cayce, Edgar, 131, 272, 274
cayenne, 139–40, 144
celery, 119, 123
Celtic sea salt, 142, 255, 259–60, 305
Chai Yu-hua, 152
chakras, 57, 90–91, 91, 93–94, 198
Chang San-feng, 110
Chang Tsung-cheng, 152
Cheng Yuan-lin, 96
chewing food, 245, 255
chi brushing massage, 67–68
chi gung, 27, 55, 69, 74, 82, 87, 87, 88, 91, 94, 96–102
antioxidant effect of, 101
cerebral benefits of, 98
as daily routine, 294
effect of, on digestion, 100
effect of, on pH balance, 101
hypertension and, 99–100
immune system and, 98–99
Chinese tui-na massage, 57–59
chiropractic, 64
chlorine, 33, 34, 122
chlorophyll in food, 140, 135, 136

chronic fatigue syndrome, 217
chronic pain syndrome, 33
cigarettes, 274–75
See also smoking
cigars, 276
See also smoking
cinnamon, 51, 192
Clarke, Dr. Hulda, 216–17
Cleanse (psyllium product), 139
See also Appendix 2 for products and suppliers
coal tar, 285
Colbin, Annemarie, 252
cold turkey and electro-acupuncture, 218–20
colds, 9, 109
Colema Board, 164–67, 165, 316
See also Appendix 1 for products and suppliers
colon, 24
Deal on, 154–55
Fasciolopsis buskii in, 216
flatulence in, 190
herbs for, 189–90
irrigation of, 24–26, 152–54, 162–67, 165
worms and parasites in, 194–95
Colon Health: the Key to Vibrant Life (Walker), 25
combining food (trophology), 231, 234–36
See also food
The Complete Guide to Chi Gung (Reid), 74, 102
Connors, Dr. C. Keith, 257
coriander, 146, 192–93

cortisone, 297, 299

Cousins, Norman, 296–97

CRON diet, 244–45

dairy products, 251–53

Dance Verse (Fu), 96

dao yin, 95

Dead Sea, 46–47

  mineral mud from, 46–47

  salt from, 46

  Scrolls, 152

Deal, Dr. Grady, 154–55

deep-tissue massage, 56, 293

dehydration, 32–33, 36, 281

  microwater and, 36

  See also water

depression, 9, 32, 40, 184, 205, 206, 228, 299

detox daily menus, 141–48

  See also Appendix 2 for products and suppliers; food

Detox Diet and Wellness Lifestyle (Deal), 154

detox/retox cycles, 289–90, *290*

  daily, 294–95

  monthly, 292–93

  weekly, 293–94

  yearly, 291–92

Deuterium sulphate, 21

diaphragm, 21, 27, 65, 73, 77, 78–83, *79*, 92, 99, 230

diaphragmatic breathing, stages of, 82

  See also breathing

Diet for New America (Robbins), 246

diet, *see* food

digestion, 100

Diogenes, 269

dioxin, 273, 274

dopamine, 98

drugs, 282

  medicinal and recreational, advice on, 282–88

  synthetic versus natural, 285–86

  withdrawal from, using electro-acupuncture, 218–20

Duffy, William, 256

Eat Right or Die Young (Ingram), 250, 299

electro-acupuncture and cold turkey, 218–20

electro-detox, 197–98

  with BEFE bio-electric bath, 215–16

  devices for, 210–23

  with electro-acupuncture, 218–20

  with Jai electro-pressure regeneration therapy, 210–11

  with SE-5 bio-field analyzer, 221

  with NET (neural electric therapy), 29, 218–20

  with radionics, 220–22

  with the Zapper (Neuro Muscle Stimulator), 216–18, 223

  See also Appendix 2 for products and suppliers; bio-energy

electromagnetic fields, 37, 105, 199–201, 207

  from appliances, 201–3

emotions, *see* mind upon body

encephalins, 98

environment, pollution of, 1
Enzyme Nutrition (Howell), 263
  alkalization, supplements for,
    264–66
enzymes, 3, 20, 44, 83, 100–102,
    113–15, 122, 263–65
  activity of, on meat, 237
  amylase, 264
  cellulase, 264
  in fermented food, 255–56
  killed by pasteurization, 251
  lipase, 264
  peroxidase, 261, 263
  preservation of, in cooking, 248
  protease, 264
  ptyalin, 237, 238, 239, 255
ESF (Everett Storey Formula), 21, 44
Essene Gospel of Peace, The, 152,
    172
essential oils, 47, 63, 110
excretory systems, 10, 22
  colon, 24–26
  kidneys and bladder, 23–24
  lungs, 23
  skin, 22–23
exercise, 26–28
  breathing and, 73–74, 81
  chi gung, *see* main entry
  dao yin, 95
  soft, 72–75
  tai chi, *see* main entry
  See also breathing
exhalation, types of, 92–93
  See also breathing
eyes and optical system, 173–74, 178,
    180

fascia, 33
fasting, 8, 114, 149–51, 154–59
  seven-day, day-by-day description
    of, 168–71
  supplements for, 159–62
fat in food, 238–39
  See also food
fatigue, 9, 32, 33, 65, 157, 168, 174,
    230
fight or flight response, 4, 26, 59,
    77–79, 99, 141, 226
  and breathing, 77–78
fish and seafood, 236, 245–47, 249
  See also food
flatulence, 190, 312
fluoride, 33, 34, 53
food:
  acid in, 114–17
  alkaline- and acid-forming, list of,
    242
  animal sources of, 113–15, 234,
    236, 237, 293
  artificial sweeteners in, 258, 267
  asparagus, 121–22, 147, 242
  avocado, 143
  beetroot, 20
  beverages for detox, 131–33
  butter in, 238–39, 242, 249–50
  and calorie-nutrient ratio, 244–45
  cancer and, 7–9, 17, 115
  cayenne, 139–40, 144
  celery, 119, 123
  Celtic sea salt in, 142, 255,
    259–60, 305
  chewing, 245, 255
  chlorophyll in, 140, 135, 136

combining (trophology), 231, 234–36

concentrated nutritional supplements to, 260–65

coriander, 146, 192–93

in CRON diet, 244–45

dairy products in, 251–53

fat in, 238–39

fermented, 255–56

fish and seafood in, 236, 245–47, 249

fruit and vegetables, 117–29, 163, 234

garlic, 119, 120, 144, 145, 185, 195

genetically modified, 118, 166, 243

glucose in, 127, 287

grains, nuts and seeds, 129–31

green, 134–37

green tea, 262

High Mountain Oolung tea, 262, 281, 320

hydrogenated vegetable oil in, 244, 249–51

junk, toxic chemicals in, 243

lemon, 140, 160–61, 312

"live," 242–43

milk, goat's versus cow's, 253

miso, 120, 144, 256

oil in, 47

organic, 118, 119, 124, 125, 243, 250, 284, 286

packaged dry cereal, 238

preparation of, 119–22, 302–12

processed, 114, 116, 226, 233, 243, 264

pumpkin, 119, 121, 148, 195

putrefactive protein in, 115, 129, 236–38

raw and lightly cooked, 119, 142, 240–41, 243

for retox, 233–42

salt in, 259–60

starch in, 115–16, 234, 237, 238

stevia in, as natural sweetener, 258, 267, 318

substitutes for, 243–44, 249

sugar in, 21, 114, 116–17, 127, 234, 239, 256–58

supplements, for detox, 265–66

teas, 24, 132, 142, 146, 184, 186, 187, 319, 320

watermelon, 128, 147, 242

wheat products in, 129, 136, 253

yin and yang considerations of, 234–35

See also Appendix 1 for recipes; detox menus; herbs; retox: diet and supplements for

Food Combining Made Easy (Shelton), 254

Food and Healing (Colbin), 252

The Food Revolution (Robbins), 246–47

four-stage breathing exercise, 82

free radicals, 34, 35, 36, 50, 101–2, 105, 121, 250, 261–62

singlet oxygen, 261

Freibott, Dr. George, 44

fruit and vegetables, 117–29, 163, 234

Fu Yi, 96

fungal infections, 6, 9, 217

galanga root, 51, 302, 303

garlic, 119, 120, 144, 145, 185, 195

gastritis, 9, 127

genetically modified produce, 118, 166, 243

GEOMED Activated Air System, 108, 209, 223, 230

   See also Appendix 2 for products and suppliers

ginger root, 51, 120, 304

   See also food

Glenn, John, 106

glucose in food, 127, 287

   See also food

Goulet, Brian, 42–43

grains, nuts and seeds, 129–31

   See also food

Grander Living Water System, 36–37

   See also Apendix 2 for products and suppliers; water

green food, 134–37

   See also food

Green Life (green food), 136

   See also Appendix 2 for products and suppliers

green tea, 262

hemoglobin, 135, 288

Hagman, Larry, 296

hair loss, 9

A Handbook of Chinese Healing Herbs (Reid), 186, 189, 196

A Handbook of Native American Herbs (Hutchens), 196

headaches, 9, 33, 65, 66, 103, 117, 168, 205, 213, 228

healing crisis, 155, 156–57, 169, 170, 229, 293

health resorts and spas, 104, 177

heart, 19, 26, 70, *70*, 71, 73, 74, 79, 80, 83, 86, 99–100, 145

heartburn, 9

Herbal Fiber Blend, 139, 189

   See also Appendix 2 for products and suppliers

herbs, 182–96

   aloe vera, 144, 190, 319

   anthelmintic, 194, 195

   bitter, 183

   for blood and lymph, 186–87

   for brain and nerves, 192–93

   for colon, 189–90

   coriander, 146, 193

   Gingko biloba, 146

   for kidneys and bladder, 187–88

   liver and, 184–85

   for lungs and bronchia, 190–91

   nervine, 193–94

   parsley, 123

   as the "people's medicine," 195–96

   sage, 47, 132–33

   as tea, 132–33

   for worms and parasites, 194–95

   See also food

High Mountain Oolung tea, 262, 281, 320

hot herbal oil massage, 63–64

Howell, Dr. Edward, 263

Hua To, 95–96

human energy system (HES), 198–201, 203, 210–11, 216, 221–22

chakras within, 198
and electromagnetic fields, 201–2
guardian energy within, 199
meridians within, 198
pollution of, 201–3
See also bio-energy
human growth hormone, 151
Hung Yi-hsiang, 76
hydration, 31–34
See also water
hydrogen, 44
hydrogenated vegetable oil, 244,
249–51
See also oil for cooking
hydrogen peroxide, 43, 261
hydrotherapy, 30, 31–53
in seawater, 48–49
See also water
hyperactivity and anxiety, 9
hypoxia, See under oxygen

immune system, 37, 43, 99, 187, 207,
250, 257
chi gung's effect upon, 98–99
oxygen and, 42
infrarared sauna, 179
Igram, Dr. Cass, 250, 299
insulin, 257, 258
Internal Medicine Classic, 298
Irons, V. E., 17, 25, 136, 150,
163–70, 316–17

Jacobs, Dr. Karl, 221, 222
Jacuzzi, 47
Jai electro-pressure regeneration
therapy, 210–11

See also Appendix 2 for products
and suppliers
Japanese shiatsu massage, 60
Jensen, Dr. Bernard, 135, 152
Jesus (of Nazareth), 152–53, 172
jing-yi ("vital fluids"), 17
Job's Tears (Coix lacryma-jobi),
129–30, 305
See also menus; recipes and
formulas
Johns Hopkins University, 241
junk food, toxic chemicals in, 243

kaffir, 51
Keaton, Kathy, 99
Kellogg, Dr. Harvey, 25, 163,
166
kidneys, 20, 187
herbs for, 187–88
Kipling, Rudyard, 276
Ko Hung, 95

lactic acid, 3, 26, 27, 73, 74, 95, 141,
226
lactobacteria, 161–62, 171, 246, 255,
288, 313
homemade, 162
Langre, Dr. Jacques de, 259
Lao Tze, 31
lavender, 47, 110, 193, 194, 303,
311, 318
lemon, 140, 160–61, 312
lemon balm, 146
lemongrass, 51, 302, 303
Levine, Dr. Stephen, 43
L'Hopital (Valent), 109–10

light, 180–81
  full-spectrum indoor, 175, 179, 180
  infrared, as sauna, 179
  quality, reduction in, 174
Lights Out, 194, 317
  See also Appendix 2 for products
    and suppliers
lime, 51, 140, 302, 303
Liu I-ming, 110–11
"live" food, 241, 243–44
  See also food
liver, 20
  "flush" for, 185
  herbs for, 184–85
livestock, 246, 249
  chickens, 248–49
  hormones fed to, 248
lungs, 23
  diaphragmatic breathing's effect
    upon, 81
  herbal steam bath for, 23
lymphatic system, 18, 47, 162, 215,
    310
  exercise for, 26–27
  herbs for, 186–87

magnesium, 20, 40–41, 46, 48, 121,
    135, 259–60, 303
  chloride, 41, 46, 48, 134, 260, 293,
    303, 304
marrow, 68, 97, 98, 99, 187
massage, 13, 27, 30, 49, 54–72
  acupressure, 65–67
  with chi brushing, 67–68
  Chinese tui-na, 58–59
  chiropractic, 64

deep-tissue, 55, 56, 58, 59, 60, 62
  with hot herbal oil, 63–64
  Japanese shiatsu, 60
  Nei-dzang internal-organ, 63
  reflexology, 60
  self-administered, 64–65
  by squeezing and rubbing, 67
  by tapping, 68–72, 69, 70,
  traditional Asian foot, 60–62
  traditional Thai, 56–57
Maximum Immunity (Weiner), 298
Mayo, Dr. Charles, 6, 233
Mayo clinic, 233
McCullum, Dr. E. V., 242
menus, 141–48
  for bowels and digestive tract, 144
  for brain and nervous system, 146
  for general tissue detox, 143
  for heart and circulatory system,
    145
  for kidneys and bladder, 147
  for liver and blood, 148
  See also Appendix 1 for recipes and
    formulas; Appendix 2 for prod-
    ucts and suppliers; food
meridians, 55, 56, 57, 58, 59, 60, 61,
    64, 65, 66, 68, 69, 86, 90, 92,
    93, 95, 108, 198, 211
  bladder, 58
  intestine, 65
  kidney, 67
  liver, 65–66
Michel, Dr., 101
microwater, 34–37
microwaves, 201–3
  See also electromagnetic fields

milk, goat's versus cow's, 253
mind upon body, effects of, 298
   and attitude, 300–1
   and negative emotion, 298–99
   and placebo effect, 298
   and positive thinking, 297–98, 301
minerals and trace elements, 20, 36,
      37, 38, 39, 46, 119
   calcium, 20, 21, 116, 255
   magnesium, 20, 255
   selenium, 101, 120, 231, 261, 262
   zinc, 101, 231, 261, 262
mint, 51
miso, 120, 144, 256
Moscow Research Institute of Psy-
      chiatry, 154
Moses (Old Testament), 237
mucus, 9, 22, 126, 128, 129, 161,
      165–67
mud, 46–47

neck lock during breathing exercises,
      85–86
negative emotion, 298
   See also mind upon body
negative ions, 102–7, 263
   air travel and, 106–7
   generator of, 106-7
nei-dzang internal-organ massage,
      63
nervous exhaustion, 4
Neti nasal douche, 41–42, 108
Neural electric therapy (NET), 29,
      218–20
   See also Appendix 2 for products
      and suppliers

Neuro Muscle Stimulator (Zapper),
      216–18
   See also Appendix 2 for products
      and suppliers
neuropeptides, 99, 297, 298
neurotransmitters, 78, 81, 98, 99,
      172, 205, 273
nuts, grains and seeds, 129–31

oculo-endocrine system, 173–75,
      177, 179
oil for cooking, 250
Omni, 99
opium, 219, 273–74, 284, 286
   See also smoking
organic food, 118, 119, 124, 125,
      243, 250, 284, 286
osteoporosis, 21, 116, 252, 257
Ott, John, 178–79
oxygen, 42–44
   immune system and, 42–43
   lack of (hypoxia), 6, 7, 17, 19, 23,
      194
   See also alkalization; oxygenation
oxygenation, 9, 11, 12, 20, 21, 27,
      230
   hydrogen peroxide for, 21
   supplements for, 21
ozone, 21, 43

packaged dry cereal, 238
parasites and worms, 194–95
parasympathetic ("rest and relax-
      ation") circuit, 4–5, 11, 12, 27,
      30, 58, 59, 65, 74, 196, 294
parsley, 123

Pasteur, Louis, 6–7

Patterson, Dr. Margaret (Meg), 218–19

Peace & Quiet, 194, 317

  See also Appendix 2 for products and suppliers

pepper, 51

pepsin, 81, 83, 100, 237, 239

Peschier, Dr. Charles Gaspard, 101

pesticides, 16, 118, 125, 233, 243, 246

pharmaceutical cartels, 9

pH balance, 18–21, 35, 38, 101, 126, 203, 230, 231, 259

photobiology, 173

pineal gland, 93, 173

pipes, 277

  See also smoking

pituitary gland, 71, 151, 175, 177, 180, 257

placebo effect, 298

  See also mind upon body

Plutarch, 159

pneumonia, 162–63

positive thinking, 297–98, 301

  See also mind upon body

Precious Recipes (Sun), 72, 78

preparation of food, 119–22, 302–12

preservatives, x, 16, 233, 241, 243, 279

processed foods, 114, 116, 226, 233, 243, 264

psoriasis, 9

psychoneuroimmunology (PNI), 99, 298

psyllium, 24, 138–39, 143, 144, 160–61, 168, 189–90, 292

pumpkin, 119, 121, 148, 195

putrefactive protein, 115, 129, 236–38

radionics, 220–22

raw and lightly cooked vegetables, 119, 142, 240–41, 243

Reagan, President (Ronald), 163–64

Recipes and formulas: 302–15

  bladder- and urinary-tract-cleansing tea, 309

  Breuss kidney tea, 307

  Carminative herbal tea for gas and flatulence, 312

  Chinese herbal constipation formula, 310–11

  clear vegetable broth, 304

  Job's Tears and Brown-Rice Porridge, 305

  Lemon flax Shake, 312

  Liver detox formula for alcohol and drug poisoning, 308–9

  Liver detox tea, 306

  Lymphatic detox tea, 310

  Nervine tea, 311

  Rejuvelac, 312–13

  Sage tea, 306

  Tai herbal steam baths, 302–3

  Tonic herbal spirits, 314–15

reflexology, 60

Rejuvelac, 162, 313

Rejuvenate Liver Regenerator, 184

  See also Appendix 2 for products and suppliers

rest and relaxation, 4–5, 12, 30, 193, 226, 292, 294, 298

Retox, xi, 4, 10, 225–32
  diet and supplements for, 233–34
  See also food
Richards, Keith, 220
Road to Wellville (novel and film),
  25, 26
Robbins, John, 246, 247
The Root of Chinese Chi Kung
  (Yang), 97
rosemary, 47, 51, 110, 293, 303,
  318

sage, 47, 132–33
Salmanoff, Dr. A., 80
salt, 259–60
  bathing in, 48–49
Dead Sea, 46–47, 152
  See also Celtic sea salt; food: salt in
  sea, bathing in, 48–49
Sea Salt's Hidden Powers (Langre),
  259
seawater and sea salt, 37–42
seeds, grains and nuts, 129–31
selenium, 101, 120, 231, 261, 262
self-administered massage, 64–65
serotonin, 98, 206
Shelton, Dr. Herbert, 254
Shen Chia-shu, 97, 102
silence, value of, 110–12
sinusitis, 9
skin, 11, 18, 22–23, 45–46, 67–68,
  189, 191, 216, 238, 303
  herbal steam bath for, 22–23,
  50–52
  and light, 176–77, 180, 181
Smithsonian Institute, 174

smoking, 4, 191, 270–77
  cannabis, 273, 284, 310
  cigarettes, 272–75
  cigars, 276
  and dioxin, 273, 274
  opium, 219, 273–74, 284, 286
  pipes, 277
  tobacco, 270–75
soft drinks, 21, 116–17, 239
  See also food
spas, *see* health resorts and spas
spine, 64, 85, 87, 89, 93–94, *94*
  energies traveling through, 89–90
Spring and Autumn Annals, 54
squeezing-and-rubbing massage, 67
starch in food, 113, 115, 234, 235,
  237, 238, 254, 257
steam baths, 23, 50–52, 302
stevia as natural sweetener, 258, 267,
  318
Storey, Everett, 44
stress hormones, 20, 29, 77, 78, 99,
  297
  cortisone, 297, 299
substitutes for food, 243–44
  See also food
Sugar Blues (Duffy), 256
sugar, 21, 114, 116–17, 127, 234,
  239, 256–58
  effect of, on children, 299, 300
  See also food
Sun Ssu-mo, 72, 78
superoxide dismutase (SOD), 101–2,
  262
supplements for detox, 265–66
Szekely, Edmond, 152

Tai Chi, 27, 55, 74, 86, 96

Tao Teh Ching, 31, 149

The Tao of Health, Sex and Longevity (Reid), xii, 74, 156

tapping massage, 68–72, *69, 70*

teas, 24, 132, 142, 146, 184, 186, 187, 319, 320

   green, 262

   High Mountain Oolung, 262, 281, 320

   See also food

thyme, 51, 303

thymus gland, 71, 213

Tilden, Dr. John, 3, 5, 12, 162, 163

Tissue Cleansing Through Bowel Management (Jensen), 152

tobacco, 270–75, 276, 277

   See also smoking

toxemia, 2–4, 6, 7, 8, 10, 54, 117

   as breeding ground, 7, 218

   chronic, 10, 32, 61, 230

   dehydration as cause of, 32, 42

   organ damage caused by, 8, 11

   Tilden's view of, 3

Toxemia (Tilden), 3

trace elements, *see* minerals and trace elements

traditional Asian foot massage, 60–62

Traditional Chinese Medicine (TCM), 16, 17, 59, 61, 63, 95, 183

   and "natural affinity," 132

traditional Thai massage, 56–57

tsai shir-tou, 62

tu na, 92, 94, *94,* 294

two-stage breathing exercises, 86

ultraviolet light, 173

vaginitis, 9

Valent, Dr. J., 109, 110

vitamins:

   alkaline C (C-salts), 137–38

   B, 130, 137, 146,

   C, 231, 261, 262, 286, 318

   D, 176–77

   E, 184, 231, 261, 262

Vit-ra-tox range, 189

   See also Appendix 2 for products and suppliers

Vortex Energizer, 36–37

   See also water

Walford, Dr. Roy, 150, 244

Walker, Dr. Norman, 24, 38, 150, 155

Warburg, Dr. Otto, 7

water, 31–53

   alkalized, 35

   chlorine in, 33, 34

   daily intake of, 18, 53, 56, 113, 159–60

   electrolysis of, 34

   energized, 33, 37

   fascia and, 33

   Fluoride in, 33, 34

   in herbal steam, 32, 50–52

   in hot springs, 49–50

   ionized, 35

   micro-clustered, 35

   oxygenated, 42–44

   polluted, 52–53

   "programming" of, 32

restructured (microwater), 34–37
salt, for bathing, 46–47
sea, 48–49
shortage of, 52–53
toxic elements in, 33–34
See also hydration; hydrotherapy
watermelon, 128, 147, 242
Weiner, Dr. Michael, 298, 299
wheat products, 129
whirlpool bath, 13, 47, 49
"winter blues," 175
World Health Organization, 195
worms and parasites, 115,
    194–95

Yang Jwing-ming, Dr., 97

*The Yellow Emperor's Classic of
    Internal Medicine,* 16
yin and yang considerations of food,
    235
yin particles, *see* negative ions
yoga, 27, 55, 56, 74, 82, 84, 90
    and deep-breathing exercises,
        90–91
    pranayama, 90
    See also breathing

Zapper (Neuro Muscle Stimulator),
    216–18, 223
    See also Appendix 2 for products
        and suppliers
zinc, 101, 231, 261, 262

BOOKS OF RELATED INTEREST

My Journey in Mystic China
Old Pu's Travel Diary
by John Blofeld

Opium Culture
The Art and Ritual of the Chinese Tradition
by Peter Lee

The Seasonal Detox Diet
Remedies from the Ancient Cookfire
by Carrie L'Esperance

The Clay Cure
Natural Healing from the Earth
by Ran Knishinsky

The Detox Mono Diet
The Miracle Grape Cure and Other Cleansing Diets
by Christopher Vasey, N.D.

The Acid–Alkaline Diet for Optimum Health
Restore Your Health by Creating pH Balance in Your Diet
by Christopher Vasey, N.D.

Optimal Digestive Health: A Complete Guide
Edited by Trent W. Nichols, M.D.,
and Nancy Faass, MSW, MPH

Addiction-Free Naturally
Liberating Yourself from Sugar, Caffeine, Food Addictions,
Tobacco, Alcohol, and Prescription Drugs
by Brigitte Mars

Inner Traditions • Bear & Company
P.O. Box 388
Rochester, VT 05767
1-800-246-8648
www.InnerTraditions.com

Or contact your local bookseller